Case Files:
General Surgery

NOTICE

Medicine is an ever-changing science. As new research and clinical experience broaden our knowledge, changes in treatment and drug therapy are required. The authors and the publisher of this work have checked with sources believed to be reliable in their efforts to provide information that is complete and generally in accord with the standards accepted at the time of publication. However, in view of the possibility of human error or changes in medical sciences, neither the editors nor the publisher nor any other party who has been involved in the preparation or publication of this work warrants that the information contained herein is in every respect accurate or complete, and they disclaim all responsibility for any errors or omissions or for the results obtained from use of the information contained in this work. Readers are encouraged to confirm the information contained herein with other sources. For example and in particular, readers are advised to check the product information sheet included in the package of each drug they plan to administer to be certain that the information contained in this work is accurate and that changes have not been made in the recommended dose or in the contraindications for administration. This recommendation is of particular importance in connection with new or infrequently used drugs.

Case Files:
General Surgery

EUGENE C. TOY, MD
The John S. Dunn, Senior Academic Chief
Christus-St. Joseph Hospital
Ob/Gyn Residency Program
Clerkship Director, Assistant Clinical Professor
Department of Obstetrics and Gynecology
University of Texas-Houston Medical School
Houston, Texas

TERRENCE H. LIU, MD
Assistant Professor of Surgery
Department of Surgery
Alameda County Medical Center
Oakland, California

McGraw-Hill

PROFESSIONAL

New York Chicago San Francisco
Lisbon London Madrid Mexico City
Milan New Delhi San Juan Seoul
Singapore Sydney Toronto

Case Files: General Surgery

1 2 3 4 5 6 7 8 9 0   DOC/DOC   0 9 8 8 8 7 6 5 4 3

ISBN 0-07-140252-7

This book was set in Times New Roman by ATLIS Graphics and Design.
The editors were Catherine A. Johnson and Karen G. Edmonson.
The production supervisor was Catherine H. Saggese.
The cover designer was Mary McKeon.
The index was prepared by Nancy Newman.
RR Donnelley was printer and binder.

This book is printed on acid-free paper.

Library of Congress Cataloging-in-Publication Data

Toy, Eugene C.
    Case files : general surgery / Eugene C. Toy, Terrence H. Liu.
      p. ; cm.
    Includes index.
    ISBN 0-07-140252-7 (alk. paper)
    1. Surgery—Case studies.   I. Title: General surgery.   II. Liu, Terrence H.   III. Title.
    [DNLM: 1. Surgical Procedures, Operative—methods—Case Report. WO 500 T756c 2003]
    RD34.T69 2003
    617—dc21

                                                                          2002044947

To my dear parents Chuck and Grace who taught me the importance of pursuing excellence and instilled in me a love for books, to my sister Nancy for her compassion and unselfishness, and to my brother Glen for his friendship and our fond memories growing up.

—ECT

To my wife Eileen for her love, friendship, support, and encouragement. To my parents George and Jackie for their constant loving support, and to my sons Andrew and Gabriel who show to me the importance of family values, everyday. To all my teachers and mentors, who took the time and effort to teach and serve as role models.

—THL

To the wonderful medical students of the University of Texas–Houston Medical School for whom this curriculum was developed.

—THE AUTHORS

❖ CONTENTS

◈ CONTRIBUTORS

Gildy V. Barbiera, MD
Assistant Professor, Division of Surgical Oncology
University of Texas–M.D. Anderson Cancer Center, Houston, Texas
Approach to Breast Carcinoma
Approach to Patients With Breast Cancer Risk

Gregory J. Beilman, MD
Associate Professor and Director of Surgical Critical Care
Department of Surgery
University of Minnesota Hospitals and Clinics, Minneapolis, Minnesota
Approach to Hemorrhagic Shock
Approach to Septic Shock

John E. Bertini, MD
Academic Chief, Christus–St. Joseph Hospital Urology
Assistant Clinical Professor, Department of Urology
University of Texas–Houston Medical School, Houston, Texas
Approach to Benign Prostatic Hypertrophy
Approach to Testicular Cancer

Martin L. Blakely, MD
Assistant Professor of Surgery and Pediatrics
University of Texas–Houston Medical School, Houston, Texas
Approach to Pediatric Abdominal Masses (Wilms tumor)

Karen J. Brasel, MD, MPH
Assistant Professor of Surgery
Medical College of Wisconsin, Milwaukee, Wisconsin
Approach to Closed Head Injury
Approach to Hernias

Eileen T. Consorti, MD, MS
General Surgeon
Kaiser Permanente Medical Group, Richmond, California
Approach to Right Upper Quadrant Pain

Charles S. Cox, Jr., MD
Associate Professor
Department of Surgery and Pediatrics
University of Texas–Houston Medical School
Houston, Texas
Approach to Persistent Jaundice in Childhood

Woody Denham, MD
Assistant Professor
Department of Surgery
Northwestern University School of Medicine, Chicago, Illinois
Approach to Acute Pancreatitis

Anthony L. Estrerra, MD
Assistant Professor
Department of Cardiovascular/Thoracic Surgery
University of Texas–Houston Medical School, Houston, Texas
Approach to Esophageal Perforation
Approach to Spontaneous Pneumothorax
Approach to Thymoma, Surgery for Myasthenia Gravis
Approach to Blunt Chest Trauma

Craig P. Fischer, MD, MPH
Assistant Professor of Surgery
University of Texas–Houston Medical School, Houston, Texas
Approach to Liver Tumor

Lillian S. Kao, MD
Assistant Professor
Department of Surgery
University of Texas–Houston Medical School, Houston, Texas
Approach to Gastroesophageal Reflux Disease
Approach to Diverticulitis

Karen L. Kwong, MD
Assistant Professor of Surgery
University of Oregon Health Sciences
Staff Surgeon, Portland VA Medical Center, Portland, Oregon
Approach to Nipple Discharge
Approach to Thermal Injuries

Ralph E. Ligon, MD
Assistant Professor
Department of Surgery
University of Texas–Houston Medical School, Houston, Texas
Approach to Fascia Dehiscence and Incisional Hernia

Alberto E. Madrid, MD
Assistant Professor
Department of Surgery
University of Texas–Houston Medical School, Houston, Texas
Approach to Anorectal Diseases

Christopher R. McHenry, MD
Associate Professor
Case Western Reserve University
Director of General Surgery
MetroHealth Medical Center, Cleveland, Ohio
Approach to Thyroid Masses
Approach to Pheochromocytoma and Hypercalcemia
Approach to Adrenal Masses
Approach to Hypercalcemia and Hyperparathyroidism

David W. Mercer, MD
Chief of Surgery
Lyndon B. Johnson Hospital
Associate Professor and Vice Chairman of General Surgery
Department of Surgery
University of Texas–Houston Medical School, Houston, Texas
Approach to Upper Gastrointestinal Hemorrhage
Approach to Peptic Ulcer Disease

Frank G. Moody, MD
Professor, Department of Surgery
University of Texas–Houston Medical School, Houston, Texas
Approach to Morbid Obesity

Kendrick M. Murayama, MD
Associate Professor and Director of Minimal Invasive Surgery
Department of Surgery
Northwestern University Medical School, Chicago, Illinois
Approach to Immune Thrombocytopenia Purpura and Splenic Disorders
Approach to Acute Pancreatitis

Alexander P. Nagle, MD
Assistant Professor
Department of Surgery
Northwestern University Medical School, Chicago, Illinois
Approach to Acute Pancreatitis
Approach to Immune Thrombocytopenia Purpura and Splenic Disorders

Ming Pan, MD, PhD
Assistant Professor of Surgery
Penn State University College of Medicine
Milton S. Hershey Medical Center, Hershey, Pennsylvania
Approach to Short Bowel Syndrome

Adam Riker, MD
Assistant Professor
Department of Surgery
Loyola University Medical Center, Maywood, Illinois
Approach to Melanomas

Courtney L. Scaife, MD
Fellow, Division of Surgical Oncology
University of Texas–M.D. Anderson Cancer Center, Houston, Texas
Approach to Breast Carcinoma
Approach to Patients with Breast Cancer Risk

Martin Schreiber, MD
Associate Professor
Department of Surgery
University of Oregon Health Sciences Center, Portland, Oregon
Approach to Penetrating Abdominal Trauma

Margo Shoup, MD
Assistant Professor of Surgery and Chief of GI Surgical Oncology
Department of Surgery
Loyola University Medical Center, Maywood, Illinois
Approach to Soft Tissue Sarcomas

Thomas V. Taylor, MD
Academic Chief and Program Director
Christus–St. Joseph Hospital General Surgery Residency
Professor of General Surgery
University of Texas–Houston Medical School, Houston, Texas
Approach to Carpal Tunnel Syndrome
Approach to Lumbar Prolapsed Nucleus Pulposus

Ara Vaporcyan, MD
Assistant Professor
Division of Thoracic and Cardiovascular Surgery
University of Texas–M.D. Anderson Cancer Center, Houston, Texas
Approach to Pulmonary Nodules

Henry Veldenz, MD
Associate Professor and Residency Director
Department of Surgery
University of Florida Health Sciences Center, Jacksonville, Florida
Approach to Claudication
Approach to Aortic Aneurysm
Approach to Carotid Arterial Disease
Approach to Mesenteric Ischemia

Gregory P. Victorino, MD
Assistant Professor
University of California, San Francisco
Attending Surgeon, UCSF–East Bay Residency Program, Oakland, California
Approach to Postoperative Respiratory Failure

◈ INTRODUCTION

Mastering the cognitive knowledge within a field such as general surgery is a formidable task. It is even more difficult to draw on that knowledge, procure and filter through the clinical and laboratory data, develop a differential diagnosis, and finally form a rational treatment plan. To gain these skills, the student often learns best at the bedside, guided and instructed by experienced teachers and inspired toward self-directed, diligent reading. Clearly, there is no replacement for education at the bedside. Unfortunately, clinical situations usually do not encompass the breadth of the specialty. Perhaps the best alternative is a carefully crafted patient case designed to stimulate the clinical approach and decision making. In an attempt to achieve this goal, we have constructed a collection of clinical vignettes to teach diagnostic or therapeutic approaches relevant to general surgery. Most importantly, the explanations for the cases emphasize the mechanisms and underlying principles rather than merely rote questions and answers.

This book is organized for versatility: to allow the student "in a rush" to go quickly through the scenarios and check the corresponding answers, and to provide more detailed information for the student who wants thought-provoking explanations. The answers are arranged from simple to complex: a summary of the pertinent points, the bare answers, an analysis of the case, an approach to the topic, a comprehension test at the end for reinforcement and emphasis, and a list of resources for further reading. The clinical vignettes are purposely arranged in randomly in order to simulate the way that real patients present to the practitioner. A listing of cases is included in Section III to aid the student who desires to test his or her knowledge of a certain area or to review a topic, including basic definitions. Finally, we intentionally did not primarily use a multiple-choice question format because clues (or distractions) are not available in the real world. Nevertheless, several multiple-choice questions are included at the end of each scenario to reinforce concepts or introduce related topics.

HOW TO GET THE MOST OUT OF THIS BOOK

Each case is designed to simulate a patient encounter and includes open-ended questions. At times, the patient's complaint differs from the issue of most concern, and sometimes extraneous information is given. The answers are organized into four different parts:

PART I:

1. **Summary:** The salient aspects of the case are identified, filtering out the extraneous information. The student should formulate his or her summary from the case before looking at the answers. A comparison with the summation in the answer helps to improve one's ability to focus on the important data while appropriately discarding irrelevant information, a fundamental skill required in clinical problem solving.

2. A **straightforward answer** is given to each open-ended question.

3. An **analysis of the case,** which consists of two parts:

   a. **Objectives:** A listing of the two or three main principles that are crucial for a practitioner in treating a patient. Again, the student is challenged to make educated "guesses" about the objectives of the case after an initial review of the case scenario, which helps to sharpen his or her clinical and analytical skills.

   b. **Considerations:** A discussion of the relevant points and a brief approach to a **specific** patient.

PART II:

An **approach to the disease process,** consisting of two distinct parts:

   a. **Definitions:** terminology pertinent to the disease process

   b. **Clinical approach:** a discussion of the approach to the clinical problem in general, including tables, figures, and algorithms.

PART III:

Comprehension questions: Each case includes several multiple-choice questions, that reinforce the material or introduce new and related concepts. Questions about material not found in the text are explained in the answers.

PART IV:

Clinical Pearls: A listing of several clinically important points, which are reiterated as a summation of the text and to allow for easy review, such as before an examination.

◆ ACKNOWLEDGMENTS

The curriculum that evolved into the ideas for this series was inspired by two talented and forthright students, Philbert Yau and Chuck Rosipal, who have since graduated from medical school. It has been a tremendous joy to work with my friend since medical school, Terry Liu, a brilliant surgeon, and the many excellent contributors. I am greatly indebted to my editor, Catherine Johnson, whose exuberance, experience, and vision helped to shape this series. I appreciate McGraw-Hill's believing in the concept of teaching through clinical cases, and I would especially like to acknowledge John Williams, the director of editing and Karen Edmonson, the supervisor of editing. I am also grateful to Catherine Saggese for her excellent production expertise. At Christus–St. Joseph Hospital, I applaud the finest administrators I have encountered: Sally Jeffcoat, Jeff Webster, Mark Mullarkey, and Dr. Benton Baker, III, for their commitment to medical education, and Dorothy Mersinger for her sage advice and support. I would especially like to acknowledge the excellent proofreading and review of the manuscript by Dr. Benton Baker, III, and Melissa L. Wilson, MS IV. Without my dear colleagues, Drs. Robert Morris, Konrad Harms, and Faith Whittier, this book could not have been written. Most of all, I appreciate my loving wife, Terri, and my four wonderful children, Andy, Michael, Allison, and Christina, for their patience and understanding

Eugene C. Toy

How to Approach Clinical Problems

PART 1.   APPROACH TO THE PATIENT

The transition from textbook or journal article learning to an application of the information in a specific clinical situation is one of the most challenging tasks in medicine. It requires retention of information, organization of the facts, and recall of a myriad of data with precise application to the patient. The purpose of this text is to facilitate this process. The first step is gathering information, also known as establishing the database. This includes recording the patient's history; performing the physical examination; and obtaining selective laboratory examinations, special evaluations such as breast ductograms, and/or imaging tests. Of these, the historical examination is the most important and most useful. Sensitivity and respect should always be exercised during the interview of patients.

◈ CLINICAL PEARL

The history is usually the single most important tool in reaching a diagnosis. The art of obtaining this information in a nonjudgmental, sensitive, and thorough manner cannot be overemphasized.

History

1. Basic information:
   a. Age: must be recorded because some conditions are more common at certain ages; for instance, age is one of the most important risk factors for the development of breast cancer.
   b. Gender: some disorders are more common in or found exclusively in men such as prostatic hypertrophy and cancer. In contrast, women more commonly have autoimmune problems such as immune thrombocytopenia purpura and thyroid nodules. Also, the possibility of pregnancy must be considered in any woman of childbearing age.
   c. Ethnicity: some disease processes are more common in certain ethnic groups (such as diabetes mellitus in the Hispanic population).

CLINICAL PEARL

The possibility of pregnancy must be entertained in any woman of childbearing age.

2. Chief complaint: What is it that brought the patient into the hospital or office? Is it a scheduled appointment or an unexpected symptom such as abdominal pain or hematemesis? The duration and character of the complaint, associated symptoms, and exacerbating and/or relieving factors should be recorded. The chief complaint engenders a differential diagnosis, and the possible etiologies should be explored by further inquiry.

CLINICAL PEARL

The first line of any surgical presentation should include *age, ethnicity, gender,* and *chief complaint.* Example: A 32-year-old Caucasian male complains of lower abdominal pain over an 8-hour duration.

3. Past medical history:
    a. Major illnesses such as hypertension, diabetes, reactive airway disease, congestive heart failure, and angina should be detailed.
        i.   Age of onset, severity, end-organ involvement
        ii. Medications taken for a particular illness, including any recent change in medications and the reason for the change.
        iii. Last evaluation of the condition (eg, When was the last echocardiogram performed in a patient with congestive heart failure?)
        iv. Which physician or clinic is following the patient for the disorder?

    b.   Minor illnesses such as a recent upper respiratory tract infection may impact on the scheduling of elective surgery.

    c.   Hospitalizations no matter how trivial should be detailed.

4. Past surgical history: Date and type of procedure performed, indication, and outcome. Laparoscopy versus laparotomy should be distinguished. Surgeon and hospital name and location should be listed. This information should be correlated with the surgical scars on the patient's body. Any complications should be delineated, including anesthetic complications, difficult intubations, and so on.

5. Allergies: Reactions to medications should be recorded, including severity and temporal relationship to administration of medication. Immediate hypersensitivity should be distinguished from an adverse reaction.

6. Medications: A list of medications, including dosage, route of administration and frequency, and duration of use should be developed. Prescription, over-the-counter, and herbal remedies are all relevant.

7. Social history: Marital status, family support, alcohol use, use or abuse of illicit drugs, and tobacco use, and tendencies toward depression or anxiety are important.

8. Family history: Major medical problems, genetically transmitted disorders such as breast cancer, and important reactions to anesthetic medications, such as malignant hyperthermia (an autosomal dominant transmitted disorder) should be explored.

9. Review of systems: A system review should be performed focusing on the more common diseases. For example, in a young man with a testicular mass, trauma to the area, weight loss, neck masses, and lymphadenopathy are important. In an elderly woman, symptoms suggestive of cardiac disease should be elicited, such as chest pain, shortness of breath, fatigue, weaknesses, and palpitations.

◈ **CLINICAL PEARL**

Malignant hyperthermia is a rare condition inherited in an autosomal dominant fashion. It is associated with a rapid rise in temperature up to 40.6°C (105°F), usually on induction by general anesthetic agents such as succinylcholine and halogenated inhalant gases. Prevention is the best treatment.

Physical Examination

1. General appearance: Note whether the patient is cachetic versus well nourished, anxious versus calm, alert versus obtunded.

2. Vital signs: Record the temperature, blood pressure, heart rate, and respiratory rate. Height and weight are often included here. For trauma patients, the Glasgow Coma Scale (GCS) is important.

3. Head and neck examination: Evidence of trauma, tumors, facial edema, goiter and thyroid nodules, and carotid bruits should be sought. With a closed head injury, pupillary reflexes and unequal pupil sizes are important. Cervical and supraclavicular nodes should be palpated.

4. Breast examination: Perform an inspection for symmetry and for skin or nipple retraction with the patient's hands on her hips (to accentuate the pectoral muscles) and with her arms raised. With the patient supine, the breasts should be palpated systematically to assess for masses. The nipples should be assessed for discharge, and the axillary and supraclavicular regions should be examined for adenopathy.

5. Cardiac examination: The point of maximal impulse should be ascertained, and the heart auscultated at the apex as well as at the base. Heart sounds, murmurs, and clicks should be characterized. Systolic flow murmurs are fairly common in pregnant women because of the increased cardiac output, but significant diastolic murmurs are unusual.

6. Pulmonary examination: The lung fields should be examined systematically and thoroughly. Wheezes, rales, rhonchi, and bronchial breath sounds should be recorded.

7. Abdominal examination: The abdomen should be inspected for scars, distension, masses or organomegaly (ie, spleen or liver), and discoloration. For instance, the Grey–Turner sign of discoloration on the flank areas may indicate an intra-abdominal or retroperitoneal hemorrhage. Auscultation should be performed to identify normal versus high-pitched, and hyperactive versus hypoactive, bowel sounds. The abdomen should be percussed for the presence of shifting dullness (indicating ascites). Careful palpation should begin initially away from the area of pain, involving one hand on top of the other, to assess for masses, tenderness, and peritoneal signs. Tenderness should be recorded on a scale (eg, 1 to 4, where 4 is the most severe pain). Guarding and whether it is voluntary or involuntary should be noted.

8. Back and spine examination: The back should be assessed for symmetry, tenderness, or masses. The flank regions are particularly important in assessing for pain on percussion that may indicate renal disease.

9. Genital examination:
   a. **Female:** The external genitalia should be inspected, and the speculum then used to visualize the cervix and vagina. A bimanual examination should attempt to elicit cervical motion tenderness, uterine size, and ovarian masses or tenderness.
   b. **Male:** The penis should be examined for hypospadias, lesions, and infection. The scrotum should be palpated for masses and, if present, transillumination should be used to distinguish between solid and cystic masses. The groin region should be carefully palpated for bulging (hernias) on rest and on provocation (coughing). This procedure should optimally be repeated with the patient in different positions.

  c. **Rectal examination:** A rectal examination can reveal masses in the posterior pelvis and may identify occult blood in the stool. In females, nodularity and tenderness in the uterosacral ligament may be signs of endometriosis. The posterior uterus and palpable masses in the cul-de-sac may be identified by rectal examination. In the male, the prostate gland should be palpated for tenderness, nodularity, and enlargement.

10. Extremities and skin: The presence of joint effusions, tenderness, skin edema, and cyanosis should be recorded.

11. Neurologic examination: Patients who present with neurologic complaints usually require thorough assessments including evaluation of the cranial nerves, strength, sensation, and reflexes.

CLINICAL PEARL

A thorough understanding of anatomy is important to optimally interpret the physical examination findings.

12. Laboratory assessment depends on the circumstances:
  a. A complete blood count: to assess for anemia, leukocytosis (infection), and thrombocytopenia.
  b. Urine culture or urinalysis: to assess for hematuria when ureteral stones, renal carcinoma, or trauma is suspected.
  c. Tumor markers: for example, in testicular cancer, β-human chorionic gonadotropin, α-fetoprotein, and lactate dehydrogenase values are often assessed.
  d. Serum creatinine and serum urea nitrogen levels: to assess renal function, and aspartate aminotransferase (AST) and alanine aminotransferase (ALT) values to assess liver function.

13. Imaging procedures:
  a. An ultrasound examination is the most commonly used imaging procedure to distinguish a pelvic process in fe-

male patients, such as pelvic inflammatory disease. It is also very useful in diagnosing gallstones and measuring the caliber of the common bile duct. It can also help to discern solid versus cystic masses.

b. Computed tomography (CT) is extremely useful in assessing fluid and abscess collections in the abdomen and pelvis. It can also help determine the size of lymph nodes in the retroperitoneal space.

c. Magnetic resonance imaging identifies soft tissue planes and may assist in assessing prolapsed lumbar nucleus pulposus and various orthopedic injuries.

d. Intravenous pyelography uses dye to assess the concentrating ability of the kidneys, the patency of the ureters, and the integrity of the bladder. It is also useful in detecting hydronephrosis, ureteral stones, and ureteral obstructions.

PART 2.   APPROACH TO CLINICAL PROBLEM SOLVING

There are typically four distinct steps that a clinician takes to systematically solve most clinical problems:

1. Making the diagnosis
2. Assessing the severity or stage of the disease
3. Proposing a treatment based on the stage of the disease
4. Following the patient's response to the treatment.

Making the Diagnosis

A diagnosis is made by a careful evaluation of the database, analyzing the information, assessing the risk factors, and developing the list of possibilities (the differential diagnosis). Experience and knowledge help the physician to "key in" on the most important possibilities. A good clinician also knows how to ask the same question in several different ways and use different terminology. For example, a patient may deny having been treated for "cholelithiasis" but answer affirmatively when asked if he has been hospitalized for "gallstones." Reaching a diagnosis may be achieved by systematically reading about each possible cause and disease.

Usually a long list of possible diagnoses can be pared down to two or three that are the most likely, based on selective laboratory or imaging tests. For example, a patient who complains of upper abdominal pain *and* has a history of nonsteroidal anti-inflammatory drugs use may have peptic ulcer disease; another patient who has abdominal pain, fatty food intolerance, and abdominal bloating may have cholelithiasis. Yet another individual with a 1-day history of periumbilical pain localizing to the right lower quadrant may have acute appendicitis.

CLINICAL PEARL

The first step in clinical problem solving is **making the diagnosis**.

Assessing the Severity of the Disease

After establishing the diagnosis, the next step is to characterize the severity of the disease process, in other words, describing "how bad" a disease is. With malignancy, this is done formally by staging the cancer. Most cancers are categorized from stage I (least severe) to stage IV (most severe). With some diseases, such as with head trauma, there is a formal scale (the GCS) based on the patient's eye-opening response, verbal response, and motor response.

CLINICAL PEARL

The second step is to **establish the severity or stage of the disease**. There is usually prognostic or treatment significance based on the stage.

Treating Based on the Stage

Many illnesses are stratified according to severity because the prognosis and treatment often vary based on the severity. If neither the prognosis nor the treatment were affected by the stage of the disease process, there would be no reason to subcategorize the illness as mild or severe. For example, obesity is subcategorized as moderate (body mass index [BMI] 35 to 40 kg/m^2) or severe (BMI greater than 40 kg/m^2), with different prognoses and recommended interventions. Surgical procedures for obesity such as gastric bypass are only generally considered when a patient has severe obesity and/or significant complications such as sleep apnea.

◈ **CLINICAL PEARL**

The third step in most cases is tailoring the treatment to the extent or stage of the disease.

Following the Response to Treatment

The final step in the approach to disease is to follow the patient's response to the therapy. The "measure" of response should be recorded and monitored. Some responses are clinical, such as improvement (or lack of improvement) in a patient's abdominal pain, temperature, or pulmonary examination. Other responses can be followed by imaging tests such as a CT scan to determine the size of a retroperitoneal mass in a patient receiving chemotherapy, or with a tumor marker such as the level of prostate-specific antigen in a male receiving chemotherapy for prostatic cancer. For a closed head injury, the GCS is used. The student must be prepared to know what to do if the measured marker does not respond according to what is expected. Is the next step to treat again, to reassess the diagnosis, to pursue a metastatic workup, or to follow up with another more specific test?

◈ **CLINICAL PEARL**

The fourth step is to monitor treatment response or efficacy, which can be measured in different ways. It may be symptomatic (the patient feels better) or based on a physical examination (fever), a laboratory test (prostate-specific antigen level), or an imaging test (size of a retroperitoneal lymph node on a CT scan).

PART 3.   APPROACH TO READING

The clinical problem-oriented approach to reading is different from the classic "systematic" research of a disease. A patient's presentation rarely provides a clear diagnosis; hence, the student must become skilled in applying textbook information to the clinical setting. Furthermore, one retains more information when one reads with a purpose. In other words, the student should read with the goal of answering specific questions. There are several fundamental questions that facilitate **clinical thinking:**

1.   What is the most likely diagnosis?
2.   How can you confirm the diagnosis?
3.   What should be your next step?
4.   What is the most likely mechanism for this disease process?
5.   What are the risk factors for this disease process?
6.   What are the complications associated with this disease process?
7.   What is the best therapy?

◈ **CLINICAL PEARL**

Reading with the purpose of answering the seven fundamental clinical questions improves retention of information and facilitates the application of book knowledge to clinical knowledge.

What Is the Most Likely Diagnosis?

The method of establishing the diagnosis has been covered in the previous section. One way of attacking this problem is to develop standard approaches to common clinical problems. It is helpful to understand the most common causes of various presentations, such as "The most common cause of serosanguinous nipple discharge is an intraductal papilloma."

The clinical scenario might be "A 38-year-old woman is noted to have a 2-month history of spontaneous blood-tinged right nipple discharge. What is the most likely diagnosis?"

With no other information to go on, the student notes that this woman has a unilateral blood-tinged nipple discharge. Using the "most common cause" information, the student makes an educated guess that the patient has an **intraductal papilloma.** If instead the patient is found to have a discharge from more than one duct and a right-sided breast mass is palpated, it is noted: "The bloody discharge is expressed from multiple ducts. A 1.5-cm mass is palpated in the lower outer quadrant of the right breast."

Then student uses the clinical pearl: "The most common cause of serosanguinous breast discharge in the presence of a breast mass is breast cancer."

◈ **CLINICAL PEARL**

The most common cause of serosanguinous unilateral breast discharge is intraductal papilloma, but **the main concern is breast cancer.** Thus, the first step in evaluating the patient's condition is careful palpation to determine the number of ducts involved, an examination to detect breast masses, and mammography. If more than one duct is involved or a breast mass is palpated, the most likely cause is breast cancer.

How Can You Confirm the Diagnosis?

In the scenario above, it is suspected that the woman with the bloody nipple discharge has an intraductal papilloma, or possibly cancer.

Ductal surgical exploration with biopsy would be a confirmatory procedure. Similarly, an individual may present with acute dyspnea following a radical prostatectomy for prostate cancer. The suspected
process is pulmonary embolism, and a confirmatory test would be a
ventilation/perfusion scan or possibly a spiral CT examination. The student should strive to know the limitations of various diagnostic tests,
especially when they are used early in a diagnostic process.

What Should Be Your Next Step?

This question is difficult because the next step has many possibilities;
the answer may be to obtain more diagnostic information, stage the illness, or introduce therapy. It is often a more challenging question than,
"What is the most likely diagnosis?" because there may be insufficient
information to make a diagnosis and the next step may be to obtain
more data. Another possibility is that there is enough information for a
probable diagnosis and that the next step is staging the disease. Finally,
the most appropriate answer may be to begin treatment. Hence, based
on the clinical data, a judgment needs to be rendered regarding how far
along one is in the following sequence.

**(1) Make a diagnosis → (2) Stage the disease →
(3) Treat based on stage → (4) Follow the response**

Frequently, students are taught to "regurgitate" information that they
have read about a particular disease but are not skilled at identifying the
next step. This talent is learned optimally at the bedside in a supportive
environment with the freedom to take educated guesses and receive
constructive feedback. A sample scenario might describe a student's
thought process as follows.

1. **Make a diagnosis:** "Based on the information I have, I believe
    that Mr. Smith has a small bowel obstruction from adhesive dis-
    ease *because* he presents with nausea, vomiting, and abdominal
    distension and has dilated loops of bowel on radiography."
2. **Stage the disease:** "I do not believe that this is severe disease
    because he does not have fever, evidence of sepsis, intractable
    pain, leukocytosis, or peritoneal signs."

3. **Treat based on stage:** "Therefore, my next step is to treat with nothing per mouth, nasogastric tube drainage, and observation."
4. **Follow the response:** "I want to follow the treatment by assessing his pain (asking him to rate the pain on a scale of 1 to 10 every day); recording his temperature; performing an abdominal examination; obtaining a serum bicarbonate level (to detect metabolic acidemia) and a leukocyte count; and reassessing his condition in 24 hours."

In a similar patient, when the clinical presentation is unclear, perhaps the best next step is a diagnostic one such as performing an oral contrast radiologic study to assess for bowel obstruction.

◈ **CLINICAL PEARL**

The vague question, "What is your next step?" is often the most difficult one because the answer may be diagnostic, staging, or therapeutic.

What Is the Likely Mechanism for This Disease Process?

This question goes further than making the diagnosis and requires the student to understand the underlying mechanism of the process. For example, a clinical scenario may describe a 68-year-old male who notes urinary hesitancy and retention and has a large, hard, nontender mass in his left supraclavicular region. This patient has bladder neck obstruction due to benign prostatic hypertrophy or prostatic cancer. However, the indurated mass in the left neck area is suggestive of cancer. The mechanism is metastasis in the area of the thoracic duct, which drains lymph fluid into the left subclavian vein. The student is advised to learn the mechanisms of each disease process and not merely to memorize a constellation of symptoms. Furthermore, in general surgery it is crucial for students to understand the anatomy, function, and how a surgical procedure will correct the problem.

What Are the Risk Factors for This Disease Process?

Understanding the risk factors helps the practitioner to establish a diagnosis and to determine how to interpret test results. For example, understanding the risk factor analysis may help in the treatment of a 55-year-old woman with anemia. If the patient has risk factors for endometrial cancer (such as diabetes, hypertension, anovulation) and complains of postmenopausal bleeding, she likely has endometrial carcinoma and should undergo endometrial biopsy. Otherwise, occult colonic bleeding is a common etiology. If she takes nonsteroidal anti-inflammatory drugs or aspirin, peptic ulcer disease is the most likely cause.

CLINICAL PEARL

A knowledge of the risk factors can be a useful guide in testing and in developing the differential diagnosis.

What Are the Complications of This Disease Process?

Clinicians must be cognizant of the complications of a disease so that they can understand how to follow and monitor the patient. Sometimes, the student has to make a diagnosis from clinical clues and then apply his or her knowledge of the consequences of the pathologic process. For example, a 26-year-old male complains of a 7-year history of intermittent diarrhea, lower abdominal pain, bloody stools, and tenesmus and is first diagnosed with probable ulcerative colitis. The long-term complications of this process include colon cancer. Understanding the types of consequences also helps the clinician to become aware of the dangers to the patient. Surveillance with colonoscopy is important in attempting to identify a colon malignancy.

What Is the Best Therapy?

To answer this question, the clinician not only needs to reach the correct diagnosis and assess the severity of the condition but also must weigh the situation to determine the appropriate intervention. For the student, knowing exact dosages is not as important as understanding the best medication, route of delivery, mechanism of action, and possible complications. It is important for the student to be able to verbalize the diagnosis and the rationale for the therapy.

◈ **CLINICAL PEARL**

Therapy should be logical based on the severity of the disease and the specific diagnosis. An exception to this rule is in an emergent situation such as shock, when the blood pressure must be treated even as the etiology is being investigated.

SUMMARY

1. There is no replacement for a meticulous history and physical examination.
2. There are four steps in the clinical approach to the patient: making the diagnosis, assessing the severity of the disease, treating based on severity, and following the patient's response.
3. There are seven questions that help to bridge the gap between the textbook and the clinical arena.

REFERENCES

Jeffrey RB. Imaging the surgical patient. In: Niederhuber JE, ed. Fundamentals of surgery. New York: Appleton & Lange, 1998:68–75.
Niederhuber JE. The surgical service and surgery training. In: Niederhuber JE, ed. Fundamentals of surgery. New York: Appleton & Lange, 1998:3–9.

Clinical Cases

A 46-year-old woman presents to the outpatient clinic for evaluation of a breast mass that was discovered by her primary care physician during a physical examination. The patient does not perform breast self-examination, and she has never noticed the mass prior to this time. Her past medical history is unremarkable. She has not had any prior history of breast complaints or trauma. The findings from the physical examination are unremarkable except for the breast examination. A hard, nontender, 4-cm mass is noted in the upper outer quadrant of her left breast. The left axilla is without abnormalities. Examination of the right breast reveals no dominant mass or axillary adenopathy.

 What is your next step?

 What is the likely therapy for this patient if she is concerned about breast cosmetic appearance and preservation?

ANSWERS TO CASE 1: Breast Cancer

Summary: A 46-year-old female has a 4-cm palpable left breast mass. The findings from an examination of the left axilla and of her right breast are normal.

◆ **Next step:** Obtain tissue for diagnosis, and if a malignancy is confirmed, proceed with cancer staging. Bilateral mammography may be helpful.

◆ **Likely therapy:** If a biopsy confirms breast carcinoma, the disease is likely in clinical stage IIa (Table 1–1), which is generally best managed by (1) first surgery and then adjuvant therapy or (2) initially systemic therapy (chemotherapy) to shrink the tumor, followed by locoregional surgical therapy (neoadjuvant). Neoadjuvant therapy is probably the best choice in this case because the patient is concerned about cosmetic appearance and desires breast conservation.

Analysis

Objectives

1. Review the initial workup and staging process for a patient with newly diagnosed breast cancer.
2. Be familiar with the options for locoregional and systemic therapy of breast cancer and the basis for selecting neoadjuvant therapy for certain patients.

Considerations

The initial workup for this patient requires confirmation of breast cancer, including bilateral mammography and core needle or excisional biopsy. If carcinoma is confirmed, an additional metastatic workup should include a complete blood count (CBC), liver function tests, and chest radiography (CXR). If a biopsy confirms breast carcinoma, it is

Table 1–1
BREAST CANCER STAGING

Stage 0	Tis	N0	M0	Tx: Cannot assess
				T0: No evidence of primary tumor
Stage I	T1	N0	M0	Tis: In situ
				T1: ≤2 cm
Stage IIA	T0–T1	N1	M0	T1a: ≤0.5 cm
				T1b: >0.5 cm, ≤1 cm
	T2	N0	M0	T1c: >1 cm, ≤2 cm
				T2: >2 cm, ≤5 cm
Stage IIB	T2	N1	M0	T3: >5 cm
				T4: Extension to chest wall or skin
	T3	N0	M0	T4a: Extension to chest wall
				T4b: Edema or ulceration of the skin
Stage IIIA	T0–T2	N2	M0	T4c: Both chest wall extension and skin involvement
	T3	N1–N2	M0	T4d: Inflammatory carcinoma
				Nx: Cannot assess
Stage IIIB	T4	N0–N2	M0	N0: No regional nodal metastases
				N1: Mobile ipsilateral axillary nodal metastases
	T$_{any}$	N3	M0	N2: Fixed ipsilateral axillary nodal metastases
				N3: Ipsilateral internal mammary nodal metastases
Stage IV	T$_{any}$	N$_{any}$	M1	
				Mx: Cannot be assessed
				M0: No distant metastases
				M1: Distant metastases

likely to be stage IIa (Table 1–1), which is best managed by surgery and adjuvant therapy or by systemic therapy (neoadjuvant) prior to locoregional therapy. This patient is a candidate for mastectomy or breast conservation therapy because the extent of local surgery does not impact her overall survival. Because she desires breast conservation therapy, neoadjuvant therapy is probably the best choice. The breast/tumor size ratio is another reason for providing systemic therapy before surgery.

APPROACH TO BREAST CARCINOMA

Definitions

Fine-needle aspiration (FNA):   A diagnostic procedure using a small-gauge needle and a syringe under vacuum for cytologic analysis, with or without image guidance. FNA can identify cancer but cannot differentiate invasive cancers from in situ cancers.

Core needle biopsy: Large-bore needle (usually 10- to 14-gauge) biopsy that provides a histologic diagnosis. This procedure can be done with image guidance via stereotactic techniques (Figure 1–1).

Neoadjuvant chemotherapy: Chemotherapy given *prior* to surgery to shrink the tumor and provide a better cosmetic result. Adjuvant therapy is chemotherapy or radiotherapy *following* surgery.

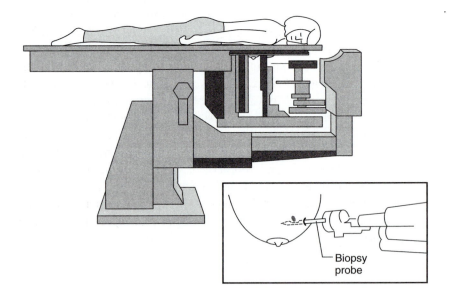

Figure 1–1.   Stereotactic core breast biopsy. The patient is prone on a table undergoing a biopsy with image guidance.

Level 1, 2, and 3 axillary nodes: Level 1 nodes are lateral to the pectoral minor muscles; level 2 nodes are deep to the pectoral minor muscles; and level 3 nodes are medial to the pectoral minor muscles.

Clinical Approach

The steps in breast cancer management include diagnosis, locoregional therapy, and systemic therapy. The history, physical examination, imaging, and tissue biopsy are involved in the diagnosis in most cases. Breast imaging for most patients consists primarily of mammography, although in selective cases ultrasound or magnetic resonance imaging (MRI) can also be considered. A tissue diagnosis can be obtained with FNA, core needle biopsy, or excisional biopsy. Once the tissue diagnosis confirms cancer, the extent of disease and metastasis must be defined, including evaluation of the ipsilateral and contralateral breasts. Stage I and II tumors should be staged with a CBC, liver function tests, and a chest radiograph (CXR). Individuals with bone pain or abdominal symptoms should be evaluated with a bone scan or an abdominal computed tomography (CT) scan to image the liver. Stage III disease should be evaluated with a CBC, liver function tests, a CXR, a bone scan, an abdominal CT scan, and brain CT or MRI if the patient has headaches or neurologic complaints (Figure 1–2).

The surgical options are individualized. If the patient desires breast conservation therapy, feasibility is based on the likely cosmetic outcome, the ability to safely obtain negative margins without a total mastectomy, and the patient's compliance with postoperative radiation therapy and follow-up breast cancer surveillance. Large lesions requiring partial mastectomy may cause significant cosmetic distortion; in such cases patients commonly undergo neoadjuvant chemotherapy to shrink the tumor to obtain better cosmetic results. Alternatively, with a more favorable tumor/breast size ratio, it is often possible to perform a partial mastectomy and obtain a good cosmetic result without the use of neoadjuvant chemotherapy.

Management

1.   The first step is obtaining a tissue diagnosis and staging the breast cancer.

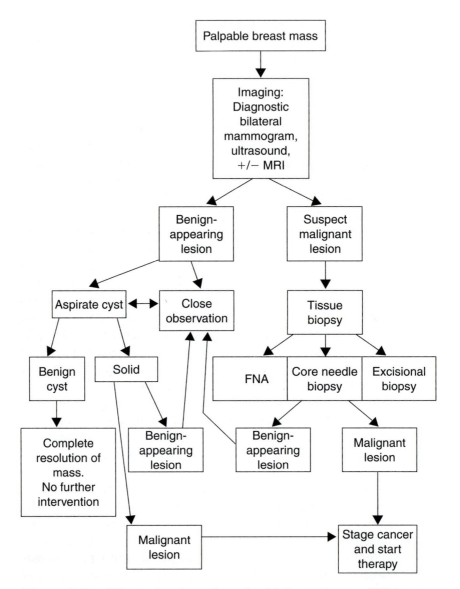

Figure 1–2.   The evaluation of a palpable breast mass. MRI, magnetic resonance imaging; FNA; fine-needle aspiration.

2. **Locoregional therapy:** Breast conservation therapy and mastectomy offer equivalent survival benefits with proper patient selection and follow-up. In addition to resection of the primary tumor, assessment of the regional lymph node basin for local control, complete staging, and determination of the appropriate adjuvant therapy (such as chemotherapy and/or radiation therapy) are undertaken. **Options for nodal staging include levels 1 and 2 axillary dissection versus sentinel lymph node biopsy.** The rationale for sentinel node sampling is to identify the primary lymphatic drainage of the tumor and perform a biopsy on only these nodes. The primary nodal drainage is identified by injecting radiotracers and blue dye at the site of the primary tumor. A gamma probe is used to identify the location of the sentinel node. A small incision is then made over the targeted node, which is further identified with the gamma probe as well as being stained with the blue dye. A biopsy of the sentinel nodes allows for a smaller incision and less axillary morbidity compared to complete nodal basin dissection. However, if the sentinel node is positive for metastatic disease, a complete dissection of the nodes level 1 and 2 axillary should be performed. A sentinel node biopsy can also be used to assess the axillary basin following neoadjuvant chemotherapy.

3. **Systemic therapy:** Systemic therapy is given to patients who are at risk for or who have known distant metastases (stage IV). The options for treatment include surgery followed by chemotherapy, or preoperative (neoadjuvant) chemotherapy followed by surgery. **Patients with stage II breast cancer have a 33% to 44% risk of recurrence of the disease at 20 years with locoregional control only. For this reason, the majority of patients with stage II disease or greater are offered systemic chemotherapy** in addition to locoregional control, with radiation therapy for breast-conserving surgery. Chemotherapy options include doxorubicin, paclitaxel, and antiestrogen-based therapies. The most common chemotherapy regimens currently used in the United States include 5-fluorouracil/doxorubicin (Adriamycin)/cyclophosphamide (FAC) and cyclophosphamide/methotrexate/5-fluorouracil (CMF). CMF is often reserved for patients with comorbidities that preclude the use of

doxorubicin-based therapy. **Generally, antiestrogen therapy is given for 5 years to patients with estrogen and/or progesterone receptor–positive tumors.** This therapy is offered after adjuvant chemotherapy if adjuvant therapy is required based on the stage of the disease. Tamoxifen is the most commonly used antiestrogen therapy, but recent trials with aromatase inhibitors have shown equivalent efficacy in the treatment of postmenopausal breast cancer and a similar or slightly improved side effects profile.

Additionally, there must be consideration of neoadjuvant versus adjuvant chemotherapy. The advantages of neoadjuvant chemotherapy include in vivo determination of tumor sensitivity to therapy, an improved breast conservation rate, and therefore likely improved cosmetic results. The disadvantages of neoadjuvant therapy may be difficulty in assessing the actual pathologic stage after therapy and difficulty in accurately assessing the pretreatment stage without a tissue assessment of the axillary nodal basin or tumor size at the initial presentation. **Current evidence has not demonstrated a survival difference between patients treated with neoadjuvant versus adjuvant therapy.**

Comprehension Questions

[1.1] A 42-year-old woman with a 2-cm mobile lesion and a single palpable 2-cm mobile node in the axilla has what clinical stage of cancer?

A. Ia
B. IIa
C. IIb
D. IIIc

[1.2] Which of the following most accurately describes a sentinel lymph node?

A. A lymph node containing cancer metastases
B. The lymph node that is most likely to become infected postoperatively

    C. The first lymph node in the lymph node basin draining a
       tumor

    D. The surgical margins of an axillary dissection

[1.3] A 45-year-old woman undergoes breast-conserving surgery (a
     lumpectomy) for a 1.5-cm tumor. The axillary lymph nodes are
     negative. Which of the following is the best therapy?

    A. Radiation therapy to the affected breast
    B. No further therapy and observation
    C. Combined chemotherapy such as the CMF regimen
    D. A radical mastectomy

[1.4] A 62-year-old woman complains of painful enlargement of her
     right breast. She has no family history of breast cancer. The right
     breast reveals warmth, redness, and right axilla nontender
     adenopathy. Which of the following is the most likely diagnosis?

    A. Mastitis
    B. Cellulitis
    C. Breast abscess
    D. Breast cancer

Answers

[1.1] **B.** T1 N1 disease in this patient puts her disease at stage IIA.

[1.2] **C.** The sentinel node is the first lymph node in the lymph node
     basin draining a tumor.

[1.3] **A.** Radiation therapy is indicated for a patient with stage I disease
     treated with breast conservation therapy. The addition of radia-
     tion therapy reduces the local recurrence rate from approximately
     30% to 9%, and it is an integral part of the treatment program.

[1.4] **D.** A postmenopausal or nonlactating woman who presents with
     red and/or tender breasts should be assumed to have breast can-
     cer until it is proven otherwise. Inflammatory breast cancer is

characterized by edema, redness, and tenderness due to tumor occlusion of the dermal lymphatic channels.

CLINICAL PEARLS

◈ Tamoxifen therapy is associated with the development of uterine cancer.
◈ The initial workup for a dominant breast mass generally involves obtaining tissue to identify the breast mass and
  mammography to assess for other nonpalpable masses.
◈ A sentinel node biopsy can eliminate the need for axillary
  node dissection in selected patients.
◈ Systemic therapy (chemotherapy) is given when widespread
  metastasis is diagnosed or when the patient is at high risk
  for distant metastasis.

REFERENCES

Krag D, et al. The sentinel node in breast cancer: a multicenter validation study.
   N Engl J Med 1998;339:941–946.
Rosen PP, Groshen S, Kinne DW. Prognosis in T2 N0 M0 stage 1 breast carcinoma:
   a 20-year follow-up study. J Clin Oncol 1991;9:1650–1661.

CASE 2

A 48-year-old man presents for an evaluation of burning epigastric and substernal pain that has recurred almost daily for the past 4 months. He says that these symptoms seem to be worse when he lies down and after meals. He denies difficulty swallowing or weight loss. The patient has been taking a proton pump inhibitor (PPI) on a regular basis over the past 12 weeks with partial resolution of his symptoms. His past medical history is significant for frequent early morning wheezing and hoarseness that have been present for the past few months. The patient has no other known medical problems, and he has had no prior surgeries. He consumes alcohol occasionally but does not use tobacco. On examination, he is moderately obese. No abnormalities are identified on the cardiopulmonary or abdominal examination.

◆ **What is the most likely diagnosis?**

◆ **What are the mechanisms contributing to this disease process?**

◆ **What are the complications associated with this disease process?**

ANSWERS TO CASE 2: Gastroesophageal Reflux Disease

Summary: A 48-year-old man complains of a 4-month history of daily burning epigastric pain. It is worse after eating and lying down and improves slightly with the use of a proton pump inhibitor. He also has symptoms of reactive airway disease and hoarseness.

◆ **Most likely diagnosis:** Gastroesophageal reflux associated with silent aspiration and pharyngitis.

◆ **Mechanisms contributing to this disease process:** Abnormalities of the lower esophageal sphincter (LES), impaired esophageal clearance, and abnormal esophageal barriers to acid exposure.

◆ **Complications associated with the disease process:** Peptic stricture, Barrett's esophagus, and extraesophageal complications.

Analysis

Objectives

1. Describe the physiologic mechanisms that prevent and the pathologic processes that lead to gastroesophageal reflux disease (GERD).
2. Understand a rational diagnostic and therapeutic approach to suspected GERD.

Considerations

This patient's history of substernal chest pain associated with meals is typical for GERD. Hoarseness and wheezing are somewhat atypical symptoms but suggest pharyngeal reflux with silent aspiration. Although this patient denies dysphagia or weight loss, the presence of these symptoms should prompt a further workup for a malignancy.

The next step should be to confirm the diagnosis of GERD and to assess the adequacy of the medical regimen. Endoscopy should be performed to evaluate for esophagitis. The use of 24-hour pH monitoring while the patient is off medication can correlate the symptoms with episodes of reflux and quantify the severity of the reflux. Pharyngeal pH monitoring, which measures proximal esophageal acid exposure, may help to support a diagnosis of silent aspiration.

While H$_2$ blockers can provide symptomatic relief for mild reflux, PPIs may be superior for decreasing acid production. However, patients with extraesophageal symptoms and pharyngeal reflux may be less responsive to medical treatment. Surgical therapy is an alternative to medical therapy and is recommended if the patient does not respond to medical therapy, cannot tolerate the medications, or prefers surgical intervention.

APPROACH TO GASTROESOPHAGEAL REFLUX DISEASE

Definitions

Gastroesophageal reflux disease: Symptoms of heartburn caused by acid regurgitation from the stomach into the distal esophagus.

Barrett's esophagus: Replacement of the normal squamous epithelium of the distal esophagus with columnar epithelium with intestinal metaplasia, which places the patient at risk for esophageal adenocarcinoma.

Manometry: A procedure in which a small electronic pressure transducer is swallowed by the patient to be positioned in the vicinity of the LES. The most commonly used technique involves a 24-hour ambulatory device.

Clinical Approach

Gastroesophageal reflux, or heartburn, occurs in about 20% to 40% of the adult population. However, abnormal GERD occurs in only 60% of patients with reflux symptoms. About half of patients with abnormal reflux develop complications such as peptic strictures, Barrett's esophagus, and extraesophageal complications. **Barrett's esophagus** is

associated with an **increased risk for esophageal adenocarcinoma.
Extra-esophageal complications,** postulated to be due to pharyngeal
reflux and silent aspiration, include **laryngitis, reactive airway disease, recurrent pneumonia, and pulmonary fibrosis.**

Pathophysiology

Normal physiologic mechanisms are important in preventing abnormal
gastroesophageal reflux. For example, abnormalities in the resting pressure, intra-abdominal length, or number of relaxations of the **LES** can
contribute to abnormal reflux. The LES normally serves as a zone of increased pressure between the positive pressure in the stomach and the
negative pressure in the chest. A hypotensive or incompetent LES can result in increased reflux. The **crural diaphragm,** which is attached to the
esophagus by the phrenoesophageal ligament, also contributes to the normal barrier against reflux. **When the LES is abnormally located in the
chest, as with a hiatal hernia, the antireflux mechanism may be compromised at the gastroesophageal (GE) junction.** Also, the esophagus
normally undergoes transient relaxations, but patients with abnormal
GERD experience an increased number and duration of relaxations.
Other proposed contributory factors include abnormal esophageal clearance of acid and decreased mucosal resistance to acid injury.

Workup   Patients with self-limiting or mild GERD symptoms do not
automatically require a further workup. Those with long-standing or
atypical symptoms (wheezing, cough, hoarseness), recurrence of disease after the cessation of medical therapy, or unrelieved symptoms
when taking maximal-dose PPIs should undergo diagnostic testing to
confirm the diagnosis and to rule out complications of GERD. Also,
patients who are being considered for a surgical antireflux procedure
should undergo further evaluation. While not all surgeons routinely
perform all four studies, a standard workup prior to a surgical antireflux
procedure includes endoscopy, manometry, 24-hour pH probe testing,
and barium esophagography (Table 2–1).

Treatment   The initial treatment of patients with GERD consists of be-
havioral modifications (Table 2–2) and medications as needed. However, for patients with esophagitis or significant symptoms, **the main-**

Table 2–1
DIAGNOSIS OF GASTROESOPHAGEAL REFLUX DISEASE

TEST	PURPOSE OF TEST
Endoscopy	Evaluates for erosive esophagitis or Barrett's esophagus, or alternative pathology. Biopsy for suspected dysplasia or malignancy.
Barium esophagogram	Identifies the location of the gastroesophageal junction in relation to the diaphragm. Identifies a hiatal hernia or shortened esophagus. Evaluates for gastric outlet obstruction (in which case fundoplication is contraindicated). Can demonstrate spontaneous reflux.
pH monitoring for 24 h	Correlates symptoms with episodes of reflux. Quantitates reflux severity.
Pharyngeal pH monitoring	Correlates respiratory symptoms with abnormal pharyngeal acid exposure.
Manometry	Evaluates the competency of the lower esophageal sphincter. Evaluates the adequacy of peristalsis prior to planned antireflux surgery. Partial fundoplication may be indicated if aperistalsis is noted. Can diagnose motility disorders such as achalasia or diffuse esophageal spasm.
Nuclear scintigraphy	May confirm reflux if pH monitoring cannot be performed. Evaluates gastric emptying.

stay of medical acid suppression is PPI therapy. High-dose PPI therapy may be required for severe symptoms or refractory esophagitis. A lack of any symptomatic relief with PPIs suggests the possibility of an alternative diagnosis.

Surgical therapy is an alternative to medical therapy and is **indicated in patients with documented GERD who have persistent symptoms when taking maximal-dose PPIs, are intolerant to PPIs, or who do not wish to take lifelong medications.** Although several antireflux operations are available, the standard operation is laparoscopic Nissen fundoplication, which involves performing a 360-degree

Table 2–2

TREATMENT OF GASTROESOPHAGEAL REFLUX DISEASE

Behavioral therapy	Avoidance of caffeine, alcohol, and high-fat meals Avoidance of meals within 2–3 h of bedtime Elevation of the head of the bed Weight loss in obese individuals Smoking cessation
Medical therapy	Antacids Histamine-2 blockers Proton pump inhibitors Prokinetic agents
Surgical therapy	Laparoscopic or open antireflux procedure
Endoscopic therapy	Radiofrequency energy directed to the gastroesophageal junction Endoscopic endoluminal gastroplication

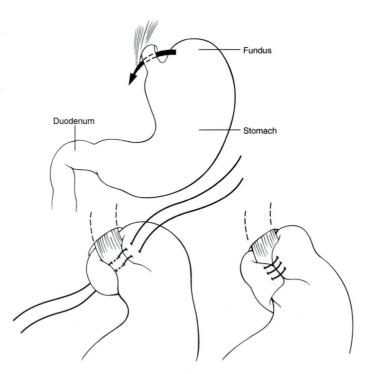

Figure 2–1.   Nissen fundoplication. The fundus of the stomach is wrapped around the distal esophagus and sutured.

wrap of the fundus of the stomach around the GE junction to create a valve effect (Figure 2–1). Long-term success with antireflux surgery exceeds 90%. Recently, two newer endoscopic endoluminal techniques have been developed to treat reflux: delivery of radiofrequency energy to the GE junction and endoluminal suturing of the GE junction. Further prospective data are required.

Comprehension Questions

[2.1] A 62-year-old man with congestive heart failure and emphysema has symptoms of substernal chest pain and regurgitation after meals and at bedtime. He obtains incomplete relief of his symptoms with ranitidine. An endoscopy confirms mild esophagitis. Which of the following is the most appropriate next step?

A. Reassure him that continued occurrence of symptoms while receiving therapy is normal.
B. Prescribe a PPI.
C. Schedule him for 24-hour pH monitoring, manometry, and a barium esophagogram for further evaluation.
D. Schedule him for laparoscopic Nissen fundoplication.

[2.2] A 51-year-old woman has a 6-month history of substernal chest pain and vague upper abdominal discomfort. She has been taking antacid therapy with minimal relief and has had a negative upper endoscopy. Which of the following is the best next step in her work-up?

A. Barium esophagogram to evaluate for a hiatal hernia
B. Performing manometry to rule out a motility disorder such as diffuse esophageal spasm or achalasia
C. Refer the patient for cardiac work-up as a potential cause of her chest pain
D. Refer to psychiatrist for possible conversion reaction.

[2.3] A 45-year-old male has had a diagnosis of GERD for 3 years with treatment with H-2 blocking agents. Recently, he has complained of epigastric pain. An upper endoscopy was performed showing Barrett's esophagus at the distal esophagus. Which of the following is the best next step in the treatment of this individual?

A. Initiate a PPI
B. Advise the patient to continue to take the H-2 blocker
C. Advise surgical therapy involving gastrectomy and esophageal bypass
D. Discontinue the H2-blocker and initiate antacids

[2.4] A 24-year-old man with long-standing GERD, currently taking PPIs, is being evaluated for possible surgical therapy. Which of the following is an indication for surgery?

A. Inability to tolerate PPIs
B. Incomplete relief of symptoms despite a maximum dosage of medical therapy
C. The patient's desire to discontinue medication
D. All of the above

Answers

[2.1] **B.** Given the patient's comorbidities, he is not a good candidate for surgical therapy. PPIs are the medication of choice and should be the next step after the failure of H2 blockers in this patient.

[2.2] **C.** When chest or epigastric pain does not respond to antacid therapy, and especially with a negative upper endoscopy, etiologies other than GERD (such as cardiac pain) should be considered. Documentation of a hiatal hernia does not necessarily correlate causally to her symptoms.

[2.3] **A.** The next step in medical therapy for GERD is the addition of a PPI. The patient has been symptomatic and developed Barrett's esophagitis on an H2-blocker and therefore additional therapy is needed for relief of symptoms and to decrease the progression of the Barrett's esophagitis to adenocarcioma. An anti-reflux surgery (such as the Nissen fundoplication) is an option, but not gastrectomy and esophageal bypass. This patient also needs endoscopic surveillance of the Barrett's esophagus.

[2.4] **D.** The indications for surgery are relative and are determined in part by the patient; thus, inability to tolerate or a desire to discontinue medical therapy is a reason for operative management.

CLINICAL PEARLS

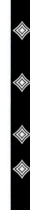

◈ Diagnostic endoscopy should be performed when patients have long-standing GERD symptoms and when patients' symptoms are refractory to medical treatment.

◈ Patients with GERD may develop pulmonary and laryngeal symptoms.

◈ Adenocarcinoma of the esophagus is a complication of long-standing GERD.

◈ Surgical therapy for GERD is indicated in patients with documented GERD who have persistent symptoms while taking maximal-dose PPIs, cannot tolerate PPIs, or do not wish to take lifelong medications.

REFERENCES

Castell DO. Medical, surgical, and endoscopic treatment of gastroesophageal reflux disease and Barrett's esophagus. J Clin Gastroenterol 2001;33(4):262–266.

Hinder RA. Gastroesophageal reflux disease. In: Bell RH, Rikkers LF, and Mulholland MW, eds. Digestive tract surgery: a text and atlas. Philadelphia: Lippincott-Raven, 1996:3–26.

Oelschlager BK, Pellegrini CA. Minimally invasive surgery for gastroesophageal reflux disease. J Laparosc Endosc Adv Surg Tech 2001;99:341–349.

Orlando RC. Overview of the mechanisms of gastroesophageal reflux. Am J Med 2001;111:174S–177S.

A 43-year-old man presents to the emergency room with severe abdominal pain and substernal chest pain. The patient's symptoms began approximately 12 hours earlier after he returned from a party where he consumed a large amount of alcohol that made him ill. Subsequently, he vomited several times and then went to sleep. A short time thereafter, he was awakened with severe pain in the upper abdomen and substernal area. His past medical history is unremarkable, and he is currently taking no medications. On physical examination, the patient appears uncomfortable and anxious. His temperature is 38.8°C (101.8°F), pulse rate 120/min, blood pressure 126/80, and respiratory rate 32/min. The findings from an examination of his head and neck are unremarkable. The lungs are clear bilaterally with decreased breath sounds on the left side. The cardiac examination reveals tachycardia and no murmurs, rubs, or gallops. The abdomen is tender to palpation in the epigastric region, with involuntary guarding. The results of a rectal examination are normal. Laboratory studies reveal that his white blood count is 26,000/mm^3 and that his hemoglobin, hematocrit, and electrolyte levels are normal. The serum amylase, bilirubin, AST, ALT, and alkaline phosphatase values are within normal limits. A 12-lead electrocardiogram shows sinus tachycardia. His chest radiograph reveals moderate left pleural effusion, a left pneumothorax, and pneumomediastinum.

◆ **What is the most likely diagnosis?**

◆ **What is your next step?**

ANSWERS TO CASE 3: Esophageal Perforation

Summary: A 43-year-old man presents with a spontaneous thoracic esophageal perforation (Boerhaave syndrome). The patient has a left pneumothorax and exhibits a septic process from the mediastinitis.

◆ **Most likely diagnosis:** A spontaneous esophageal rupture (Boerhaave syndrome).

◆ **Next step:** Management of the airway, breathing, and circulation (ABC's), including the placement of a left chest tube, fluid resuscitation, and the administration of broad-spectrum antibiotics, followed by a water-soluble contrast study of the esophagus.

Analysis

Objectives

1. Recognize the clinical settings, early signs and symptoms, and complications of esophageal perforation.
2. Understand the diagnostic and therapeutic approach to a suspected esophageal perforation.

Considerations

This patient's clinical presentation is classic for a spontaneous esophageal perforation; however, delay in diagnosis and treatment can still occur because many physicians do not have extensive experience in the evaluation and treatment of this problem. Maintaining a high index of suspicion and pursuing an early diagnosis and early treatment are essential.

APPROACH TO SUSPECTED ESOPHAGEAL PERFORATION

Esophageal perforation remains a surgical emergency. A delay in diagnosis leads to increased morbidity and mortality; therefore, a high index of suspicion should be maintained. Most esophageal perforations are iatrogenic and occur during a diagnostic or therapeutic procedure. Spontaneous esophageal perforation, also referred to as Boerhaave syndrome, accounts for about 15% of all causes of esophageal perforation.

The development of an **acute onset of chest pain after an episode of vomiting** is typical of Boerhaave syndrome. Other symptoms that may be present include shoulder pain, dyspnea, and midepigastric pain. Findings from a physical examination, screening radiographs, and laboratory results depend on (1) the integrity of the mediastinum, (2) the location of the perforation, (3) and the time elapsed since the perforation. Seventy-five percent of patients present with a **pleural effusion** indicating disruption of the mediastinal pleura. Contamination of the mediastinum with esophageal luminal contents often leads to **mediastinitis and chest pain.** A delay in treatment leads to sepsis with signs of systemic infection (tachycardia, fever, and leukocytosis). Perforation into the mediastinum leads to pneumomediastinum that can be seen on a chest radiograph and subcutaneous emphysema that can be demonstrated by physical examination. Because **most spontaneous esophageal ruptures occur in the distal third of the esophagus** above the gastroesophageal junction, **two-thirds of patients present with a left pleural effusion.** The time from perforation to the time of diagnosis is of paramount importance to the ultimate outcome (see Table 3–1).

Diagnosis

The best initial diagnostic test for an esophageal rupture is a water-soluble contrast esophagogram, which identifies perforation in 90% of cases. Water-soluble contrast is preferred during the initial examination because it causes less mediastinal irritation than barium if a large leak is discovered. If no leak is encountered with the water-soluble

Table 3–1
CLINICAL PROGRESSION OF SPONTANEOUS ESOPHAGEAL PERFORATION

SIGN OR SYMPTOM	TIME OF OCCURRENCE	COMMENTS
Chest pain	Immediate, persistent	Most common presenting symptom; less specific are shoulder and abdominal pain.
Subcutaneous emphysema	1 h after perforation	Occurs more frequently with iatrogenic cervical perforation; may not be present with lower esophageal perforation.
Pleural effusion on chest radiograph	May be immediate or late (>6 h)	Occurs in 75% of cases; most often on left side (66%) but may occur on right side (20%).
Fever, leukocytosis	>4 h	Sepsis from mediastinitis.
Death	Diagnosis made <24 h, 15% Diagnosis made >24 h, >40%	Outcome is dependent on early diagnosis and treatment.

medium, a barium contrast must be utilized to be assured that no leak is present. After the diagnosis is confirmed and the initial treatment measures have been performed (ie, ABC's, resuscitation, a tube thoracostomy, and the administration of intravenous antibiotics), the patient is prepared for surgical intervention. **The treatment principles for spontaneous esophageal perforation include surgical drainage, debridement, repair, and diversion** (Figure 3–1).

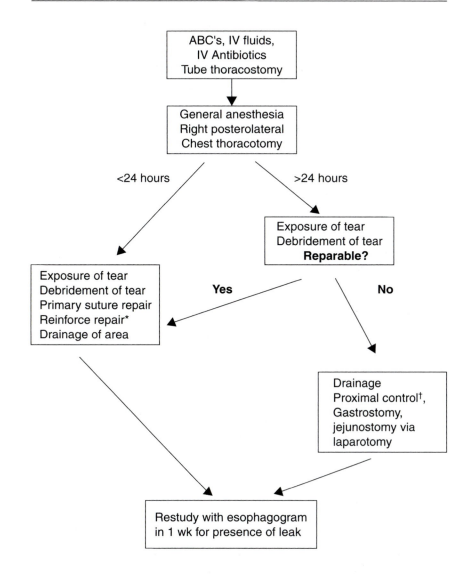

*Reinforce with flap (eg, intercostal, pleural).
†Proximal control refers to diversion (eg, nasogastric tube drainage, cervical stoma).

Figure 3–1.   An algorithm for managing esophageal perforation.
ABC's, airway, breathing, circulation; IV, intravenous.

Comprehension Questions

[3.1] Which of the following is the most common cause of esophageal perforation?

A. Trauma
B. Iatrogenic (endoscopy)
C. Spontaneous rupture (Boerhaave syndrome)
D. Caustic injury

[3.2] Which of the following is the most sensitive diagnostic examination for diagnosing esophageal perforation?

A. A barium esophagogram
B. A Gastrografin esophagogram
C. Esophagoscopy
D. Computed tomography

[3.3] Which of the following is the most important factor that determines the outcome in esophageal perforation?

A. The size of the perforation
B. Whether a meal has been ingested recently
C. The duration between the event and the corrective surgery
D. Leukocytosis

[3.4] After eating some stale pizza, a 21-year-old college student presents to the emergency room with a 24 hour history of nausea, vomiting, and severe chest pain. A esophageal perforation is diagnosed by a contrast study, with the best clinical impression of its onset occurring about 12 hours previously. Which of the following is the best treatment?

A. Primary surgical repair
B. Endoscopic repair
C. Gastrostomy tube and observation
D. Continued observation for spontaneous healing

Answers

[3.1] **B.** Diagnostic endoscopy is associated with the risk of cervical esophageal perforation, and therapeutic endoscopy (pneumatic dilatation) is most commonly associated with perforation at the gastroesophageal junction.

[3.2] **A.** 90% of the time, a Gastrografin (water-soluble) esophagogram is accurate in identifying a perforation, but a barium study remains the most sensitive method.

[3.3] **C.** The outcome for an esophageal perforation is directly related to the amount of time that elapses between the diagnosis and the treatment.

[3.4] **A.** Primary esophageal repair is generally performed when the perforation is less than 24 hours in duration. In patients in good physiologic condition, surgical repair is generally employed regardless of the duration of perforation.

CLINICAL PEARLS

◈ Spontaneous esophageal perforation should be suspected in a patient with chest pain after vomiting, subcutaneous emphysema found on physical examination, and left-sided effusion demonstrated on a chest radiograph.

◈ A high index of suspicion is needed because a delay in diagnosis often leads to a worse outcome.

◈ Most spontaneous esophageal ruptures occur in the distal third of the esophagus.

◈ Most iatrogenic esophageal perforations are associated with endoscopy.

REFERENCES

Chang CH, Lin PJ, Chang JP, Hseih MJ, Lee MC, Chu JJ. One-stage operation for treatment after delayed diagnosis for thoracic esophageal perforation. Ann Thorac Surg 1992;53:617–620.

Jones WG II, Ginsberg RJ. Esophageal perforation: a continuing challenge. Ann Thorac Surg 1992;53:534–543.

Pate JW, Walker WA, Cole FH, Owen EJ, Johnson WH. Spontaneous rupture of the esophagus: a 30-year experience. Ann Thorac Surg 1989;47:689–692.

During a routine physical examination of a 30-year-old, fair-complex-ioned Caucasian man, you discover a 1.5-cm, pigmented skin lesion on the posterior aspect of his left shoulder. This lesion is nonindurated, has ill-defined borders, and is without surrounding erythema. Examination of the patient's left axilla and neck reveals no identifiable abnormalities. No other pigmented skin lesions are observed during your thorough physical examination. According to the patient's wife, this skin lesion has been present for the past several months, and she believes that it has increased in size and become darker during this time. The patient is otherwise healthy.

◆ **What is your next step?**

◆ **What is the most likely diagnosis?**

◆ **What is the best treatment for this problem?**

ANSWERS TO CASE 4: Malignant Melanoma

Summary: A 30-year-old man has a suspicious pigmented skin lesion on his left shoulder.

◆ **Next step:** Perform an excisional biopsy.

◆ **Most likely diagnosis:** Malignant melanoma.

◆ **Best treatment for this problem:** If this proves to be melanoma, wide local excision with an appropriate clear margin is the best initial treatment. Additionally, evaluation and excision of the regional lymph nodes may be appropriate depending on the depth of invasion of the tumor.

Analysis

Objectives

1. Be familiar with the clinical presentation of malignant melanomas.
2. Appreciate the principles involved in performing biopsies of suspected melanomas.
3. Learn about the treatment and prognosis associated with melanomas.

Considerations

Melanoma should be considered whenever a patient presents with a pigmented skin lesion, and lesions should be assessed with the following ABCDE approach. **A: asymmetry; B: border irregularity; C: color change; D: diameter increase; E: enlargement or elevation.**
    All suspicious lesions should undergo a diagnostic biopsy and be assessed for depth of tumor invasion. A simple excision can be used to perform a biopsy on small lesions on the extremities. Lesions that are large or involve cosmetically important areas require an incisional biopsy.

During the initial biopsy, no attempts are made to achieve a wide margin. Once the melanoma has been confirmed and microstaged via biopsy, the patient will require a thorough examination for locoregional metastases and distant metastasis prior to treatment of the primary melanoma.

APPROACH TO PIGMENTED SKIN LESIONS

Clinical Approach

The incidence of cutaneous melanoma is increasing at an alarming rate. In the year 2000, there were 60,000 new cases and 7700 deaths. Melanoma accounts for 4% of all newly diagnosed cancers in the United States and for 1% of all cancer deaths. It is responsible for 6 out of 7 deaths caused by skin cancer. The site of occurrence is evenly distributed among the head and neck, trunk, and upper and lower extremities. Risk factors can be divided into environmental, genetic, and others (Table 4–1), with an associated increase in the overall relative risk. Melanocytes, dendritic cells found at the dermal/epidermal junction, are found in the skin, choroids of the eye, mucosa of the respiratory and

Table 4–1
RISK FACTORS FOR MELANOMA

GENETIC*	ENVIRONMENTAL FACTORS	OTHER
Fair skin (2.1)	Sunlight (especially	Age
Red hair (3)	ultraviolet-B)	Gender
Caucasian (5–10)	Areas near the equator	Tanning lamps?
More than 20 nevi on	First sunburn at young age	Ultraviolet-A?
body (3.4)		Higher socioecoeconomic class
Blue eyes (4.5)		Immunosuppression
Easily burned and		Halogenated compounds
unable to tan (4.5)		Alcohol/tobacco?
Familial cases (4–10)		Coffee/tea?
Prior history of		
melanoma (900)		

*Relative risk is shown in parentheses.

gastrointestinal tracts, lymph node capsules, and substantia nigra in the brain. The **four types of melanoma are (1) superficial spreading, (2) nodular sclerosis, (3) lentigo maligna, and (4) acral lentiginous.** By far the most common is **superficial spreading,** which accounts for 70% of all cases. It has a slight female predominance and typically has a prolonged radial growth phase (1 to 10 years) and a late vertical growth phase. In comparison to that for the other types of melanoma, the prognosis is favorable. **Nodular sclerosis** is the second most common form, accounting for 15% to 30% of all cases. It has no radial growth phase but has an aggressive vertical growth phase that spreads quickly, partially explaining its poorer prognosis. **Lentigo maligna** occurs in about 4% to 10% of patients and has a relatively long radial growth phase (5 to15 years) and a good prognosis. **Acral lentiginous** melanoma represents 35% to 60% of cases occurring in **African Americans, Asians, and Hispanics** and appears primarily on the palms and soles of the hands and feet and in the nail beds. Similar to nodular sclerosis, it has a very aggressive vertical growth phase and is associated with a poor prognosis.

The incidence of melanoma is directly related to sun exposure, and patients should be educated about the dangers of spending an excessive amount of time in the sun. Commonsense tips include staying out of the sun during the hours of 10 AM to 4 PM, seeking shade at all times, and using sunscreen liberally to protect against ultraviolet (UV) radiation, primarily UVB. Other measures include the use of titanium dioxide or zinc oxide for UVA protection, a wide-brimmed hat, sunglasses, darker clothes, and the avoidance of tanning booths and sunlamps.

In melanoma the treatment and prognosis are determined by the microstage and the pathologic stage of the tumor. The Melanoma Task Force of the American Joint Committee on Cancer has recently revised the staging system for melanoma. Some important changes include the following: (1) Thickness and ulceration continue to be used for the T classification, however, the level of invasion is no longer used except for T1 lesions. (2) The number of metastatic lesions (rather than the largest dimension) is now used for the N classification as well as whether the nodes are microscopic versus macroscopic. (3) The site of distant metastases and the serum lactate dehydrogenase levels are used for the M classification. (4) All patients with stage I, II, or III disease with an associated primary lesion that is **ulcerated should be upstaged.** (5) Satellite and in-transit metastases are all combined under stage III disease. (6) The information gained from a sentinel lymph node (SLN) biopsy for staging is utilized in making clinical management decisions. Table 4–2 contains the new melanoma TNM classification and AJCC stage grouping.

The two methods of microstaging were originally described by Clark and by Breslow in the early 1970s. The Clark method of microstaging is based on the level of invasion of the dermal layers (i.e., intraepithelial, into or filling the papillary dermis, into the reticular dermis). The Breslow method of microstaging level is based on the depth of invasion, which is the vertical height of the melanoma from the granular layer to the area of deepest penetration. Most studies have shown that, compared to the Clark method, Breslow depths of invasion are more accurate prognostic indicators; the overall 5-year survival correlates with tumor thickness. **The 5-year survival rate for stage I melanoma with a thickness of less than 0.75 mm is greater than 96%.**

Table 4–2
TMN CLASSIFICATION

T CLASSIFICATION

Thickness	Ulceration status
T1: 1.0 mm	a: level II/III and without; b: level IV/V or with
T2: 1.01–2 mm	a: without; b: with ulceration
T3: 2.01–3 mm	a: without; b: with ulceration
T4: >4.0 mm	a: without; b: with ulceration

N CLASSIFICATION

Metastatic nodes	Nodal Metastatic Mass
N1: 1 node	a: micro; b: macro
N2: 2–3 nodes	a: micro; b: macro; c: in-transit or satellite
N3: ≥4 nodes or in-transit lesions	

M CLASSIFICATION

Site	
M1: Distant skin, subcutaneous, or nodal	Normal lactate dehydrogenase level
M2: Lung metastsis	Normal lactate dehydrogenase level
M3: Any other distant site	Elevated lactate dehydrogenase level

Revised AJCC Classification, 2002

Treatment

Primary Tumor

The surgical treatment of melanoma begins with proper management of the primary lesion. There are three studies (two are large, prospective, randomized trials, and the third is a retrospective analysis) that help to define the requirements for surgical margins. A treatment plan is summarized in Table 4–3. Since wide local excision is performed to achieve adequate margins, the re-excision of the previous biopsy scar is the usual approach. Therefore, the orientation of the initial biopsy is important to consider to avoid excessive tissue removal and morbidity.

Lymph nodes

The role of therapeutic nodal dissection in melanoma has been heavily debated for many years. In the presence of palpable adenopathy, it is recommended that complete lymphadenectomy of the involved lymph node basin be performed. However, an attempt should be made to obtain a tissue diagnosis (either with fine-needle aspiration or excisional biopsy) prior to this procedure. Patients with **intermediate-depth melanoma (0.76 to 4 mm) seem to have a longer survival after prophylactic lymph node dissection,** suggesting that some patients without clinically evident lymph node involvement may also benefit from regional lymphadenectomy. Because of the morbidity associated with lymphadenectomy, prophylactic dissection is not usually routinely done, but instead the lymph node basins are generally assessed by an SLN biopsy. The SLN is the first node in the lymphatic channel through

Table 4–3
SUGGESTED SURGICAL MARGINS

MINIMUM MARGIN WIDTH	CLINICAL SITUATION
0.5 cm	Melanoma in situ
1.0 cm	Lesions <1.5 mm in thickness
2 cm	Lesions 1.5–4 mm in thickness
At least 2 cm	Lesions >4 mm in thickness

which the primary melanoma drains and can be identified with more than 90% accuracy by using the combined technique of vital blue dye and radiolymphoscintigraphy. This approach offers the advantages of identifying patients with regional nodal metastases who may benefit from therapeutic lymph node dissection and avoids exposing patients without regional lymph node metastases to the morbidity associated with a lymphadenectomy. Additionally, the histologic analysis results from an SLN biopsy can be utilized to more accurately stage the disease process.

All patients with confirmed lymph node metastases should undergo a thorough workup to exclude or identify extranodal spread. **Surgery is the primary therapy for patients with nodal** involvement, and adjuvant therapy provides minimal benefits for stage I and II disease and only limited benefits for stage III disease. Currently, the only **treatment option approved by the Food and Drug Administration (FDA) is interferon-2A** (Intron-A), which has been shown to provide marginal overall and disease-free survival. However, these results must be weighed against the adverse reactions and outcomes associated with this therapy. Multiregimen chemotherapy and radiation therapy have achieved limited success.

The prognosis for patients with stage IV disease remains dismal, with a median survival of 6 to 9 months. Again, it is essential that a thorough workup be performed to develop a therapeutic plan for all sites of disease involvement. Therapeutic options for patients with stage IV disease are limited. The most promising treatment, now **FDA-approved for stage IV melanoma patients, is high-dose interleukin-2,** which has a known complete, durable response rate of 9% and a partial response rate of 8%.

Comprehension Questions

[4.1] Which of the following is the most common form of melanoma?

 A. Superficial spreading
 B. Nodular sclerosis
 C. Acral lentiginous
 D. Lentigo maligna

[4.2] According to the new TNM classification, what is the classification of a patient with a 2.5-mm-deep primary lesion with two positive lymph nodes and no evidence of other disease on metastatic workup?

A. T1 N2 N1
B. T3 N1 M0
C. T3 N2 M0
D. T4 N3 M1

[4.3] Which of the following is the most accurate prognostic indicator during microstaging of a melanoma?

A. Breslow depth of invasion
B. Clark level of invasion
C. T-cell infiltration
D. Size of the primary tumor

[4.4] Based on the current consensus, which of the following is the most appropriate surgical margin for a 2.0-mm-depth melanoma?

A. 0.5 cm
B. 1 cm
C. 2 cm
D. 4 cm

Answers

[4.1] **A.** Superficial spreading is the most common form of melanoma.

[4.2] **C.** Between 2.01 and 3 mm is a T3 tumor; two positive lymph nodes is N2.

[4.3] **A.** Although Breslow staging and Clark staging both use depth of invasion, the Breslow criterion is considered more accurately reflective of prognosis.

[4.4] **C.** 2-cm margins are considered adequate for a tumor with between 1.5- and 4-mm invasion.

CLINICAL PEARLS

◈ A biopsy should be performed on all suspicious pigmented lesions.

◈ *A*symmetry, *B*order irregularity, *C*olor change, *D*iameter increase, and *E*nlargement or *E*levation is more suspicious for malignant melanoma.

◈ The staging systems for malignant melanoma are based on the depth of invasion.

◈ Although interleukin therapy has been found to be somewhat helpful, surgical therapy remains the best treatment for melanoma.

REFERENCES

Balch CM, Urist MM, Karakousis CP, et al. Efficacy of 2-cm surgical margins for intermediate thickness melanomas (1–4 mm). Results of a multi-institutional randomized surgical trial. Ann Surg 1993;218:262–267.

Kanzler MH, Marz-Gernhard S. Treatment of primary cutaneous melanoma. JAMA 2001;285:1819–1821.

Rivers JK. Melanoma. Lancet 1996;347(9004):803–806.

Veronesi U, Cascinelli N. Narrow excision (1-cm margin): a safe procedure for thin cutaneous melanoma. Arch Surg 1991;126:438–441.

A 63-year-old male complains of a 6-month history of difficulty voiding and feeling as though he cannot empty his bladder completely. After voiding, he often feels as though he needs to urinate again. He denies a urethral discharge. He has mild hypertension and takes a thiazide
diuretic. His only other medication is ampicillin prescribed for two urinary tract infections during the past year. On examination, his blood
pressure is 130/84 and his pulse rate 80/min; he is afebrile. Findings
from examinations of the heart and lungs are normal, and the abdomen
reveals no masses.

◆ **What is the most likely diagnosis?**

◆ **What is the best therapy for this patient?**

ANSWERS TO CASE 5: Benign Prostatic Hypertrophy

Summary: A 63-year-old hypertensive male complains of a 6-month history of difficulty voiding and feeling as though he cannot empty his bladder completely. He has experienced two episodes of cystitis. He denies dysuria or urgency and does not have a urethral discharge.

◆ **Most likely diagnosis:** Benign prostatic hypertrophy (BPH).

◆ **Best therapy:** Transurethral prostatectomy (TURP).

Analysis

Objectives

1. Know the clinical presentation of BPH.
2. Know the differential diagnosis for urinary outlet obstruction in males and when a biopsy is appropriate.

Considerations

The prostate gland is the male reproductive organ that is positioned at the base of the bladder and completely encircles the urethra as it exits the bladder and before it becomes part of the penile urethra. The physiologic function of the prostate is to produce the ejaculate, which serves as a vehicle for spermatozoa. As the male ages, the prostate increases in size. This increase in size can have consequences, as the human prostate is the only mammalian prostate with a capsule. The capsule restricts expansion of the prostate gland as BPH progresses. The bladder neck and prostatic urethra become compromised in their function, leading to a condition known as bladder outlet obstruction.

Symptoms of BPH, known as **prostatism,** include irritative and obstructive symptoms. They can **include frequent urination of small amounts,** a feeling of **incomplete voiding** with subsequent attempts to urinate to achieve the feeling of bladder emptying, **slow urinary flow, voiding at night** after sleep (nocturia), **hesitancy** at the beginning of urinary flow, and in its extreme form, **complete urinary retention.** Several conditions that produce similar symptoms mimic BPH. Urethral stricture disease (a narrowing of the urethra with scarring), urinary tract infection, including infection of the prostate (prostatitis), prostate cancer, and neurologic conditions affecting the control and strength of bladder contraction all mimic and may be indistinguishable from BPH. When there is **nodularity or an elevation in the prostate-specific antigen (PSA), biopsy of the prostate is generally indicated.**

APPROACH TO URINARY OUTLET OBSTRUCTION

Definitions

Micturition: The physiologic act of voiding. This involves contraction of the detrusor (bladder muscle) followed by relaxation of the bladder neck and other urinary sphincters to allow unrestricted, complete emptying of the bladder in a single setting.

Digital rectal examination (DRE): The prostate is palpated with a gloved examining finger inserted into the rectum. The normal prostate has the "feel" of the thenar eminence of the thumb (Figure 5–1).

Prostate-specific antigen: A blood protein normally produced by the prostate. PSA is specific to the prostate but not to a particular condition of the prostate because age, size, infection, and cancer are among the several reasons why PSA values can be elevated.

Urodynamics: Testing performed on the function of the bladder in both its filling and emptying phases, which may be as simple as voiding into a specially developed toilet to measure the voiding flow rate to as complicated as the placement of a catheter into the urinary bladder to measure pressures and volumes during filling and emptying.

Clinical Approach

When faced with the vague symptomatology of prostatism, the initial duty of the physician is to exclude other etiologies because the treatment would differ. This exclusion process begins with obtaining a history and looking for associated signs and symptoms of other disease

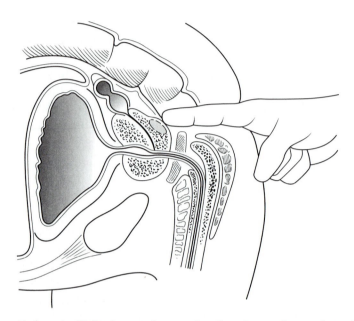

Figure 5–1.   A digital rectal examination is performed to detect nodularity in the prostate gland.

processes. A **review of systems** should entail a search for **neurologic abnormalities.** A **urinalysis** is the cornerstone of laboratory testing to exclude the presence of a **urinary tract infection or microscopic hematuria** that might indicate a **bladder tumor. PSA blood testing** should be performed as well as determination of the **serum creatinine** level to rule out severe prostatism with renal compromise. A **DRE** not only characterizes the **size of the prostate** but also is performed to exclude the **presence of a palpable nodule suggestive of prostate cancer** (Figure 5–1). Even the best history and physical and laboratory testing may not discriminate between bladder outlet obstruction secondary to BPH and a urethral stricture because both of these pathologic entities are secondary to restriction of the urethra. If a patient requires urodynamic testing in cases where the diagnosis is not clear, consultation with a urologist is generally helpful. Making matters more difficult, prostatism may coexist with a urinary tract infection and/or a neurologic disease such as Parkinson disease. Evidence of **renal compromise,** an **elevated serum creatinine value** and/or **urinary retention,** multiple small voids with incomplete emptying, and/or a **palpable bladder** on physical examination call for **urgent urologic intervention.**

Once the correct diagnosis of BPH has been made, **initial treatment is often medical.** Two classes of medication are available for the management of prostatism. The first class are alpha agonist agents, which cause relaxation of the prostate smooth muscle, thereby increasing the functional diameter of the urethra. Another class of medication used in the management of prostatism causes a reduction in prostate size by blocking a metabolite of testosterone, thus leading to the involution of prostate glandular tissue and shrinkage of the overall prostate size. When medical therapy fails, surgical intervention, which serves to destroy prostate obstructing tissue, is used. The **standard operative procedure** is known as transurethral resection of the prostate, or **TURP.** This procedure is carried out transurethrally using a specially developed scope that has attached to it a cutting element with water irrigation. "Chips" of the prostate are carved out from within the prostate urethra and removed via the scope. Alternative methods to destroy prostate tissue include the use of a laser, radiofrequency waves, or microwaves. Rarely, the prostate enlarges to such a size that open surgical removal known as a suprapubic prostatectomy is required. Regardless of the method of therapy chosen to manage BPH, the patient needs to be monitored thereafter for response to therapy as residual glandular tissue will continue to grow.

Comprehension Questions

[5.1] A 57-year-old asymptomatic male is noted to have a prostate that is normal in shape and size on rectal examination. His PSA level is 18 ng/mL (normal < 2.5 ng/mL). What is the best next step for this patient?

   A. Observation
   B. Transrectal ultrasound examination with a prostate biopsy
   C. Repeated PSA testing in 6 months
   D. Initiate finasteride therapy

[5.2] A 72-year-old man has a lower abdominal mass and constantly dribbles urine. Which of the following is the best next step?

A. Computed tomography (CT) scan of the pelvis
B. Enema
C. Placement of a Foley catheter
D. Referral to a general surgeon and a neurologist

[5.3] A 58-year-old commercial airline pilot has confirmed prostatism. He is being treated by a doctor but seeks emergency room treatment for dizziness, which precludes his flying. What is the most likely problem?

A. Unrecognized Parkinson disease
B. Undiagnosed metastatic prostate cancer
C. Drug side effect
D. Silent renal failure

[5.4] A 42-year-old male requests prostate "testing" because his father has recently been given a diagnosis of prostate cancer. You perform a digital rectal examination, which reveals a normal-sized, smooth prostate gland. A PSA test is then performed and is run stat because the patient insists on knowing the results before leaving the office. The PSA result is 3.2 ng/mL (normal < 2.5 ng/mL). Which of the following is the best next step?

A. CT scan of the abdomen and pelvis for a workup for prostatic cancer
B. Sonographically directed prostate biopsy
C. Repeated PSA test
D. Prostatectomy with possible lymphadenectomy

Answers

[5.1] **B.** A substantially elevated PSA value in this patient generally requires a prostate biopsy to assess for prostate cancer. Transrectal sonography is performed to help determine the location of the biopsy.

[5.2] **C.** Overflow incontinence occurs when the urinary bladder is filled to capacity. As the pressure rises, with standing and coughing, a small amount of urine leaks out of the bladder through the restricted bladder outlet in a dribbling fashion. A small amount of urine is seen to squirt from the penis as the Valsalva maneuver pushes on the massively distended bladder. Immediate urinary drainage and hospitalization are in order.

[5.3] **C.** The alpha agonist class of medications, originally developed for blood pressure control, relax the smooth muscle within the arterial wall, leading to a decrease in blood pressure that may result in dizziness and/or syncope (fainting). Patients must be warned of this side effect. Titration and nighttime dosing are often required.

[5.4] **C.** Mild elevations of the PSA value may be seen immediately after a DRE. The best course in this case is to repeat the PSA test several days to 1 week later.

CLINICAL PEARLS

◈ Patients with symptoms suggestive of BPH should undergo a renal function test (creatinine), a PSA test, urinalysis, and a digital rectal examination.

◈ The International Prostate Symptom Score can characterize voiding symptoms based on a patient's report of incomplete emptying, frequency, intermittency, urgency, weak stream, straining, and nocturia.

◈ Although there is no physiologic relationship between BPH and prostate malignancy, the age of onset of these two clinical entities overlaps.

◈ Distinguishing characteristics of prostate cancer include a firm, hard, and/or misshapened prostate gland on examination and/or an elevated or elevating PSA value. Both PBH and prostate malignancy can coexist in the same patient.

◈ The diagnosis of prostate cancer is made with transrectal biopsy of the prostate.

REFERENCES

Walsh PC, Wein AJ, Dorracott E, Retik AB, eds. Campbell's urology, 8th ed. Philadelphia; Saunders, 2002.

Tanagho EA, McAninch JW, eds. Smith's general urology, 15th ed. New York; McGraw-Hill, 2000.

A 43-year-old man presents with a 16-hour history of intermittent, crampy abdominal pain and bilious vomiting. He states that the symptoms began approximately 3 hours after lunch on the previous day, improved after vomiting, but returned after 1 to 2 hours. He had a bowel movement shortly after the onset of the pain, but there has been no passage of flatus or stool since then. The patient denies any similar episodes previously and has no current medical problems. He underwent exploratory laparotomy for a gunshot wound to the abdomen 3 years previously. On examination, his temperature is 100.5°F, pulse rate 105/min, blood pressure 140/80, and respiratory rate 24/min. The abdomen is distended, with a well-healed midline surgical scar. The abdomen is tender throughout with no masses or peritonitis. The bowel sounds are hypoactive with occasional high-pitched rushes. No hernias are identified. A rectal examination reveals no masses and no stool in the rectal vault. Laboratory studies reveal normal electrolyte levels. His white blood cell (WBC) count is 16,000/mm^3 with 85% neutrophils, 4% bands, 10% lymphocytes, and 1% monocytes; the hemoglobin and hematocrit values are 18 g/dL and 48%, respectively. The serum amylase value is 135 IU/L. An abdominal radiograph was obtained (Figure 6–1).

◆ **What is your next step in management?**

◆ **What are the complications associated with this disease process?**

◆ **What is the probable therapy?**

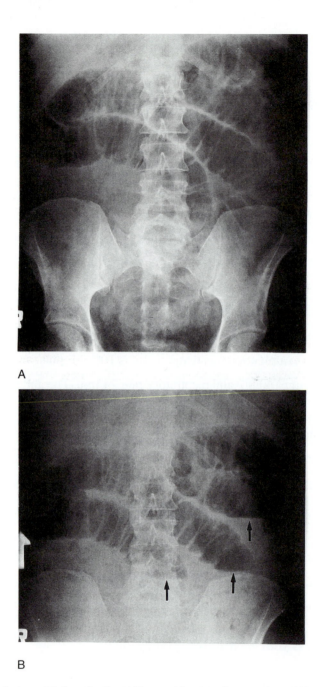

Figure 6–1. Abdominal radiographs in the supine (A) and upright (B) positions show a dilated small bowel with air-fluid levels. (Reproduced, with permission, from Kadell BM, Zimmerman P, Lu DSK. Radiology of the abdomen, Zinner MJ, Schwarz SI, Ellis H, et al, eds. Maingot's abdominal operations, 10th ed. New York: McGraw-Hill, 1997:24.)

ANSWERS TO CASE 6: Small Bowel Obstruction

Summary: A patient has signs, symptoms, and radiographic evidence of a high-grade mechanical small bowel obstruction.

◆ **Next step in management:** Place a nasogastric (NG) tube to decompress the stomach, begin fluid resuscitation, and place a Foley catheter to monitor urine output and assess his response to the fluid resuscitation.

◆ **Complications associated with this disease process:** Mechanical small bowel obstruction may lead to strangulation, bowel necrosis, and sepsis. Vomiting may result in aspiration pneumonitis. When unrecognized or untreated, intravascular fluid loss (from third-space fluid loss and vomiting) can lead to prerenal azotemia and acute renal insufficiency.

◆ **Probable therapy:** Exploratory laparotomy after fluid resuscitation.

Analysis

Objectives

1. Learn the clinical and radiographic features associated with mechanical small bowel obstruction and strangulating or complicated disease processes.
2. Learn the management strategy for mechanical small bowel obstruction.

Considerations

An otherwise healthy 43-year-old man who has undergone previous abdominal surgery presents with typical signs and symptoms associated with mechanical small bowel obstruction. Because of the previous abdominal operation, the cause of the obstruction is most likely related to postoperative adhesions. The change in pain pattern from intermittent to persistent is a concern. **Persistent pain** in this setting can be produced by severe bowel distension (which may produce venous congestion, decreased bowel perfusion, and necrosis) or **bowel ischemia secondary to strangulation.** Other features of this patient's presentation suggesting the presence of a complicated bowel obstruction include **fever, tachycardia, leukocytosis, an elevated serum amylase level, and radiographic signs of a high-grade small bowel obstruction.** Mechanical obstruction of the bowel results in the accumulation of fluid in the bowel lumen and bowel wall, in addition to extravasation of fluid into the peritoneal cavity. The net result of these fluid shifts is a depletion of intravascular volume and decreased perfusion of all organs. Therefore, **one of the most vital aspects of treatment is early recognition of the problem and restoration of the intravascular volume to reestablish organ perfusion.** Restoration of intravascular volume is critical in this patient prior to operative therapy because the induction of general anesthesia in a volume–depleted individual may lead to profound hypotension. Nonoperative therapy is frequently successful for mechanical small bowel obstruction due to adhesions, however, this approach is inappropriate in a patient exhibiting signs and symptoms consistent with existing or impending bowel ischemia and/or necrosis. The most appropriate management in this case consists of NG tube placement to prevent further vomiting and potential aspiration, fluid resuscitation, administration of broad-spectrum antibiotics, and urgent laparotomy.

APPROACH TO SMALL BOWEL OBSTRUCTION

Definitions

Strangulating small bowel obstruction: Mechanical obstruction leading to bowel ischemia and/or necrosis. This process may result from strangulation due to an abdominal wall hernia or an internal hernia, with high-grade and/or complete obstruction.

Ileus: Distension of the small bowel and/or colon from nonobstructive causes. Common causes include local or systemic inflammatory or infectious processes, a variety of metabolic derangements, recent abdominal surgery, and adverse effects of medications.

Internal hernia: A congenital or acquired defect within the peritoneal cavity that can lead to small bowel obstruction.

Gallstone ileus: Mechanical obstruction of the small bowel due to large gallstone(s) in the bowel lumen. This condition generally occurs when a stone or stones in the gallbladder enter the adjacent duodenum. The typical clinical presentation is characterized by intermittent bowel obstruction for several days until the stone lodges in the distal small bowel and causes complete obstruction.

Clinical Approach

Mechanical small bowel obstruction is a common clinical problem. The cause of the obstruction, treatment considerations, and the approach to the disease differ based on the patient's age, the duration of symptoms, and whether or not the patient has a history of abdominal operation or trauma. An obstruction in a neonate, an infant, or a young **child** is most likely the result of a **hernia, malrotation, meconium ileus, Meckel diverticulum, intussusception, or intestinal atresia.** In contrast, a small bowel obstruction in an **adult** is most frequently due to an **adhesion, a hernia, Crohn's disease, gallstone ileus, or a tumor.** As a mechanical small bowel obstruction prevents the passage of small bowel luminal contents, the patient develops cramplike abdominal pain, nausea, and bilious vomiting. It is not uncommon for patients to describe the occurrence of a bowel movement at the onset of an acute obstruction, and this is generally due to the stimulation of peristalsis with evacuation of the distal gastrointestinal tract contents. Hence, **the presence of a bowel movement does not rule out bowel obstruction.** Whenever the small bowel obstruction is nearly complete or complete (high grade) there may be a cessation of flatus and stool passage following the initial bowel movement. The recommended approach to patient evaluation and treatment is outlined in Figure 6–2.

Physical Examination

The physical examination of a patient with small bowel obstruction may initially reveal a low-grade fever and tachycardia as a result of dehydration and inflammatory changes. The persistence of tachycardia

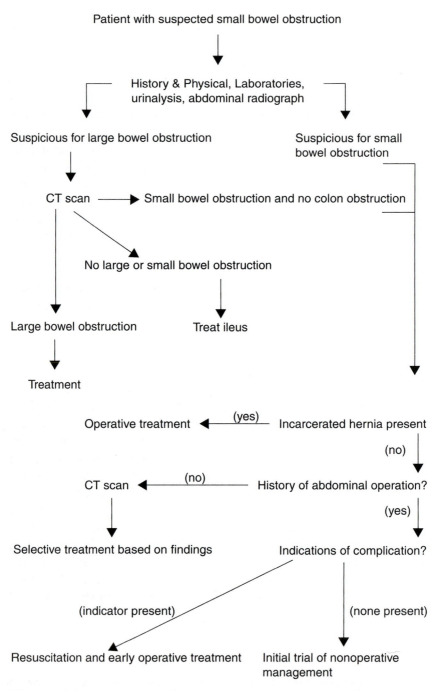

Figure 6–2. Algorithm for the management of small bowel obstruction. CT, computed tomography.

after the completion of fluid resuscitation may suggest unresolved inflammation from small bowel ischemia and/or necrosis. Similarly, the early presence of a high fever should raise a suspicion of bowel ischemia or pulmonary complications due to aspiration. In most patients abdominal examinations will reveal mild, diffuse tenderness. Nonspecific tenderness that improves following successful decompression by the placement of an NG tube is observed commonly in patients with an uncomplicated obstruction. Localized tenderness directly over distended bowel loops suggests the presence of severe distension or bowel ischemia; although a worrisome finding, this localized tenderness is not specific for ischemia. A digital rectal examination of patients with small bowel obstruction often reveals little or no stool in the rectal vault, which is due to continued peristalsis and evacuation of stool from the distal bowel. The finding of a large amount of stool in the rectum is unusual and may suggest ileus rather than mechanical obstruction as the cause of distension.

Pathophysiology

Mechanical obstruction of the small bowel leads to diminished absorptive function and the accumulation of luminal fluid. Additionally, there is a fluid shift into the extravascular space due to local inflammatory stimulation and venous congestion. As the obstruction continues, transudative fluid loss into the peritoneal cavity occurs. These losses, along with vomiting, generally produce tremendous intravascular volume depletion and place untreated patients at risk for the development of remote organ dysfunction due to hypoperfusion. Generally, patients with **proximal small bowel obstruction have more frequent vomiting, and those with more distal obstruction have more distension and less vomiting.** With long-standing distal small bowel obstruction, bacterial overgrowth can develop and lead to feculent vomitus. Prolonged distal small bowel obstruction can lead to further intra-abdominal and pulmonary (aspiration) infectious complications.

Laboratory and Radiographic Evaluations

The initial laboratory evaluation should include a complete blood count with a differential count, serum electrolyte and amylase determinations, urinalysis, and arterial blood gas studies (for selected patients). With dehydration and a physiologic response to bowel obstruction, patients with uncomplicated small bowel obstruction may initially present with mild leukocytosis (WBC count 10,000 to 14,000/μL) and a left-shifted differential. Generally, the leukocytosis resolves with therapy. **Persistent leukocytosis after hydration should raise a suspicion of complications** and may mandate early surgical intervention or an additional diagnostic evaluation. An elevation in the serum amylase level is most commonly associated with pancreatitis but may also develop with complicated small bowel obstruction.

Plain radiographs of the abdomen are generally obtained to evaluate all patients with suspected bowel obstruction. These usually reveal dilated small bowel with or without colonic air. These findings are not pathopneumonic for obstruction and may also be observed in the setting of ileus. Not uncommonly, radiographs of an advanced obstruction demonstrate a fluid-filled bowel with a paucity of air rather than a dilated bowel. Similarly, patients with an obstruction involving the proximal small bowel may have radiographs showing little or no air-filled bowel.

Additional Radiographic Studies

A **computed tomography (CT) scan may be useful** for patients in whom the **etiology is obscure, such as those with a functional obstruction (ileus), inflammatory bowel disease, a tumor, or gallstone ileus.** CT scans can reliably identify the transition from dilated to decompressed bowel, which is diagnostic for mechanical obstruction. In addition, CT imaging may be useful in visualizing peritoneal tumor spread (carcinomatosis), primary small bowel tumors, Crohn's disease, gallstone ileus, and clinically obscure hernias. Alternatively, contrast radiography such as **upper gastrointestinal and small bowel follow-through (UGI/SBFT) can be used to differentiate between mechanical obstruction and ileus** or to assist in determining the location and severity of a bowel obstruction. It is important to bear in mind that CT scanning and UGI/SBFT require the administration of contrast into the bowel lumen and can aggravate patient vomiting and may contribute to aspiration. **The goals in patient evaluation are to diagnose the bowel obstruction and to identify factors that may indicate the presence**

of a strangulated bowel. Table 6–1 lists some of the more commonly used indicators to identify bowel strangulation.

Treatment

Patients with **uncomplicated partial small bowel obstruction** from adhesions can be initially treated with a trial of **nonoperative therapy** consisting of nothing by mouth (NPO), placement of an NG tube, close monitoring of fluid status, serial clinical examinations, and laboratory and radiographic follow-up. Most patients who are successfully treated non-operatively demonstrate improvement within 6 to 24 hours after the initiation of treatment. These improvements include a decrease in abdominal discomfort and distension, a decrease in the volume of NG aspirate, and radiographic resolution of bowel distension. The absence of early improvement with nonoperative treatment should prompt further evaluation with a CT scan or UGI/SBFT to confirm the diagnosis and/or further define the obstruction for possible surgical therapy. When operative treatment is determined to be necessary, perioperative broad-spectrum antibiotics are administered to prevent wound and intra-abdominal infectious complications. Operative therapy for

Table 6–1

INDICATORS SUGGESTIVE OF STRANGULATED
SMALL BOWEL OBSTRUCTION

HISTORY	PHYSICAL EXAMINATION	LABORATORY FINDINGS	RADIOGRAPHY[‡]
Constant pain[*]	Localized	Leukocytosis[*]	Complete obstruction[*,†]
Constipation[*]	tenderness[*]	Elevated amylase	Fluid-filled bowel[*]
	Fever[*,†]	level[†]	Thickened bowel wall[*]
	Tachycardia[*,†]	Elevated lactate	Mesentery edema (CT)[*,†]
	Peritonitis[†]	level[†]	Free-fluid (CT)[*,†]
	Tender mass[*,†]		

[*]Nonspecific (ie, may occur without strangulation).
[†]Not sensitive (ie, may not occur with strangulation).
[‡]CT, computed tomography.

adhesive small bowel obstruction consists of careful exploration and identification of the obstruction source. Adhesive bands responsible for the obstruction are divided, and ischemic or necrotic bowel is resected.

Early Postoperative Small Bowel Obstruction

Early postoperative small bowel obstruction is characterized by symptoms developing within 30 days following an abdominal operation. This condition can result from narrowing of the lumen because of mechanical causes or ileus. An exact determination of the cause is generally not necessary because nonoperative observation is the usual treatment for both. A CT scan may be useful in some patients to identify or rule out an intra-abdominal infection as the cause.

Outcome

The mortality associated with small bowel obstruction has improved over the past 50 years with improved medical technology and supportive care. Despite this overall improvement in patient outcome, there continues to be a significant increase in morbidity and mortality associated with complicated small bowel obstruction. Therefore, one of the major goals in patient treatment is early diagnosis and treatment of uncomplicated small bowel obstruction to prevent a progression to strangulation and bowel necrosis. Patients with a **high-grade bowel obstruction or suspected of having strangulated bowel should undergo prompt resuscitation and early operative therapy,** which may prevent the development and/or progression of bowel necrosis.

Comprehension Questions

[6.1] A 79-year-old woman who has had no previous abdominal surgery presents with intermittent bowel obstruction symptoms of 1 week's duration and persistent vomiting for the past 1 day. Her physical examination does not reveal any hernias and is consistent with that of distal small bowel obstruction. She is afebrile. Her WBC count is 4000/μL. What is the most appropriate next step?

A. Attempt nonoperative treatment for 48 hours.
B. Perform upper gastrointestinal tract endoscopy.
C. Proceed with an immediate exploration laparotomy.
D. Perform a CT scan.

[6.2] Which of the following situations is most likely to respond to non-surgical management?

A. A 72-year-old woman with a bowel obstruction due to mid-gut volvulus
B. Small bowel obstruction due to gallstone ileus
C. A 45-year-old female who has small bowel obstruction after open gall bladder surgery 20 days previously
D. A 2-day-old male who has small bowel obstruction due to jejunal atresia

[6.3] A 67-year-old white male arrives in the emergency room with nausea and vomiting following an appendectomy performed 25 days previously. He is afebrile. The abdomen is slightly tender and distended. The WBC count is 18,000/μL. Electrolyte studies reveal a sodium level of 140 mEq/L, potassium 4.2 mEq/L, chloride 105 mEq/L, and bicarbonate 14 mEq/L. Which of the following is the best therapy for this patient?

A. Placement of an NG tube and observation
B. Colonoscopy for possible intussusception
C. A barium enema to relieve a volvulus
D. Surgical therapy

Answers

[6.1] **D.** Patients without previous abdominal surgery or hernias who present with symptoms and signs of bowel obstruction may benefit from CT imaging (to identify possible malignancy, gallstone ileus, or internal hernia).

[6.2] **C.** Early small bowel obstruction (within 30 days) following abdominal surgery is generally due to adhesions or persistent inflammation that frequently resolves with non-surgical therapy (hospitalization, nothing by mouth, intravenous hydration).

[6.3] **D.** The patient has anion gap acidosis as evidenced by the low bicarbonate level, which is probably caused by lactic acid, reflecting ischemic bowel or severe fluid depletion. Elderly patients often have a minimum of symptoms and are afebrile. Surgical therapy may be indicated if CT imaging confirms intraabdominal sepsis or high grade obstruction.

CLINICAL PEARLS

◈ A significant proportion of patients with small bowel obstruction can be treated conservatively (NPO, placement of an NG tube, close monitoring of fluid status, serial clinical examinations, and laboratory and radiographic follow-up), while constantly being assessed for bowel ischemia or strangulation.

◈ Persistent pain, fever, tachycardia, leukocytosis, an elevated serum amylase level, and radiographic signs of high-grade small bowel obstruction are often signs of complicated bowel obstruction and the need for surgical therapy.

◈ Computed tomography imaging plays an important role in patient evaluation. The exceptions to this rule include patients with simple adhesive obstruction and an absence of indicators of complicated small bowel obstruction (Table 6–1), as well as patients in whom early operative intervention is clinically indicated.

REFERENCE

Hodin RA, Mathews JB. Small intestine. In: Norton JA, Bollinger RR, Chang AE, Lowery SF, Mulvihill SJ, Pass HI, Thompson RW, eds. Surgery: basic science and clinical evidence. New York: Springer, 2001:617–646

A 34-year-old diabetic woman complains of a 6-month history of progressive numbness and pain in her right hand that wakes her up at night. She states that her thumb is especially affected. She says that she is beginning to drop objects she is carrying in her right hand. She denies a history of trauma, exposure to heavy metals, or a family history of multiple sclerosis. The only medication she takes is an oral hypoglycemic agent.

◆ **What is the most likely diagnosis?**

◆ **What is the mechanism of the disorder?**

◆ **What is your next step?**

ANSWERS TO CASE 7: Carpal Tunnel Syndrome

Summary: A 34-year-old diabetic woman complains of a 6-month history of progressive numbness and pain in her right hand occurring especially at nighttime and affecting her thumb. She states that she is beginning to drop objects that she carries in her right hand.

◆ **Most likely diagnosis:** Carpal tunnel syndrome.

◆ **Mechanism of the disorder:** Median nerve compression.

◆ **Next step in therapy:** Nighttime splint and nonsteroidal anti-inflammatory drugs (NSAIDs).

Analysis

Objectives

1. Know the clinical presentation, pathophysiology, and risk factors for carpal tunnel syndrome.
2. Know the medical and surgical options for treating carpal tunnel syndrome.

Considerations

The distribution of the progressive numbness and pain is suggestive of median nerve compression. In addition, exacerbation of the patient's symptoms at night is typical of carpal tunnel syndrome. The mechanism of this disorder is compression of the median nerve as it passes within the carpal tunnel. This causes axonal damage and narrowing of the nerve. Median nerve compression causes numbness and pain in the thumb, index finger, and middle and lateral aspects of the ring finger. The median nerve may be compressed anywhere along its length from the brachial plexus down to the hand, but the most common site of compression is within the carpal tunnel, where it is dorsal to the transverse carpal ligament. The carpal canal is a rigid structure that causes physiologic dysfunction by producing median nerve ischemia. The best initial management is a nighttime splint for the wrist and avoidance of excess activity with the hand.

APPROACH TO CARPAL TUNNEL SYNDROME

Definitions

Carpal tunnel syndrome: Median nerve compression at the wrist leading to paresthesias of the radial three fingers and sometimes hand weakness.

Tinel sign: Reproduction of the patient's symptoms by percussion of the median nerve at the wrist.

Electrophysiologic studies: Investigation of nerve conduction and muscle innervation.

Clinical Approach

The carpal canal serves as a mechanical conduit for the digital flexor tendons. The walls and floor on the dorsal surface of the canal are formed by the carpal bones, and the ventral aspect is confined by the strong, inelastic, transverse carpal ligament. The smallest cross-sectional area of the canal is created by extremes of flexion and extension of the wrist (Figure 7–1). Exacerbation of symptoms at night is thought to be caused by edema; tenosynovitis may also be present. Carpal tunnel syndrome has been associated with endocrine conditions, diabetes, myxedema, hyperthyroidism, acromegaly, and pregnancy. Other causes are autoimmune disorders, lipomas of the canal, bone abnormalities, and hematomas. The etiology is often multifactorial. Females are more commonly affected in a ratio of approximately three to one.

The diagnosis of carpal tunnel syndrome is clinical, and the symptoms are typical. The exertion of direct digital pressure by the examiner over the median nerve at the carpal tunnel frequently reproduces the symptoms in about 30 seconds. In the Phalen maneuver, gravity-induced wrist flexion also produces the classic symptoms of this condition. A positive Tinel sign is present when direct percussion over the

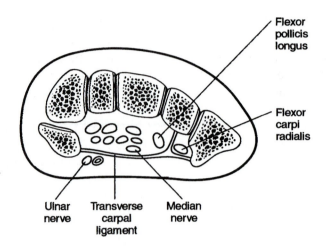

Figure 7–1. The carpal tunnel. The wrist in cross section reveals that the median nerve is susceptible to impingement.

nerve reproduces paresthesia. Sensory loss, particularly vibration sense, and motor loss may be present with thenar muscle wasting and decreased abductor muscle resistance. Electrophysiologic studies may be helpful. A comparison of median and ulnar or median and radial sensory stimulation values at the wrist is useful in confirming the diagnosis. Radiographs, including a "carpal tunnel view" are recommended in order to detect arthritis or fractures. Computed tomography and magnetic resonance imaging are rarely needed.

Conservative therapy consists of the use of splints and nonsteroidal anti-inflammatory agents. Splints should be light and should hold the wrist in a neutral or slightly extended position. Local steroid injections are effective in 80% to 90% of patients, but symptoms tend to return after months or sometimes years. Injections should not be given more frequently than on two or three occasions per year. Care must be taken not to inject directly into the median nerve. Surgery is indicated for intractable symptoms that are refractory to medical management. It consists of complete division of the transverse carpal ligament extending distally from the ulnar side of the median nerve. The results of surgery are generally good. Poor results are usually associated with either a misdiagnosis or failure to completely divide the ligament. The surgery can be performed with an open or an endoscopic approach. A tourniquet is used to exsanguinate the limb, and the operative field is infiltrated with a local anesthetic agent such as Xylocaine; in addition, intravenous sedation can be used. The Palmer fascia and the ligament are divided vertically from the proximal end of the carpal tunnel to its most distal point, and a wide separation of the ends of the ligament is observed (Figure 7–2). The underlying median nerve is carefully protected. A small tissue flap is left attached to the hook of the hamate, and

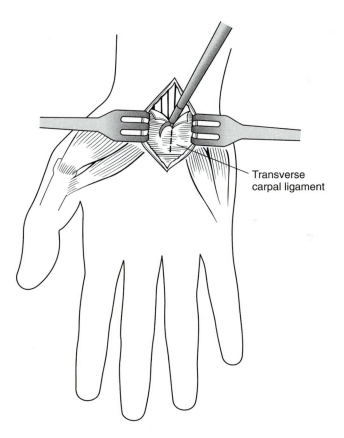

Transverse
carpal ligament

Figure 7–2.   Carpal tunnel release. The transverse carpal ligament is incised.

the skin is closed. Postoperatively the wrist is splinted in slight extension for about 2 weeks.

The potential advantages of the endoscopic approach are less discomfort, minimal scarring, a shorter period of immobilization, and a
more rapid recovery. Persistent or recurrent symptoms should be investigated by repeated electrophysiologic studies and by exclusion of other
causes of nerve compression. Occasionally, the ulnar nerve is compressed at the wrist, but more commonly compression of this nerve occurs in the fibromuscular groove posterior to the medial epicondyle.

Comprehension Questions

[7.1] A 24-year-old medical student notes some numbness and tingling
      of her right hand. She states that primarily her little finger is af-
      fected. Which of the following is most likely to be the etiology?

      A. Median nerve
      B. Radial nerve
      C. Ulnar nerve
      D. Long thoracic nerve

[7.2] Which of the following is most likely to be a risk factor for the
      development of carpal tunnel syndrome?

      A. Diabetes insipidus
      B. Hypothyroidism
      C. Addison's syndrome
      D. Fibromyalgia

Answers

[7.1] **C.** The sensory innervation of the little finger and the ulnar side
      of the ring finger is achieved with the ulnar nerve.

[7.2] **B.** Hypothyroidism (as well as diabetes mellitus, hyperthy-
      roidism, pregnancy, acromegaly), is associated with carpal tunnel
      syndrome.

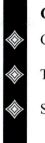

CLINICAL PEARLS

Carpal tunnel syndrome usually involves pain to the radial three fingers, especially at night.

The initial treatment of carpal tunnel syndrome includes administration of NSAIDs and the use of a wrist splint.

Surgery is indicated when severe pain or progressive motor weakness occurs despite conservative measures.

REFERENCES

Peimer CA. Surgery on the hand. In: Schwarz SI, Shires TG, Daly JM, et al, eds. Principles of surgery, 7th ed. New York: McGraw-Hill, 1999:2062–2067.

Watts MC, Brem H. Neurosurgery. In: Niederhuber JE, ed. Fundamentals of surgery. New York: Appleton & Lange, 1998:721–739.

A 46-year-old woman presents with a 24-hour history of abdominal pain that began approximately 1 hour after a large dinner. The pain initially began as a dull ache in the epigastrium but then localized in the right upper quadrant (RUQ). She describes some nausea but no vomiting. Since her presentation to the emergency center, the pain has improved significantly to the point of her being nearly pain-free. She describes having had similar pain in the past with all previous episodes being self-limited. Her past medical history is significant for type II diabetes mellitus. On physical examination, her temperature is 38.1°C (99°F), and the rest of her vital signs are normal. The abdomen is nondistended with minimal tenderness in the RUQ. Findings from the liver examination appear normal. The rectal and pelvic examinations reveal no abnormalities. Her complete blood count reveals a white blood cell (WBC) count of 13,000/mm^3. Serum chemistry studies demonstrate total bilirubin 1.8 mg/dL, direct bilirubin 0.6 mg/dL, alkaline phosphatase 140 U/L, AST 45 U/L, and ALT 30 U/L. Ultrasonography of the RUQ demonstrates stones in the gallbladder, a thickened gallbladder wall, and a common bile duct diameter of 4.0 mm.

◆ **What is the most likely diagnosis?**

◆ **What is the best therapy?**

◆ **What are the complications associated with this disease process?**

ANSWERS TO CASE 8: Gallstone Disease

Summary: A 46-year-old woman presents with a 1-day history of RUQ
abdominal pain and a physical examination and laboratory findings
suggestive of gallstone disease.

◆ **Diagnosis:** Cholecystitis, likely acute and chronic.

◆ **Best therapy:** Laparoscopic cholecystectomy is the preferred
  treatment for all patients with a reasonable life expectancy and
  no prohibitive risks for general anesthesia and abdominal
  surgery.

◆ **Complications:** Complications from gallstone disease include
  acute and chronic cholecystitis, pancreatitis, choledocholithiasis,
  cholangitis, and gallstone ileus.

Analysis

Objectives

1. Know the etiology of gallstone disease and learn the differences
   among biliary colic, acute cholecystitis, and chronic cholecystitis.
2. Know the basic diagnostic and therapeutic plans for patients
   with gallstone disease.
3. Become aware of the complications arising from gallstone
   disease.

Considerations

This patient provides a good history of recurrent RUQ abdominal pain
episodes following meals, consistent with biliary colic. Although she
demonstrates minimal tenderness to palpation in her right upper ab-

domen on physical examination, the **elevated leukocyte count and ultrasound findings of gallbladder wall thickening are consistent with acute or chronic cholecystitis**. If this patient had a normal WBC count and an ultrasound examination demonstrating stones in the gallbladder and no other abnormalities, the presentation would be consistent with biliary colic, which can be treated by elective cholecystectomy. For cholecystitis, the appropriate treatment consists of hospital admission, administration of intravenous antibiotics, and laparoscopic cholecystectomy prior to discharge from the hospital.

APPROACH TO GALLSTONE DISEASE

Definitions

Biliary colic: Also known as symptomatic cholelithiasis, it is characterized by waxing and waning postprandial epigastric or RUQ pain radiating to the back and normal transaminase levels. It is caused by gallbladder contraction stimulated by cholecystokinin secretion following food ingestion, gallstone obstruction at the gallbladder neck, or less commonly gallbladder dysfunction.

Acute cholecystitis: In 95% of patients, acute cholecystitis results from a stone or stones obstructing the cystic duct. Bacterial infection is thought to occur via the lymphatics, with the most commonly found organisms being *Escherichia coli, Klebsiella, Proteus,* and *Streptococcus faecalis.* Patients generally present with persistent RUQ pain, with or without fever, gallbladder tenderness, leukocytosis, and often mild, nonspecific elevated liver enzyme levels, which may or may not indicate common bile duct stones. Treatment includes hospital admission, administration of intravenous fluids, nothing by mouth, antibiotics directed at the above-listed organisms, and cholecystectomy during the hospitalization.

Acalculous cholecystitis: Gallbladder inflammation due to biliary stasis (in 5% of patients with acute cholecystitis) leading to gallbladder distension, venous congestion, and decreased perfusion; it nearly always occurs in patients hospitalized with a critical illness.

Chronic cholecystitis: Results from repeated bouts of biliary colic and/or acute cholecystitis leading to gallbladder wall inflammation and fibrosis. The patient may present with persistent or recurrent localized RUQ pain without fever or leukocytosis. Sonography may demonstrate a thickened gallbladder wall and a contracted gallbladder.

Cholangitis: **Infection within the bile ducts,** most commonly due to complete or partial obstruction of the bile ducts by gallstones or strictures. The classic **Charcot triad (RUQ pain, jaundice, and fever)** is seen in only 70% of patients. This condition may lead to life-threatening sepsis and multiple-organ failure. Treatment consists of antibiotic therapy, and supportive care; in cases of severe cholangitis, endoscopic decompression of the bile duct by endoscopic retrograde cholangiopancreatography (ERCP) or surgery is indicated.

Right upper quadrant ultrasonography: This technique has a 98% to 99% sensitivity in identifying gallstones in the gallbladder. The examination is also useful for measuring the diameter of the common bile duct, which can indicate the possible presence of stones in the common bile duct (choledocholithiasis). When present, common bile duct stones are visualized only 50% of the time with this imaging modality.

Biliary scintigraphy: The study of gallbladder function and biliary patency using an intravenous radiotracer. Normally the liver is visualized, followed by the gallbladder, followed by emptying of the radiotracer into the duodenum. Nonvisualization of the gallbladder in a patient with RUQ pain indicates gallbladder dysfunction due to acute or chronic cholecystitis.

Endoscopic retrograde cholangiopancreatography: Endoscopic common bile duct cannulation and direct injection of contrast material to visualize the duct. An endoscopic sphincterotomy in the duodenum during the procedure may facilitate bile drainage and the clearance of bile duct stones, which is especially useful in treating cholangitis and choledocholithiasis. The procedure requires sedation and may be associated with complication rates of 8% to 10%.

Pathophysiology

At least 16 million Americans have gallstones, and 800,000 new cases occur each year. Most stones are composed of pure cholesterol, mixed cholesterol, phospholipids, or pigmented stones. Patients with cholesterol stones can be shown to have supersaturated bile. The proportion of cholesterol, lecithin, and bile salts determines whether the cholesterol is maintained in solution or precipitates and results in stone formation. A small fraction, only about 20%, of all patients with gallstones have symptoms related to stones. While it is unknown why some patients with gallstones develop symptoms whereas others do not, it is clear that those who develop symptoms are at risk for the subsequent development of complications, including acute or chronic cholecystitis, choledocholithiasis, pancreatitis, and cholangitis.

Patient Evaluation and Treatment

The evaluation in every patient should consist of a history, a physical examination, a complete blood count, liver function studies, a serum amylase determination, and RUQ ultrasonography (Table 8–1). It is important to differentiate patients with biliary colic from patients with complicated gallstone disease, such as acute or chronic cholecystitis, choledocholithiasis, cholangitis, and biliary pancreatitis, because the management varies for these conditions. For example, a patient with **choledocholithiasis may present with symptoms identical to those of biliary colic, but the condition may be differentiated on the basis of an elevation in serum liver enzyme levels and dilatation of the common bile duct by ultrasound.** In contrast to patients with biliary colic, who are treated by elective cholecystectomy, patients with choledocholithiasis require in-hospital observation for the development of cholangitis and early endoscopic clearance of common bile duct stones, in addition to cholecystectomy. A major goal in patient evaluation is to make an accurate diagnosis without using unnecessary imaging and invasive diagnostic studies. **Choledocholithiasis should be suspected if** the RUQ ultrasound findings include a **common bile duct diameter greater than 5 mm in the presence of elevated liver enzyme levels. Gallstone pancreatitis** should be considered in the presence of **significantly elevated amylase and lipase values.**

Table 8–1

GALLSTONE DISEASE PRESENTATIONS*

DISEASE	SYMPTOMS	PHYSICAL EXAMINATION	ULTRASONOGRAPHY	LABORATORY STUDIES
Biliary colic	Postprandial pain, usually <6 h in duration	Afebrile, mild tenderness over gallbladder	Gallstones in gallbladder but no wall thickening, no CBD dilatation	Normal WBC count, normal LFT values, normal serum amylase level
Acute cholecystitis	Persistent epigastric or RUQ pain lasting >8 h	May be febrile or afebrile; usually localized gallbladder tenderness	Gallstones in gallbladder; may have pericholecystic fluid; may or may not have CBD dilatation	Normal or elevated WBC count; may have normal or mildly elevated LFT values
Chronic cholecystitis	Persistent recurrent RUQ pain	Afebrile; may have localized tenderness over a palpable gallbladder	Stones in gallbladder, thickened gallbladder wall; in advanced cases contracted gallbladder	Normal WBC count; may have mild elevation in LFT values
Choledo-cholithiasis	Postprandial abdominal pain that improves with fasting	May or may not be clinically jaundiced; nonspecific RUQ abdominal tenderness	Gallstones in gallbladder; CBD usually dilated	Elevation in LFT values; the pattern of elevation is dependent on the chronicity and partial versus complete obstruction
Biliary pancreatitis	Persistent epigastric and back pain	Epigastric tenderness to deep palpation is present	Gallstones in gallbladder; CBD dilatation may occur because of pancreatitis (does not always indicate CBD stones)	Leukocytosis, serum amylase level frequently >1000 U/L, LFT values may be transiently elevated, but persistence may indicate CBD stones

*CBD, common bile duct; WBC, white blood cell; LFT, liver function test; RUQ, right upper quadrant.

Sometimes, acute and chronic cholecystitis may be difficult to differentiate clinically because in both cases patients may have localized tenderness over the gallbladder. When this situation arises, the patient should be treated as if they had acute cholecystitis. The treatment for both acute and chronic cholecystitis is cholecystectomy. The operation of choice is a laparoscopic cholecystectomy with or without cholangiography (radiopaque dye injected into the common bile duct and an radiograph taken). Some surgeons selectively perform cholangiograms if the common bile duct is dilated and liver enzyme levels are elevated. Other surgeons obtain cholangiograms with every laparoscopic cholecystectomy performed. Patients with gallstone pancreatitis are treated with bowel rest and intravenous hydration. When the pancreatitis clinically resolves, a laparoscopic cholecystectomy can be done. Generally, patients with **uncomplicated biliary pancreatitis should undergo cholecystectomy** during the same hospitalization. When cholecystectomy is delayed, 25% to 30% of patients may develop recurrent bouts of pancreatitis within a 6-week period.

Comprehension Questions

[8.1] A 65-year-old woman presents to the emergency room with postprandial RUQ pain, nausea, and emesis over the last 12 hours. The pain is persistent and radiates to her back. She is afebrile, and her abdomen is tender to palpation in the RUQ. Sonography demonstrates cholelithiasis, gallbladder wall thickening, and a dilated common bile duct measuring 12 mm. Laboratory studies reveal the following values: WBC count 13,000/mm³, AST 220 U/L, ALT 240 U/L, alkaline phosphatase 385 U/L, and direct bilirubin 4.0 mg/dL. Which of the following is the most appropriate treatment at this time?

A. Admit the patient to the hospital, provide intravenous hydration, and check hepatitis serology values.

B. Admit the patient to the hospital and perform a laparoscopic cholecystectomy.

C. Admit the patient to the hospital, provide intravenous hydration, begin antibiotic therapy, and recommend ERCP.
D. Provide pain medication in the emergency room and ask the patient to follow up in the clinic.

[8.2] A 28-year-old woman undergoing an obstetric ultrasound during the second trimester of pregnancy and is found to have gallstones in her gallbladder. She claims to have had indigestion with frequent belching throughout her pregnancy. Which of the following is the most appropriate treatment?

A. A low-fat diet until the end of her pregnancy and then a postpartum laparoscopic cholecystectomy
B. Elective laparoscopic cholecystectomy during the second trimester
C. Follow-up after completion of her pregnancy
D. Open cholecystectomy during the second trimester

[8.3] Which of the following findings is most consistent with the diagnosis of acute cholecystitis?

A. Fever, intermittent RUQ pain, and jaundice
B. Persistent abdominal pain, RUQ tenderness, and leukocytosis
C. Intermittent abdominal pain and minimal tenderness over the gallbladder
D. Epigastric and back pain

[8.4] A 69-year-old man presents with confusion, abdominal pain, shaking chills, a rectal temperature of 94°F, and jaundice. An abdominal radiograph shows air in the biliary tree. Which of the following is the most likely diagnosis?

A. Acute cholangitis
B. Acute pancreatitis
C. Acute cholecystitis
D. Acute appendicitis

Answers

[8.1] **C.** Admission to the hospital, administration of intravenous fluids and antibiotics, and ERCP. This patient's presentation is highly suggestive of cholangitis, with the presence of a significant elevation in her liver enzyme levels, common bile duct dilatation, and tenderness in the RUQ.

[8.2] **C.** Reevaluation after the completion of pregnancy is appropriate for this patient, who has stones in her gallbladder and symptoms that are most likely unrelated to gallstones and may be pregnancy-induced.

[8.3] **B.** Persistent abdominal pain, RUQ tenderness, and leukocytosis indicate acute cholecystitis. Choice A is most consistent with cholangitis; choice C is typical of biliary colic and choice D is consistent with acute pancreatitis.

[8.4] **A.** Elderly patients who present with fever (or hypothermia), jaundice, abdominal pain, and shaking chills often have acute cholangitis (purulent infection of the biliary tract). The presence of air in the biliary tree is consistent with this illness. This is a life-threatening condition and often requires urgent surgical or endoscopic decompression of the biliary system, in addition to aggressive supportive care, and broad-spectrum antibiotic therapy.

CLINICAL PEARLS

◈ Cholecystectomy is generally not indicated unless there is a clear link between the patient's symptoms and gallstones or if there is objective evidence of gallbladder dysfunction (eg, a thickened gallbladder wall on ultrasonography, nonvisualization of the gallbladder on biliary scintigraphy) or gallstone-related complications.

◈ In general, the treatment of cholecystitis is hospitalization, administration of intravenous antibiotics, and a laparoscopic cholecystectomy prior to discharge from the hospital.

◈ **Cholangitis, which can be diagnosed with the Charcot triad—RUQ pain, jaundice, and fever**—is life-threatening. Treatment consists of antibiotics therapy, supportive care, and in cases of severe cholangitis biliary duct, decompression via ERCP.

◈ Choledocholithiasis should be suspected if the RUQ ultrasound findings include a common bile duct diameter greater than 5 mm in the presence of elevated liver enzyme levels.

REFERENCES

Harris HW. Biliary system. In Norton JA, Bollinger RR, Chang AE, Lowery SF, Mulvihill SJ, Pass HI, Thompson RW, eds. Surgery: basic science and clinical evidence. New York: Springer, 2001:553–584.

Wu JS, Soper NJ. Acute and chronic cholecystitis. In: Cameron JL, ed. Current surgical therapy, 6th ed. St. Louis: Mosby-Year Book, 1998:406–410.

A 38-year-old man presents at the emergency center with tarry stools and a feeling of light-headedness. The patient indicates that over the past 24 hours he has had several bowel movements containing tarry-colored stools and for the past 12 hours has felt light-headed. His past medical and surgical history are unremarkable. The patient complains of frequent headaches due to work-related stress, for which he has been self- medicating with six to eight tablets of ibuprofen a day for the past 2 weeks. He consumes two to three martinis per day and denies tobacco or illicit drug use. On examination, his temperature is 37.0°C (98.6°F), pulse rate 105/min (supine), blood pressure 104/80, and respiratory rate 22/min. His vital signs upright are pulse 120/min and blood pressure 90/76. He is awake, cooperative, and pale. The cardiopulmonary examinations are unremarkable. His abdomen is mildly distended and mildly tender in the epigastrium. The rectal examination reveals melenotic stools but no masses in the vault.

◆ **What is your next step?**

◆ **What is the best initial treatment?**

ANSWERS TO CASE 9: Upper Gastrointestinal Tract Hemorrhage

Summary: A 38-year-old man presents with signs and symptoms of acute upper gastrointestinal (GI) tract hemorrhage. The patient's presentation suggests that he may have had significant blood loss leading to class III hemorrhagic shock.

◆ **Next step:** The first step in the treatment of patients with upper GI hemorrhage is intravenous fluid resuscitation. The etiology and severity of the bleeding dictate the intensity of therapy and predict the risk of further bleeding and/or death.

◆ **Best initial treatment:** Prompt attention to the patient's airway, breathing, and circulation is mandatory for patients with acute upper GI hemorrhage. After attention to the airway, breathing, and circulation (ABC's), the patient is prepared for endoscopy to identify the etiology or source of the bleeding and possible endoscopic therapy to control hemorrhage.

Analysis

Objectives

1. Be able to outline resuscitation and treatment strategies for patients presenting with acute upper GI tract hemorrhage and hemorrhagic shock.
2. Be familiar with most common causes of upper GI tract hemorrhage and their therapies.
3. Know the adverse prognostic factors associated with continued bleeding and increased mortality.

Considerations

The treatment of patients with suspected upper GI tract hemorrhage begins with an initial assessment to determine if the bleeding is acute or occult. Acute bleeding is recognized by a history of hematemesis, coffee-ground emesis, melena, or bleeding per rectum, whereas patients with occult bleeding may present with signs and symptoms associated with anemia and no clear history of blood loss. **A critical part of the initial evaluation is assessment of the patient's physiologic status to gauge the severity of blood loss. The sequence in the management** of acute upper GI tract hemorrhage consists of **(1) resuscitation, (2) diagnosis, and (3) treatment,** in that order. In this patient's case, his symptoms and physiologic parameters suggest severe, acute blood loss (class III hemorrhagic shock with up to 35% total blood volume loss) and should prompt immediate resuscitation with close monitoring of patient response (urine output, clinical appearance, blood pressure, heart rate, serial hemoglobin and hematocrit values, and consideration of central venous pressure monitoring). A nasogastric tube should be inserted following resuscitation to determine whether bleeding is active. The stomach should be irrigated with room-temperature water or saline until gastric aspirates are clear. For patients with **massive upper GI tract bleeding, agitation, or impaired respiratory status, endotracheal intubation is recommended prior to endoscopy.** Laboratory studies to be obtained include a complete blood count, liver function studies, prothrombin time, and partial thromboplastin time. A type and cross-match should be ordered. Platelets or fresh frozen plasma should be administered when thrombocytopenia or coagulopathy is identified, respectively. Early endoscopy has been shown to identify the bleeding source in patients with active ongoing bleeding and may achieve early control of bleeding. Given the history of nonsteroidal anti-inflammatory drug (NSAID) use, it would be appropriate to begin empirical therapy for a presumed gastric ulcer and gastric erosions with a proton pump inhibitor prior to endoscopic confirmation.

APPROACH TO UPPER GI BLEEDING

Definitions

Mallory–Weiss tear: A proximal gastric mucosa tear following vigorous coughing, retching, or vomiting. The bleeding is generally self-limiting, mild, and amenable to conservative management.

Dieulafoy's erosion: Infrequently encountered, this problem describes bleeding from an aberrant submucosal artery located in the stomach. This bleeding is frequently significant and requires prompt diagnosis by endoscopy, followed by endoscopic or operative therapy.

Arteriovenous (AV) malformation: A small mucosal lesion located along the GI tract. Bleeding is usually abrupt, but the rate of bleeding is usually slow and self-limiting.

Esophagitis: Mucosal erosions frequently resulting from gastroesophageal reflux, infections, or medications. Patients most frequently present with occult bleeding, and treatment consists of correction or avoidance of the underlying causes.

Esophageal variceal bleeding: Engorged veins of the gastroesophageal region, which may ulcerate and lead to massive hemorrhage; related to portal hypertension and cirrhosis.

Clinical Approach

The sources of upper GI tract bleeding can be categorized as variceal versus non-variceal. Common sources of non-variceal bleeding include duodenal ulcers (25%), gastric erosions (25%), gastric ulcers (20%), and Mallory–Weiss tears (7%). Up to 30% of patients have multiple etiologies of bleeding identified during endoscopy. In addition, all studies indicate that a proportion of cases have no endoscopically discernible cause, and these cases are associated with an excellent outcome. Rare causes of upper GI tract bleeding include neoplasms (both benign and malignant), AV malformations, and Dieulafoy erosions. **Bleeding tends to be self-limited in approximately 80% of all patients with acute upper GI tract bleeding.** Continuing or recurrent bleeding occurs in 20% of patients and is the major contributor to mortality. The **overall mortality associated with upper GI tract bleeding is 8% to 10%** and has not changed over the last several decades. There are striking differences in the rates of rebleeding and mortality depending on the diagnosis at endoscopy (Table 9–1). **Patient mortality with acute upper GI tract bleeding increases with rebleeding, increased age, and in patients who develop bleeding in the hospital.** A number of clinical predictors and endoscopic stigmata have been identified with the development of recurrent bleeding, and these are listed in Table 9–2.

Table 9–1

RISK OF REBLEEDING BASED ON SOURCE

SOURCE	REBLEEDING (%)
Esophageal varices	60
Gastric cancer	50
Gastric ulcer	28
Duodenal ulcer	24
Gastric erosion (gastritis)	15
Mallory–Weiss tear	7
No identified source	2.5

Source: Modified, with permission, from Silverstein FE, Gilbert DA, Tedesco FJ, et al. The national ASGE survey on upper gastrointestinal bleeding, Parts I, II, and III. Gastrointest Endosc 1981;27:73–101.

Table 9–2

FACTORS ASSOCIATED WITH INCREASED
REBLEEDING AND MORTALITY

Clinical
    Shock on admission
    Prior history of bleeding requiring transfusion
    Admission hemoglobin <8 g/dL
    Transfusion requirement ≥5 units of packed red blood cells
    Continued bleeding noted in nasogastric aspirate
    Age greater than 60 y (increased mortality but no increase in rebleeding)
Endoscopic
    Visible vessel in ulcer base (50% rebleeding risk)
    Oozing of bright blood from ulcer base
    Adherent clot at ulcer base
    Location of ulcer (worse prognosis when located near large arteries, eg, posterior duodenal bulb or lesser curve of stomach)

Source: Modified, with permission, from Silverstein FE, Gilbert DA, Tedesco FJ, et al. The national ASGE survey on upper gastrointestinal bleeding, Parts I, II, and III. Gastrointest Endosc 1981;27:73–101.

The use of NSAIDs contributes to the development of NSAID-induced gastric ulcers. All NSAIDs produce mucosal damage. The risk of developing an ulcer is dose-related. Roughly, 2% to 4 % of NSAID users have GI tract complications each year. **About 10% of patients who take NSAIDs daily develop an acute ulcer.** NSAID-induced ulcers have an increased incidence of bleeding, with gastric ulcers and duodenal ulcers having 10- to 20-fold and 5- to 15-fold risk ratios, respectively.

Upper GI tract endoscopy establishes a diagnosis in more than 90% of cases and assesses the current activity of bleeding. It aids in directing therapy and predicts the risk of rebleeding. Furthermore, it allows for endoscopic therapy. Endoscopic hemostasis can be achieved through a variety of ways, including thermotherapy with a heater probe, multipolar or bipolar electrocoagulation, and ethanol or epinephrine injections. As shown in Figure 9–1, endoscopy can demonstrate bleeding, esophageal varices, gastroduodenal bleeding, or no bleeding. For non-variceal bleeding, endoscopic hemostasis is usually achieved with the use of epinephrine injections followed by thermal therapy. Permanent hemostasis occurs in roughly 80% to 90% of patients. Once bleeding is controlled, long-term medical therapy with antisecretory agents such as histamine-2 blockers or proton pump inhibitors is utilized to treat the underlying disease. Testing for *Helicobacter pylori* should be performed, and if this organism is present, treatment should be initiated. Any NSAID use should be discontinued. If this is not possible, a prostaglandin analog (such as misoprostol) should be used or, alternatively, one of the selective COX-2 inhibitors should be used to replace nonselective COX inhibitors.

If bleeding continues or recurs, surgery may be necessary. **Surgery is indicated for complicated peptic ulcer disease with massive, persistent, or recurrent upper GI tract hemorrhage or in association with nonhealing or giant ulcers (larger than 3 cm).** For a bleeding gastric ulcer where there is a concern for possible malignancy, either gastrectomy or excision of the ulcer is indicated. For other types of ulcers, the vessel may require ligation followed by a vagotomy procedure and pyloroplasty. If the bleeding source cannot be identified but active bleeding is clearly occurring, patients may undergo selective angiography. This treatment strategy can diagnose and treat bleeding in roughly 70% of patients, as arterial embolization with gel foam, metal

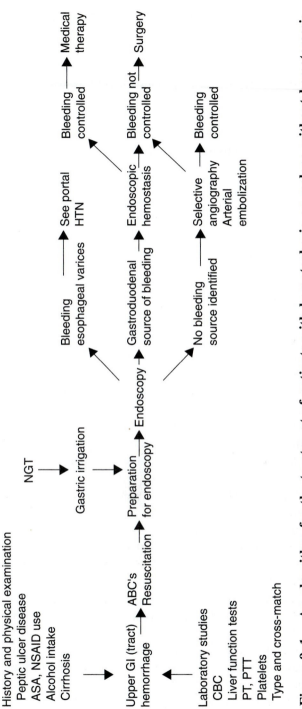

Figure 9–1. An algorithm for the treatment of patients with hematochezia or melena without hematemesis. ASA, aminosalicylate; NSAID, nonsteroidal anti-inflammatory drug; NGT, nasogastric tube; HTN, hypertension; GI, gastrointestinal; ABC's, airway, breathing, circulation; CBC, complete blood count; PT, prothrombin time; PTT, partial thromboplastin time.

coil springs, or a clot can be utilized to control bleeding. In addition, arterial vasopressin can cause bleeding to stop in some patients with peptic ulcer disease.

Comprehension Questions

[9.1] A 55-year-old male has undergone upper endoscopy. He is told by his gastroenterologist that although this disorder may cause anemia, it is unlikely to cause acute gastrointestinal hemorrhage. Which of the following is the most likely diagnosis?

A. Gastric ulcer
B. Duodenal ulcer
C. Gastric erosions
D. Esophageal varices
E. Gastric cancer

[9.2] A 32-year-old man comes to the emergency department with a history of vomiting "large amounts of bright red blood." The first step in the treatment of this patient is:

A. Obtaining a history and performing a physical examination
B. Determining hemoglobin and hematocrit levels
C. Fluid resuscitation
D. Inserting a nasogastric tube
E. Performing urgent endoscopy

[9.3] A 65-year-old male is brought into the emergency room with acute upper gastrointestinal hemorrhage. A nasogastric tube is placed with bright red fluid aspirated. After 30 minutes of saline flushes, the aspirate is clear. Which of the following is the most accurate statement regarding this patient's condition?

A. He has about a 20% chance of rebleed
B. The mortality for his condition is much lower today than 20 years ago
C. His age is a poor prognostic factor for rebleeding
D. Mesenteric ischemia is a likely cause of his condition

[9.4] A 52-year-old alcoholic male with known cirrhosis comes into the ER with acute hematemesis. Bleeding esophageal varices are found during upper GI endoscopy. Which of the following is most likely to be effective treatment for this patient?

A. Balloon tamponade of the esophagus
B. Proton pump inhibitor
C. Triple antibiotic therapy
D. Misoprostol oral therapy
E. Endoscopic sclerotherapy

Answers

[9.1] **E.** Gastric cancer is relatively asymptomatic until late in its course. Weight loss and anorexia are the most common symptoms with this condition. Hematemesis is unusual, but anemia from chronic occult blood loss is common.

[9.2] **C.** Fluid resuscitation is the first priority in order to maintain sufficient intravascular volume to perfuse vital organs.

[9.3] **A.** About 20% of patients with acute upper GI hemorrhage will have continued or rebleeding episodes. The mortality has remained the same (about 8–10%) over the past 20 years.

[9.4] **E.** Endoscopic injection of sclerosing agents directly into the varix is effective in controlling acute hemorrhage due to variceal bleeding in about 90% of cases. Balloon tamponade is a therapy used infrequently for acute esophageal variceal bleeding due to its limited effectiveness in achieving sustained control of bleeding. Other therapies include vasopressin or octreotide to decrease portal pressure.

CLINICAL PEARLS

◆ Early endoscopy has been shown to be more efficacious in identifying the bleeding sources, and in patients with active ongoing bleeding it may help in achieving early control of bleeding

◆ About 10% of patients who take daily NSAIDs develop an acute ulcer.

◆ Surgery is indicated for complicated peptic ulcer disease with massive, persistent, or recurrent upper GI tract hemorrhage or in association with nonhealing or giant ulcers (larger than 3 cm).

◆ Acute GI tract hemorrhage should be treated with aggressive fluid resuscitation, close monitoring of patient response, nasogastric tube insertion following resuscitation to determine whether bleeding is active, and gastric irrigation with room-temperature water or saline until gastric aspirates are clear.

◆ The most common cause of upper GI tract hemorrhage in a patient with cirrhosis and portal hypertension is variceal bleeding, which carries a high rate of mortality and risk of rebleeding.

◆ The most common cause of pediatric significant upper GI tract hemorrhage is variceal bleeding from extrahepatic portal venous obstruction.

REFERENCES

Morgan AG, Clamp SE. OMGE International Upper Gastrointestinal Bleeding Survey 1978–82. Scand J Gastroenterol 1984;19(suppl 95):41–58.

Silverstein FE, Gilbert DA, Tedesco FJ, et al. The National ASGE Survey on Upper Gastrointestinal Bleeding, Parts I, II, and III. Gastrointest Endosc 1981;27:73–101.

CASE 10

A 67-year-old man presented to the emergency center with a 6-hour history of bleeding per rectum. The patient's symptoms began after he developed an urge to defecate that was followed by several voluminous bowel movements containing maroon-colored stool mixed with blood clots. The patient complains of feeling light-headed just prior to arriving at the hospital but denies any abdominal pain. His past medical history is significant for borderline hypertension managed with diet control. His surgical history is significant for a right inguinal hernia repair 2 years ago. His blood pressure is 100/80, pulse rate 110/min, and respiratory rate 20/min. The results of an examination of his abdomen are unremarkable. The rectal examination revealed no masses and a large amount of maroon-colored stool in the rectal vault.

◆ **What should be your next step?**

◆ **What is the most likely diagnosis?**

◆ **How would you confirm this diagnosis?**

ANSWERS TO CASE 10: Lower Gastrointestinal Tract Hemorrhage

Summary: A 67-year-old man presents with acute lower gastrointestinal (GI) tract hemorrhage. The patient's symptoms and vital signs indicate a significant acute hemorrhage.

◆ **Next step:** The patient's presentation is highly suggestive of hypovolemic shock; therefore the initial treatment should consist of volume resuscitation with isotonic crystalloid solution and close monitoring of his response to resuscitation.

◆ **Most likely diagnosis:** Acute lower GI tract hemorrhage.

◆ **How to confirm the diagnosis:** Place a nasogastric (NG) tube to sample the upper GI tract contents; the possibility of gastric bleeding can be eliminated if nonbloody, bilious material is recovered. Esophagogastroduodenoscopy (EGD) is the definitive method of evaluation to rule out a duodenal source of bleeding.

Analysis

Objectives

1. Be able to differentiate the clinical presentations of occult and acute anorectal, nonanorectal lower GI tract, and upper GI tract bleeding.
2. Learn a diagnostic and therapeutic approach to lower GI tract bleeding.

Considerations

The passage of maroon-colored stool and blood clots generally indicates acute bleeding from a lower GI tract source (distal to the ligament of Treitz). Maroon-colored stool represents a mixture of fecal material and blood, indicating that the bleeding source is located proximal to the lower rectal segment and anus. **The passage of blood clots can occur with brisk bleeding from an upper GI tract source. Placement of an NG tube is useful during the initial evaluation for possible upper GI tract bleeding,** although up to 16% of patients may have nonbloody NG aspirate with upper GI tract bleeding originating from the duodenum. In middle-aged and older adult patients, the **most likely causes of acute lower GI tract bleeding are diverticulosis, angiodysplasia, and neoplasm,** and these lesions are generally painless. When lower GI tract bleeding occurs in the presence of **abdominal pain,** the possibility of **an ischemic bowel, inflammatory bowel disease, intussusception, and a ruptured abdominal aneurysm** should be entertained. Following resuscitation, the **primary goal in the treatment of a patient with acute and continued lower GI tract bleeding is localization of the bleeding site** (colonoscopy, mesenteric angiography, and/or an isotope-labeled red blood cell [RBC] scan).

APPROACH TO LOWER GI TRACT BLEEDING

Definitions

Occult gastrointestinal tract bleeding: Slow bleeding originating anywhere along the upper aerodigestive or lower GI tract, most commonly associated with neoplasm, gastritis, and esophagitis. Patients generally do not report bleeding and commonly present with iron-deficiency anemia, fatigue, and hemoccult-positive stool.

Overt lower gastrointestinal tract bleeding: Hematochezia or melena. The **most common causes in children and adolescents are Meckel diverticulum, inflammatory bowel disease, and polyps.** In young and middle-aged adults the most common causes are diverticulosis, neoplasm, and inflammatory bowel disease. In **older adults, the most common causes are diverticulosis, angiodysplasia, and neoplasm.**

Tagged red blood cell (RBC) scan: Nuclear medicine imaging using RBCs labeled with technetium-99m. This technique is highly sensitive in identifying active bleeding at a rate of 0.1 ml/min or greater; however, the images obtained may not accurately localize the GI tract bleeding site. Some recommend this imaging modality as an initial screening study prior to performing mesenteric angiography.

Mesenteric angiography: Selective angiography of the superior and inferior mesentery arteries can help identify bleeding from the midgut and hindgut. This procedure has greater specificity in localizing the bleeding site than a tagged RBC scan. Selective injection of vasopressin or gel foam can be applied to treat active bleeding in patients who are not suitable surgical candidates. The bleeding generally has to be greater than 0.5 to 1.0 mL/min in order to be visualized by angiography.

Rigid proctosigmoidoscopy: A simple bedside procedure in which a nonflexible endoscope is used to visualize the most distal 25-cm segment of the lower GI tract.

Diagnostic colonoscopy: Flexible fiberoptic endoscopy that evaluates the entire colon and rectum and is reserved for hemodynamically stable patients. The reported success rate in identifying the bleeding source and site is as high as 75%, but this figure is highly variable depending on the operator and the timing. The advantages of this procedure are that it can rule out the possibility of a colorectal bleeding source and that identified bleeding angiodysplasia can be treated with epinephrine injection or coagulation.

Angiodysplasia: Also known as vascular ectasia, a common degenerative vascular lesion characterized by small, dilated, thin-walled veins in the mucosa of the GI tract. It occurs most commonly in the cecum and ascending colon of individuals more than 50 years of age. Approximately 50% of patients have associated cardiac disease. Up to 25% of patients with angiodysplasia have aortic stenosis. Most patients with angiodysplasia present with low-grade, self-limiting bleeding, although approximately 15% present with massive bleeding.

Clinical Approach

A patient presenting with overt lower GI tract bleeding should be quickly assessed for intravascular volume status and hemodynamic sta-

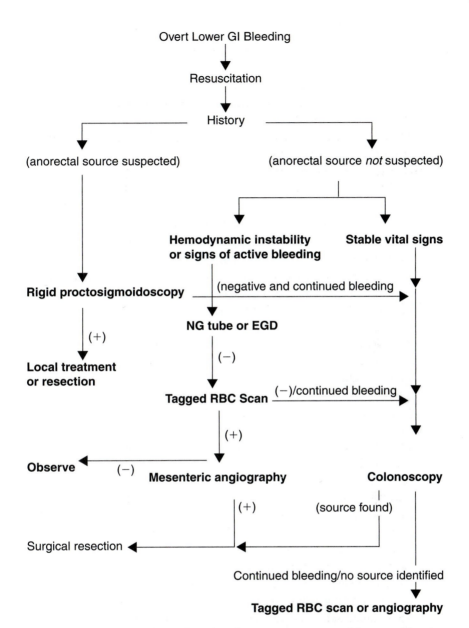

Figure 10–1. An algorithm for the management of hematochezia. Esophagogastroduodenoscopy (EGD), colonoscopy, and small bowel contrast radiography should be performed in patients whose gastrointestinal (GI) tract bleeding has resolved to eliminate the possibility of GI tract bleeding as the cause of bleeding. NG, nasogastric; RBC, red blood cell.

bility. A detailed history is important. The identification of coexisting medical problems may help identify patients whose bleeding is the result of coagulopathy or thrombocytopenia (medical causes of bleeding). **If the patient has had a previous abdominal vascular reconstruction, the possibility of an aortoenteric fistula must be strongly considered and ruled out.** The history elicited should include details regarding the quality and appearance of the bleeding. **Melena** (tarry stool) indicates the degradation of hemoglobin by bacteria and forms after blood has remained in the GI tract for more than 14 hours. **Melena is usually associated with upper GI tract or small bowel bleeding but can occur with bleeding from the ascending colon.** The passage of **maroon-colored stools** generally excludes a possible bleeding source in the rectum and anus. Bleeding from the rectum is usually characterized by the passage of formed stools streaked with blood or the passage of fresh blood at the end of a normal bowel movement. Most episodes of overt lower GI tract bleeding resolve spontaneously without specific therapy. It is important to rule out GI tract neoplasm as the source of bleeding in patients whose bleeding resolves. Patients whose bleeding creates adverse hemodynamic consequences or necessitates blood transfusion should undergo prompt evaluation to localize the source of bleeding so that operative excision can be accomplished. (See Figure 10–1 for management strategy.)

Comprehension Questions

[10.1] A 75-year-old man develops hematochezia and presents with hemodynamic instability. The patient's vital signs improve slightly with crystalloid and packed red cells infusion. Which of the following is considered the most appropriate next step(s) in management?

A. EGD, proctosigmoidoscopy, and a barium enema
B. NG tube, proctosigmoidoscopy, and a tagged RBC scan with or without mesentery angiography.
C. NG tube, mesentery angiography, and colonoscopy
D. EGD and colonoscopy

[10.2] Which of the following conditions is almost always associated with painless hematochezia?

  A. Aortoenteric fistula developing 1 year after an abdominal aortic aneurysm repair
  B. Ischemic colitis involving the descending colon
  C. Bleeding duodenal ulcer
  D. Superior mesentery artery embolus

[10.3] Which of the following diagnostic modalities has the greatest specificity in identifying the source of lower GI tract bleeding?

  A. Tagged RBC scan
  B. Barium enema
  C. Colonoscopy
  D. Surgical exploration

Answers

[10.1] **B.** NG tube, proctosigmoidoscopy, and a tagged RBC scan are most appropriate for a patient who is unstable.

[10.2] **A.** Aortoenteric fistula following aortic reconstruction is nearly always associated with painless hematochezia.

[10.3] **C.** Colonoscopy has the highest specificity in identifying the source of lower GI tract bleeding (ie, the lowest false-positive rate for bleeding source identification).

CLINICAL PEARLS

◈ The primary goal in the treatment of a patient with acute and continued lower GI tract bleeding is localization of the bleeding site.

◈ The ability to localize the bleeding during an abdominal exploration is greatly compromised. Thus, exploratory laparotomy should be avoided prior to precise localization of the bleeding site.

◈ Tagged RBC scan results should be interpreted with great caution because localization of bleeding to a region of the abdomen does not necessarily localize bleeding from a specific segment of the GI tract.

◈ Colonoscopy should be reserved for stable patients with lower GI tract bleeding.

REFERENCES

Cohen FS, Sohn N. Lower gastrointestinal bleeding. In Cameron JL, ed. Current surgical therapy, 7th ed. St. Louis: Mosby-Year Book, 2001:322–327.

Laine L. Acute and chronic gastrointestinal bleeding. In: Feldman M, Sleisenger MH, Scharschimdt BF, eds. Sleisenger and Fortran's gastrointestinal and liver disease, 6th ed. Philadelphia: Saunders, 1998:198–219.

A 32-year-old woman underwent initial screening mammography that revealed bilateral breast abnormalities shown in Figure 11–1. According to an evaluation by the radiologist, these abnormalities are probably benign (American College of Radiology category 3). The patient's past medical history is unremarkable. She has never had any previous breast mass or undergone mammography in the past. Her family history is significant in that her mother died of breast cancer at age 45 years. On examination, extensive fibrocystic changes are found to be present in both breasts, and no dominant mass is identified. The examination results for both axillary areas are unremarkable.

◆ **What is the most likely diagnosis?**

◆ **What complications are associated with these changes?**

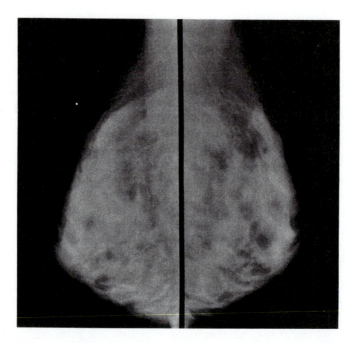

Figure 11–1.   Bilateral mammogram showing dense fibrocystic changes in the breasts. (Reproduced, with permission, from Schwarz SI, Shires GT, Spencer FC et al, eds. Principles of surgery, 7th ed. New York: McGraw-Hill, 1999:544.)

ANSWERS TO CASE 11: Breast Cancer Risk and Surveillance

Summary: The patient is a 32-year-old woman with a high-risk profile for breast cancer based on her mother's dying of breast cancer at age 45 years, an unreliable breast examination because of dense fibrocystic changes, and a normal mammogram

◆ **Diagnosis:** Benign fibrocystic changes

◆ **Complications:** These changes can lead to difficulty in detecting breast carcinoma by physical examination and mammography (Figure 11–1).

Analysis

Objectives

1. Understand the histologic features of common benign breast tissue changes and the associated risks for breast cancer (Table 11-1).
2. Understand the principles of the treatment of patients at high risk for breast cancer.
3. Know some of the treatment options for benign breast lesions.

Considerations

For this patient, whose mother developed premenopausal breast cancer and who has clinically benign, dense fibrocystic changes in both breasts and a screening mammogram showing no abnormalities, there is no uniform approach to treatment. The **ultimate decision** regarding **therapy or surveillance** is based on patient **risk factors,** her **concerns** about the threat of breast cancer, the **effectiveness of surveillance,** and the **anticipated cosmetic results** of a biopsy and/or treatment. These factors must be explored with the patient during the initial consultation. In this case, **breast ultrasonography** may provide additional information for evaluating this patient and may serve as a baseline evaluation.

Table 11–1
BENIGN BREAST LESIONS AND RELATIVE RISK OF BREAST CANCER

Benign breast histology not associated with an increased risk for breast cancer:
   Adenosis, apocrine metaplasia, cysts, ductal ectasia, fibroadenoma, fibrosis, mild hyperplasia, mastitis, squamous metaplasia

Risk increased 1.5–2.0 fold:
   Moderate or severe hyperplasia, papillomatosis

Risk increased 5-fold:
   Atypical hyperplasia

Risk increased 10-fold:
   Lobular carcinoma in situ
   Atypical hyperplasia with family history of breast cancer

For an intermediate-risk patient, it may be worthwhile to consider chemoprevention strategies ranging from dietary supplements to the administration of antiestrogens.

SURVEILLANCE AND MANAGEMENT OF HIGH-RISK PATIENTS

Definitions

Invasive lobular carcinoma: Make up only 10% to 15% of all breast cancers. They frequently do not appear as dominant breast masses but instead as focal thickening (resembling fibrocystic changes). Mammography of these lesions has a tendency to be **negative.** Detection is by physical examination, magnetic resonance imaging (MRI), and ultrasonography.

Atypical ductal hyperplasia: When this condition is diagnosed during core needle biopsy, 25% to 40% of patients have ductal carcinoma in situ diagnosed on excisional biopsy.

Screening mammography: Radiologic procedure for the examination of breast tissue with approximately 10% to 15% false-negative and 10% false-positive rates. The false-negative rate in younger patients (40 to 49 years) is higher and may approach 25%. Roughly 20% of patients undergoing a biopsy for mammographic abnormalities are found to have carcinoma.

Ultrasonography: Imaging using sound waves that can visualize small solid and cystic lesions (2 to 5 mm). It may be useful for the evaluation of cystic lesions and evaluating a low-risk patient with a palpable abnormality and a negative mammogram. When identified by ultrasound, a benign-appearing cyst characterized by the absence of septation and a solid component has a 99.5% negative predictive value for cancer.

Magnetic resonance imaging: A useful technique for defining the local extent of breast cancers. It is sensitive in identifying small cancers in the breast, but it lacks specificity in that lesions identified as abnormal may not be cancerous. For premenopausal patients, MRI is even less useful in differentiating hormone-induced changes caused by cancers.

Familial Risk Factors

The risk of developing breast cancer increases **1.8-fold** in an individual **with a mother or sister in whom breast cancer has been diagnosed.** This risk is further increased if the disease was diagnosed in the first-degree relative at a **premenopausal age (3.0-fold risk)** or if it was **bilateral breast cancer (4.0- to 5.4-fold if postmenopausal and 9.0-fold if premenopausal).** In addition, some families carry a genetic predisposition for breast cancer in the BRCA 1 or 2 gene. Whereas only 5% to 10% of cancers are attributed to mutations of the BRCA genes, the diagnosis of a BRCA 1 or 2 gene carrier significantly increases the lifetime risk of developing breast cancer by 3- to 17-fold.

Approach to Patient Treatment

Treatment options for benign breast lesions vary from patient to patient depending on each patient's **risk factors,** personal concerns regarding **cancer risk versus breast cosmesis,** and the **ability to continue close breast surveillance.** Low-risk benign lesions can be observed or excised based on the patient's clinical presentation and/or preference. A high-risk lesion or a patient with a high-risk history may opt for excision with observation and/or chemoprevention with anti-estrogen therapy and close observation. Some patients with a strong family history or a known BRCA gene mutation may consider prophylactic mastectomy. Regardless of the treatment selected, all high-risk patients should be followed with annual mammography and a physical examination and instructed on monthly breast self-examination (Table 11-2).

Screening ductal lavage: A new technology useful in the surveillance of patients with high-risk lesions or high-risk profiles. It involves aspiration of the areola to induce nipple discharge. The effluent produced is analyzed by **cytology,** specifically to identify the presence of atypical cells. Early reports on this technology show that 78% of patients screened produced an adequate sample for surveillance and that 24% of these samples were atypical, leading to further investigation. Screening duct lavage may identify patients with early lesions who should be screened with more aggressive techniques including ductography, ductoscopy, or MRI, but it currently **remains an investigational tool.**

Table 11–2

NATIONAL COMPREHENSIVE CANCER NETWORK HIGH-RISK SCREENING ALGORITHM (>25 y of Age)

Prior thoracic XRT: Annual mammogram and physical examination every 6 mo beginning 10 y after the XRT.

GAIL[†] model risk >1.67% (>35 years of age): Annual mammogram and physical examination; consider risk reduction strategies.

Family history or genetic predisposition (mutations of BRCA 1 or 2): Annual mammogram and physical examination every 6 mo starting at age 25 or 5–10 y prior to the earliest familial case; consider risk reduction strategies.

Lobular carcinoma in situ: Annual mammogram and physical examination every 6–12 mo; consider risk reduction strategies.

[*]XRT, chest radiograph.
[†]GAIL mathematical model risk factors: age, menarche, age at first live birth, number of first-degree relatives with breast cancer, number of previous benign breast biopsies, atypical hyperplasia in previous biopsy, race.

Comprehension Questions

[11.1] A 42-year-old woman has no family history of breast cancer. She undergoes a stereotactic biopsy for a suspicious mammographic lesion, which shows hyperplasia with atypia. Which of the following describes her risk of developing breast cancer?

    A. No increased risk as compared to other 42-year-old women
    B. 2-fold increase
    C. 5-fold increase
    D. 10-fold increase

[11.2] Which of the following factors is associated with the highest risk of developing breast cancer?

    A. Age of less than 25 years
    B. First-degree relative with breast cancer

C. Previous breast biopsy
D. Mutation of the BRCA 1 gene

[11.3] How often should high-risk patients undergo screening mammography?

A. Every 3 months
B. Every other year, alternating with ultrasonography
C. Every year after the age of 35 years (or 5 to 10 years prior to the index case)
D. Every 3 years

[11.4] Which of the following statements is most accurate regarding mammography?

A. The radiation has led to pulmonary malignancies.
B. Its primary role is to determine a malignant versus a benign condition of masses found on physical examination.
C. Its main role is to detect nonpalpable breast masses.
D. It is more accurate in younger patients.

Answers

[11.1] **C.** Atypical hyperplasia is associated with a 5-fold increased risk for breast cancer, and mandates an excisional biopsy.

[11.2] **D.** BRCA 1 gene carriers have a 3- to 17-fold increased risk for breast cancer development. Female carriers of the BRCA 1 gene have a 56% to 85% lifetime risk of developing breast cancer and a 15% to 45% risk of developing ovarian cancer.

[11.3] **C.** For high-risk patients, an annual examination and mammography are recommended beginning at age 35 years.

[11.4] **C.** The main purpose of mammography is to detect nonpalpable breast cancers.

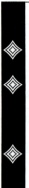

CLINICAL PEARLS

◈ The primary role of mammography is the detection of non-palpable breast masses.

◈ Having a first-degree relative with breast cancer, especially if this individual is premenopausal and the disease is bilateral, represents a risk factor for developing mammary cancer.

◈ Mammography in younger women tends to be less sensitive because of the possibility of dense fibrocystic changes.

REFERENCES

Hartmann LC, Schaid DJ, Woods JE, et al. Efficacy of bilateral prophylactic mastectomy in women with a family history of breast cancer. N Engl J Med 1999;340(2):77–84.

Hartmann LC, Sellers TA, Schaid DJ, et al. Efficacy of bilateral prophylactic mastectomy in BRCA1 and BRCA2 gene mutation carriers. J Natl Cancer Inst 2001;93(21):1633–1637.

Kinsinger LS, Harris R, Woolf SH, et al. Chemoprevention of breast cancer: a summary of the evidence from the U.S. Preventative Services Task Force. Ann Intern Med 2002;137(1):E59–E69.

Marchant DJ. Risk factors. In: Marchant DJ, ed. Breast disease. Philadelphia: Saunders; 1997:115–133.

Schrag D, Kuntz K, Garber JE, Weeks JC. Decision analysis: effects of prophylactic mastectomy and oophorectomy on life expectancy among women with BRCA 1 or BRCA 2 mutations. N Engl J Med 1997;336(20):1464–1471.

A 22-year-old man was walking past a construction site when a brick fell off the scaffold and struck him in the head. Witnesses noted that the patient was unconscious immediately after the incident and did not regain consciousness for approximately 10 minutes. The paramedics placed the patient in C-spine precautions and brought him to the emergency room. During the primary survey at the emergency center, the patient has apparently normal air exchange, a respiratory rate of 18/min, blood pressure of 138/78, and a pulse of 80/min. The patient does not open his eyes in response to voice commands but has eye opening in response to painful stimuli. He withdraws from painful stimuli. His only verbal responses are incomprehensible sounds. The secondary survey demonstrates a 3-cm scalp laceration and a contusion over the right temporal region. The right pupil is dilated 6 mm and sluggishly reactive to light; the left pupil is 4 mm in diameter and reacts normally to light. No blood is visualized behind the tympanic membranes. The results from an examination of the truncal region and extremities are within normal limits.

◆ **What is the most likely diagnosis?**

◆ **What should be your next step?**

ANSWERS TO CASE 12: Closed Head Injury

Summary: A 22-year-old man has an injury mechanism and presentation indicating an isolated severe closed head injury. He has an initial Glasgow Coma Scale (GCS) aggregate score of 8 (see Table 12–1).

Table 12–1
GLASGOW COMA SCALE

ASSESSMENT AREA	SCORE
EYE OPENING	
Spontaneous	4
To speech	3
To pain	2
None	1
BEST MOTOR RESPONSE	
Obeys commands	6
Localizes pain	5
Withdraws to pain	4
Decorticate posture (abnormal flexion)	3
Decerebrate posture (extension)	2
No response	1
VERBAL RESPONSE	
Oriented	5
Confused conversation	4
Inappropriate words	3
Incomprehensible sounds	2
None	1

Most likely diagnosis: Severe closed head injury with possible mass effect.

 Next step: Immediate endotracheal intubation to control ventilation and oxygenation.

Analysis

Objectives

1. Be able to calculate and know the significance of the GCS score.
2. Be familiar with the causes of and preventive measures for secondary brain injury.
3. Become familiar with the emergent management of intracranial mass lesions.

Considerations

This patient may have an epidural hematoma, subdural hematoma, intraparenchymal injury, subarachnoid hemorrhage, diffuse axonal injury, or any combination of these injuries. The anatomic classification of the injury is **not important** in the initial treatment of this patient. **With a patient with a severe head injury, the most important management principle is avoidance of secondary brain injury**. The injured brain is much more susceptible to hypoxia and hypotension; **in patients with both hypoxia and hypotension, mortality is approximately 75%, and hypotension alone doubles the mortality risk compared to that for normotensive patients with a severe head injury**. Definitive **airway management by endotracheal intubation** is vital in the initial treatment of this patient.

This patient also has evidence of increased intracranial pressure with localizing signs, **unequal pupils and hemiparesis.** The Monro–Kellie doctrine governs intracranial pressure and expanding mass lesions. This equation states that the volume of blood, brain, and cerebrospinal fluid within the nonexpansile cranium must remain constant in order for intracranial pressure to remain constant. If an additional substance, such as an expanding hematoma is added, the intracranial pressure will increase unless a compensatory amount of blood, brain, or cerebrospinal fluid is removed. Once the patient has been intubated and appropriately resuscitated with crystalloids and blood, the **emergent treatment of a patient with localizing signs includes hyperventilation and administration of mannitol.** Hyperventilation causes cerebral vasoconstriction, reducing the volume of blood in the cranium and allowing room for the intracranial mass lesion. It must be used cautiously, however, as prolonged use can cause cerebral ischemia secondary to this reduced blood flow. Intravenous mannitol, at a dose of 1 g/kg, is also used to decrease the volume of blood in the brain and to decrease brain volume due to edema. **Mannitol should not be used unless patients are adequately resuscitated because it can aggravate hypovolemia and cause uncompensated shock.**

APPROACH TO CLOSED HEAD INJURY

Definitions

Epidural hematoma: The collection of blood outside the dura but within the skull, most often in the temporal region (middle meningeal artery laceration). These hematomas are uncommon, occurring in 0.5% of all head injuries and 9% of severe head injuries, and have a better prognosis than other types of hematomas. They appear classically biconvex or lens-shaped on a computer tomography (CT) scan.

Subdural hematoma: The collection of blood between the brain surface and the dura, commonly as a result of the tearing of bridging veins. They are much more common than epidural hematomas, and their prognosis is worse than that for epidural hematomas because of coexisting brain injury.

Concussion: Transient loss of consciousness associated with no CT scan abnormalities.

Mild head injury: GCS of 13 to 15.

Moderate head injury: GCS of 9 to 12.

Severe head injury: GCS of 8 or less.

Coma: Severe head injury, GCS of 8 or less.

Burr hole: A hole drilled through the skull, usually on the side of the larger pupil, as an emergency procedure to decompress an intracranial mass lesion. This procedure should be performed infrequently, only by those who have been trained by a neurosurgeon, and only when timely transfer to a neurosurgeon is not possible.

Clinical Approach

As in any trauma patient, airway, breathing, and circulation concerns should be addressed first. The goals include avoidance of hypoxia and hypotension that can exacerbate head injury, and stabilization of associated spine, chest, abdomen, pelvic, and extremity injuries. A neurologic assessment should then be performed and include a pupillary examination and calculation of the GCS.

The pupillary examination determines pupil size and reactivity to light. **Dilation of a pupil with a sluggish response to light is an early sign of temporal lobe herniation.** The third nerve becomes compressed against the tentorium with herniation of the temporal lobe. **Ninety percent of the time this herniation and pupillary abnormality** occur on **the same side of the intracranial lesion.** This can direct the placement of emergency Burr holes should they become necessary. The **GCS** evaluates **eye opening, motor response, and verbal response.** The best motor response is a better indicator of prognosis than the worst response. The **trend** observed in a patient's examination is **much more important than a single examination.** The diagnostic test of choice for all patients with a head injury is CT imaging. This scan should *not* be obtained at a facility that is not able to definitively treat the head-injured patient if it will delay transfer to a qualified neurosurgeon or trauma surgeon.

Comprehension Questions

[12.1] A 46-year-old unrestrained driver was "T-boned" by another car traveling at 60 mph. He is brought to the emergency department with a pulse of 130/min, blood pressure 90/62, and respiration rate 28/min. His pupils are equal and reactive, he does not open his eyes to painful stimuli, he does not make any sound, and he withdraws from painful stimuli. What is the patient's GCS?

A. 2
B. 3
C. 5
D. 6
E. 7

[12.2] Which of the following is the most appropriate initial step in taking care of the above patient?

A. Drilling an emergency burr hole
B. Obtaining a CT scan of the head
C. Administering intravenous mannitol
D. Immediate intubation
E. Fluid resuscitation with 2 liters of lactated Ringer's solution

[12.3] An 18-year-old skier runs into a tree on a downhill run. He is initially brought to the emergency department screaming unintelligibly, not following commands, opening his eyes spontaneously, and moving all extremities spontaneously. What is his GCS?

A. 8
B. 10
C. 12
D. 14
E. 15

[12.4] After 2 hours in the emergency department the above patient does not open his eyes, mutters unintelligible sounds, and has flexor posturing. What is his GCS is now?

A. 4
B. 5
C. 6
D. 7
E. 12

[12.5] Which of the following would be considered *inappropriate* in managing the above patient?
A. Continued observation as the patient will likely wake up
B. Immediate intubation
C. Obtaining a head CT scan
D. Arranging for transfer to a neurosurgeon
E. Repeating the primary survey

Answers

[12.1] **D.** GCS 6 (eye opening 1, verbal 1, motor 4). This score corresponds to a severe head injury.

[12.2] **D.** Immediate intubation (definitive airway management) is indicated for a patient with a severe closed head injury (GCS <9).

[12.3] **C.** GCS 12 (eye opening 4, verbal 3, motor 5)

[12.4] **C.** GCS 6 (eye opening 1, verbal 2, motor 3)

[12.5] **A.** A significant deterioration in the GCS (≥2) is an indication of serious injury or a worsening condition mandating immediate reassessment and treatment.

CLINICAL PEARLS

◆ Prevention of secondary brain injury begins with optimizing the patient's oxygenation, ventilation, and brain perfusion, particularly avoiding hypoxemia and hypotension.

◆ The initial GCS determined at the emergency center and the patient's age are the most important indicators of outcome in head-injured patients.

◆ Pupillary reflex and the GCS (eye opening, motor response, and verbal response) are the cornerstones of initial neurologic assessment.

◆ The side on which the dilated pupil is located usually indicates the side on which the intracranial mass is located.

REFERENCES

American Association of Neurological Surgeons. Guidelines for the management of severe head injury. J Neurotrauma 1996;13(11):641–734.

Chestnut RM, Marshall LF, Klauber MR, et al. The role of secondary brain injury in determining outcome from severe head injury. J Trauma 1993;34:216–222.

Advanced trauma life support for doctors. American College of Surgeons, 1997.

A 63-year-old man is rescued from a house fire and brought to the emergency center. According to paramedics responding to a three-alarm fire, the victim was found unconscious in an upstairs bedroom of a house. The patient's past medical problems are unknown. His pulse is 112/min, blood pressure 150/85, and respiratory rate 30/min. A pulse oximeter registers 92% O_2 saturation with a face mask. He face and the exposed portions of his body are covered with a carbonaceous deposit. The patient has blistering and open burn wounds involving the circumference of his left arm and left leg and more than 80% of his back and buttocks. He does not respond verbally to questions and reacts to painful stimulation with occasional moans.

◆ **What is the most appropriate next step?**

◆ **What are the immediate and late complications associated with thermal injuries?**

ANSWERS TO CASE 13: Thermal Injury

Summary: A 63-year-old man presents with an approximately 40% total body surface area (TBSA) burn injury and inhalation injuries.

◆ **Next step:** Definitive airway management by intubation is appropriate in this patient with possible inhalation injuries and carbon monoxide (CO) poisoning.

◆ **Immediate and late complications:** Airway compromise and tissue hypoperfusion are common early complications, and sepsis and functional loss are possible late complications.

Analysis

Objectives

1. Be familiar with the initial assessment and treatment of patients with thermal injuries.
2. Be familiar with the assessment and management of burn wounds.
3. Be familiar with the prognosis associated with thermal injuries.

Considerations

Given the circumstances surrounding the injury (a house fire), the size of the burn, and the age of patient, all of which indicate a high likelihood of pulmonary complications, immediate intubation is clearly indicated. Persons at risk for upper airway thermal damage include this particular patient because he was found unconscious in a closed-space fire. Fluid resuscitation with lactated Ringer's solution should be initiated based on 2 to 4 mL/kg/% burn. Unless the patient is already at a facility that specializes in burn care, immediate arrangements should be made for a transfer after initial stabilization.

APPROACH TO THERMAL INJURY

The skin is the largest organ of the body. It allows the body to maintain fluid balance, temperature regulation, and protein regulation and provides a barrier against bacteria and fungi. It is a necessary organ for living. Knowledge of the initial resuscitation and treatment, along with the late complications, can help minimize the morbidity and mortality of these injuries.

Initial Assessment

The initial assessment of a burn patient is the same as for a trauma patient (attention to the airway, breathing, and circulation–the ABC's), with additional considerations. Along with their burns, patients can acquire thoracic and abdominal trauma, fractures, or head injuries from associated falls or crashes. This chapter will focus on the particulars of burn injuries, but one must be mindful that associated injuries must be managed concurrently.

Airway

As for other traumas, airway assessment is the initial consideration. Although patients do not receive "pulmonary burns" (unless they inhale live steam or explosive gases), the upper airway can be burned as it cools the hot gases from a fire. Additional signs of potential airway involvement include facial and upper torso burns and carbonaceous sputum. If **the oropharynx is dry, red, or blistered, the patient will probably require intubation.** When indicated, endotracheal intubation should be performed early, before a surgical airway is required secondary to pharyngeal and laryngeal edema. Smoke inhalation can also cause tracheobronchitis and edema from exposure to the incomplete combustion of carbon particles and other toxic fumes.

Carbon monoxide poisoning can cause hypoxia because CO has a 240-fold greater affinity for hemoglobin than O_2, thus shifting the oxyhemoglobin curve to the left. **All patients injured in closed-space fires should have their carboxyhemoglobin (COHgb) level determined. A COHgb level of greater than 30% may indicate significant central nervous system dysfunction** that may also be permanent. A **COHgb level of greater than 60% may portend coma and**

death. Note that one can develop a 30% COHgb level within 3 minutes in a moderately smoky fire. When associated with cutaneous burns, smoke inhalation doubles the risk of mortality. Patients with a COHgb greater than 10% with carbonaceous sputum from a closed-space fire have a greater than 90% chance of needing ventilator support if they have associated burns of more than 20% TBSA. The half-life of CO in the blood on room air is 250 minutes. If the patient is receiving 100% O_2, the half-life is approximately 40 to 60 minutes. Therefore, calculation of the patient's initial COHgb level is estimated by knowing the transport time and the time prior to the arterial blood draw, as well as the oxygen concentration the patient is receiving. A request for the COHgb level can be sent to the laboratory along with the request for a baseline arterial blood gas analysis. In the scenario described here, where the patient is found unconscious in a building with 40% TBSA burns, carbonaceous sputum, signs of hypoxia (abnormal oxygen saturation), and neurologic deficits (responding only to painful stimuli), intubation is needed.

Resuscitation

Cutaneous burns result in accelerated fluid loss. Mediators such as prostaglandins, thromboxane A2, and reactive oxygen radicals are released from injured tissue, which can cause local edema with increased capillary permeability, along with microvascular and end-organ dysfunction. Burn sizes exceeding 20% TBSA can result in a systemic response, with significant interstitial edema in distant soft tissues. With these large burns, an initial decrease in cardiac output is seen, followed by a hypermetabolic state. These intravascular fluid losses make resuscitation an important part of burn management. Organs, including skin, can progress from a hypoperfused state to more permanent end-organ damage if resuscitation is not accomplished.

Calculating Resuscitation Fluid Requirements

Most patients with burns involving **less than 15% TBSA can be resuscitated with oral fluids.** For larger burns, isotonic intravenous fluids such as lactated Ringer's solution should be used (large volumes of normal saline can cause hyperchloremic metabolic acidosis). Fluid needs are estimated by the Parkland or Baxter formula. Based on the

Parkland formula, for adults and children weighing more than 10 kg, the total 24-hour volume is calculated using 3 to 4 mL/kg/% burn. Half of this amount is given in the first 8 hours, and the remainder in the next 16 hours. Intravenous fluid hydration given by the paramedics en route should be considered part of this volume. Children weighing less than 10 kg should be given 2 to 3 mL/kg/% burn divided similarly over the next 24 hours. In addition, they should receive a maintenance fluid that includes 5% dextrose. Because of the increased capillary permeability, colloids such as albumin are generally avoided for the first 12 to 18 hours but can be used subsequently if resuscitation is not being achieved with the crystalloid regimen. **Inhalational injuries, extensive and/or deep burns, and delayed resuscitation usually result in larger fluid requirements than initially calculated.**

Assessing the Adequacy of Resuscitation

Measuring urine output (UOP) is a helpful way of assessing the adequacy of the resuscitation. Adults should achieve 0.5 mL/kg/h of UOP, children should produce 0.5 to 1 mL/kg/h, and infants should produce 1 to 2 mL/kg/h because they have a higher volume/surface area ratio. Generally, UOP is averaged over 2 to 3 hours before changes are made. Excess UOP should also be avoided unless one is treating myoglobinuria.

Calculating the Burn Area

The "rule of nines" is a useful guide in assessing the extent of a person's burns (Table 13–1). The body can be fairly accurately divided into anatomic regions that represent 9% or multiples of 9% of the total body surface. In estimating irregular outlines or distributions, note that the palm of a patient's hand (not including the fingers) represents approximately 1% of the patient's total body surface.

Burn Depth

When calculating the total percent of burn involvement in a patient with more serious burns, first-degree burns are not included. Different

Table 13–1
RULE OF NINES

LOCATION	ADULT (%)	INFANT (%)
Front of head with neck	4.5	9
Back of head with neck	4.5	9
Front of torso	18	18
Back of torso	18	18
Front of one arm	4.5	4.5
Back of one arm	4.5	4.5
Front of one leg (full length)	9	7
Back of one leg (full length)	9	7

burn depths (see Table 13–2) should be noted on a burn diagram form. As burns marginate, the assessment of depth may change from the value calculated initially, particularly in the case of scald burns, where the initial depth may not appear as severe.

Fourth-degree burns are those that extend through skin and subcutaneous fat, even involving deep structures.

Temporary Wound Coverings

Because the skin serves in temperature regulation and as a barrier against bacterial and fungal organisms, attention must be given to the prevention of hypothermia and monitoring for infection. **Since a burn site can become infected and allow microbes systemic access, steroids should not be used for any burn greater than 10% TBSA.** Prophylactic intravenous antibiotics are usually not recommended, as they select for resistant organisms. The different creams commonly used topically have local broad antimicrobial activity that can resist colonization. **Silver sulfadiazine** (SS) does not penetrate the eschar and so is not helpful in an infected burn. It can rarely cause leukopenia, requiring cessation of use. Patients who are allergic to sulfa are usually not affected by SS because the silver molecule is

Table 13–2

BURN DEPTH

CHARACTERISTICS AND TREATMENT	FIRST-DEGREE	SECOND-DEGREE OR PARTIAL THICKNESS	THIRD-DEGREE OR FULL THICKNESS
Location affected	Epidermis	Through epidermis and into dermis.	All the way through dermis.
Characteristics	Erythema and pain	Pink/red, weepy, swelling and blisters, very painful.	White or dark, leathery, waxy, painless.
Course	Heal in 3–4 d without scarring. The dead epidermal cells desquamate (peel). Sunburns that blister are actually superficial dermal burns.	Superficial dermal heal within 3 wk without scarring or functional impairment. Deep dermal heal in 3–8 wk but with severe scarring and loss of function.	Burns can heal only by epithelial migration from periphery and contraction. Unless they are tiny (cigarette burn size), they will need grafting.
Treatment	Lotions (like aloe) and nonsteriodal anti-inflammatory drugs.	Excise and graft deep dermal burns.	Excise and graft.

attached to the antigenic portion of the sulfadiazine molecule; however, if this cream is chosen, it is prudent to try a test patch for patients with a sulfa allergy. A rash or pain (rather than the usual soothing) will ensue if they are truly allergic to SS. **Sulfamylon (mafenide)** is less commonly used because it is painful on application. Furthermore, it can cause severe systemic metabolic acidosis through carbonic anhydrase inhibition. It penetrates the eschar and is therefore useful for full-thickness infected burns (there is less pain on application) and for unexcised burns with colonization. **Silver nitrate** does not penetrate the eschar and turns the burn area black. Usage can result in severe leaching of sodium and chloride, which can lead to profound hyponatremia and hypochloremia, particularly when used on large areas on children. **Pigskin** can be used on flat, clean wounds. Its growth factors can encourage epithelialization in partial-thickness burns.

Burn Complications

Neurologic: Transient delirium commonly occurs, but an altered mental status requires evaluation to identify other etiologies such as anoxia and metabolic abnormalities.

Pulmonary: Pneumonias and respiratory failure requiring mechanical ventilation are frequently seen.

Cardiovascular: Venous thrombosis can occur. Suppurative thrombophlebitis can lead to bacteremia, which may cause endocarditis along with the local venous abscess.

Gastrointestinal: Stomach and duodenal ulcers can develop secondary to decreased mucosal defenses resulting from the decrease in splanchnic blood flow. Early gastric tube feedings before atony occurs may help improve nutrition or prevent stress ulcers. If preventing the development of nosocomial pneumonias by inhibiting bacterial overgrowth, histamine-2 blockers may also be helpful. Critically ill patients can also develop acalculous cholecystitis or, because of hypoperfusion, pancreatitis or hepatic dysfunction.

Renal: Acute tubular necrosis can develop because of inadequate resuscitation or myoglobinuria.

Infection: Can arise from the burns themselves or from treatments used in critical care: urinary tract infections from Foley catheters and sinusitis or otitis from feeding or nasogastric tubes.

Ophthalmic: Corneal abrasions or ulcerations may been seen, resulting either from the initial injury or from exposure. Patients with

Table 13-3

AMERICAN BURN ASSOCIATION RECOMMENDATIONS
FOR TRANSFER TO BURN CENTERS

<10 years or >50 yrs with full-thickness burn >10% TBSA
Any age with TBSA burn >20%
Partial- or full-thickness burn involving face, eyes, ears, hands, genitalia, perineum, and over joints
Burn injury complicated by chemical, electrical, or other forms of significant trauma
Any patient requiring special social, emotional, and long-term rehabilitative support

potential eye injuries, particularly those caused by explosions, should be examined early in the emergency department using fluorescein for corneal abrasions, which should be treated with antibiotic lubrication. Early examination is important before edema makes the examination difficult. Eyelid problems also may require treatment.

Musculoskeletal and soft tissue: Scarring can cause functional or cosmetic defects. Physical and occupational therapy, scar releases, regrafting, and silicone prostheses can help.

Psychological: Burns can be very traumatic as well as defacing. Adequate support should be provided.

Because of the specialized care required and the multidisciplinary aspects of burn treatment, the American Burn Association recommends that certain patients receive their care at burn centers (Table 13-3).

Comprehension Questions

[13.1] Calculate the estimated intravenous fluid rates and volumes for the patient in Case 13 who has a 40% TBSA burn. Use the Parkland formula and assume a 70-kg man.

[13.2] You determine a COHgb level for this patient (Case 13) in the emergency room (ER) 1 hour after he has been given a 100% O_2 nonrebreathing mask at the site and intubated with 100% F_{IO_2} in the ER. The level is 15%. What was his probable COHgb at the fire?

Answers

[13.1] With the Parkland formula, 24-hour volume = 3 mL/kg/% burn. Total volume = 3 mL $\times$ 70 kg $\times$ 40% = 8400 mL. Half should be given over the first 8 hours, and so (8400 mL)/2 = 4200 mL. Setting the rate over 8 hours, (4200 mL)/8 h = 525 mL/h. The remainder is given over 16 hours: (4200 mL)/16 h = 263 mL/h.

[13.2] His probable COHgb level at the fire was approximately 30%, which can portend significant central nervous system dysfunction. Because the half-life of COHgb is approximately 40 to 60 minutes in the face of 100% O_2, and 1 hour has passed, the initial level is 2 $\times$ 15% = 30%.

CLINICAL PEARLS

◈ When the oropharynx is dry, red, or blistered, the patient will probably require intubation.

◈ All patients injured in closed-space fires should have their COHgb values determined in the emergency department to assess for CO poisoning.

◈ The rule of nines is a useful guide to determine the extent of a person's burns in that the body can be divided into anatomic regions that represent 9% or multiples of 9% of the total body surface.

REFERENCES

American College of Surgeons Committee on Trauma Staff. Injuries due to burns and cold. In: ATLS: advanced trauma life support program for doctors instructor course manual, 6th ed. American College of Surgeons. Chicago, IL, 1997: 337–352.

Heimbach D, Gibran N. In: Burn pearls, 18th ed. Seattle: University of Washington Burn Center at Harborview. 2000:12–57.

Sheridan RL, Tompkins RG. Burns. In: Greenfield LJ et al, eds. Surgery: scientific principles and practices, 2nd ed. Philadelphia: Lippincott-Raven, 1997:422–438.

A 62-year-old man with chronic hypertension presents with pain and fatigue in his legs that occurs whenever he walks. The patient says his symptoms have been present for the past 12 months and have progressively worsened. The patient currently has pain and tightness in both calves that develop after walking less than one block but routinely resolve after a short period of rest. His past medical history is significant for hypertension. He smokes approximately one pack of cigarettes per day. On examination, his feet are warm and without lesions. The femoral pulses are normal bilaterally. The popliteal, dorsalis pedis, and posterior tibial pulses are absent bilaterally. Doppler examination of the lower extremities reveals the presence of Doppler signals in both his feet with ankle-brachial indexes (ABIs) showing moderately severe disease: ABI 0.5 on the left, and 0.54 on the right.

◆ **What is the most likely diagnosis?**

◆ **What is the most appropriate next step?**

◆ **What is the best initial treatment for this patient?**

ANSWERS TO CASE 14: Claudication Syndrome

Summary: A 62-year-old nondiabetic man presents with bilateral leg claudication. Based on the physical examination, the patient most likely has bilateral superficial femoral artery (SFA) occlusion.

 Most likely diagnosis: Atherosclerosis with bilateral superficial artery occlusions.

 Next step: Assessment of disability and adequate counseling on the risks and benefits of therapy.

 Best initial treatment: Lifestyle modification with smoking cessation, exercise training, and risk factor control.

Analysis

Objectives

1. Know the differential diagnosis for claudication due to arterial insufficiency.
2. Be able to recognize the indications for lower extremity revascularization and the benefits and limitations of open surgical and endovascular techniques.
3. Be familiar with noninvasive modalities in the evaluation and follow-up of patients with claudication.

Considerations

This patient's presentation is similar to that of typical vascular disease patients with lower extremity peripheral arterial disease: a history of slowly increasing exertional pain in conjunction with multiple risk factors for atherosclerosis. Lower extremity peripheral vascular occlusive disease (LEPVOD) represents a continuum of regional signs and symptoms of the systemic disease state of atherosclerosis. Early presentations can and should be managed conservatively. More advanced stages require interventional treatments as limb salvage becomes the desired goal. The recommended standard of LEPOVD classification can help stratify patients according to their presentation and treatment (Table 14–1). More advanced disease generally implies more anatomic levels with occlusive or stenotic pathology. His ABIs of 0.5 and 0.54 are consistent with exertional pain.

Table 14–1

FONTAINE CLASSIFICATION OF LOWER EXTREMITY PERIPHERAL VASCULAR OCCLUSIVE DISEASE

STAGE	SYMPTOMS	SIGNS	NONINVASIVES*	TREATMENT
I	None	None	$0.8 < ABI < 1.0$	Lifestyle and risk factors
II	Claudication, exertional pain	Decreased or absent distal pulses	$0.41 < ABI < 0.8$	Stage I plus potential intervention
III	Rest pain	Stage II plus elevation pallor	$0.2 < ABI < 0.4$	Stage II plus probable bypass
IV	Ulceration	Stage III plus distal skin breakdown	$ABI < 0.2$	Stage III plus wound care
V	Minor gangrene	Stage III plus digital gangrene	$ABI < 0.2$	Stage IV plus possible minor amputation
VI	Major gangrene	Stage III plus gangrene proximal to forefoot	$ABI < 0.2$ to not obtainable	Stage IV plus possible major or minor amputation

ABI = ankle/brachial index.

APPROACH TO LOWER EXTREMITY VASCULAR DISEASE

Definitions

Lower extremity peripheral vascular occlusive disease: Ischemia in the lower extremities due to arterial stenosis. Acute ischemia is typically characterized by a sudden onset of **pain, pallor, and pulselessness.** Chronic arterial ischemia manifests as lower extremity pain with exercise and resolves with rest.

Arterial bypass: Surgical procedure in which one artery is connected to another artery with a conduit (such as a saphenous vein or prosthetic material).

Ankle-brachial index: Ratio of Doppler signals of the ankle systolic blood pressure to those of the brachial artery, normally greater than 0.95; intermittent disease correlates with 0.5 to 0.95, and severe disease with less than 0.5.

Clinical Approach

An understanding of the arterial circulation helps one to localize the pathology in LEPVOD. More levels of arterial involvement usually suggest a greater need for interventional therapy. One must also keep in mind that patients with LEPVOD are patients with systemic atherosclerosis; thus, there is a higher probability of concomitant coronary artery and carotid artery disease. The other manifestations of atherosclerosis impact long-term survival in patients with LEPVOD. Diabetes is important in LEPVOD, both because of its presence as an independent risk factor and because it can alter the clinical presentation. Neuropathy can confound an impression of ischemic rest pain. Additionally, the susceptibility of a diabetic patient to infection can enhance the risk of tissue loss.

Lifestyle therapy is essential for all patients. Because **any intervention can cause complications that may be limb- or life-threatening, the clinician needs to weigh the risks and benefits of intervention for a patient with claudication differently than for a patient with digital gangrene.** The patient with claudication should be severely disabled and not merely inconvenienced by having either angioplasty or a potential bypass. On the other hand, the patient with digital gangrene is in a limb-threatening situation, requiring definitive revascularization if a limb is to be salvaged. Tissue loss is a limb-threatening presentation that requires revascularization. True ischemic rest pain with multilevel LEPVOD also requires revascularization for definitive treatment. A patient with claudication with severe lifestyle limitations (such as the loss of a job) may be a candidate for revascularization if the risk profile is not too unfavorable.

All interventional therapy carries a spectrum of risks and benefits. Angioplasty techniques work best for proximal vessels with short, focal, concentric, noncalcified atherosclerotic stenosis. The more unfavorable the lesion is with respect to length, number, placement, and morphology, the less successful percutaneous therapy will be. As a general rule, outright arterial occlusions require bypass to achieve revascularization. More proximal level bypasses at the aortoiliac level can achieve 90% 5-year patency, whereas even distal femoral tibial bypasses can achieve only 65% 5-year patency.

Comprehension Questions

[14.1] A 57-year-old man who works as a deliveryman is able to walk only 40 yd before stopping because of right calf and thigh cramping. He is worried that he will lose his job. He is a diabetic and takes an oral hypoglycemic agent, a long-acting beta-blocker, and a statin-class lipid-lowering agent. He smokes one pack of cigarettes a day. He has normal right leg pulses, but no pulses in the left leg. Which of the following is the most likely site of arterial occlusion?

A. His left aortoiliac system
B. His left SFA
C. His right SFA
D. His left internal carotid artery

[14.2] A patient has the symptoms described above, as well as non-healing ulcers between his left third and fourth toes. He probably has which of the following? (More than one answer may be correct.)

A. An occlusion in his left aortoiliac system
B. An occlusion in his left SFA

C. An occlusion in his right SFA

D. An occlusion in his right aortoiliac artery

[14.3] A patient has the symptoms and ulcers described above, as well as documented left iliac artery occlusion for the entire left external iliac artery and full-length occlusion of his left SFA with reconstitution of his popliteal artery just below the adductor hiatus. How should he be treated?

A. Lifestyle counseling and risk factor control

B. A femoral-femoral bypass from the left leg to the right leg

C. A femoral popliteal bypass with a reversed saphenous vein if available

D. All of the above

Answers

[14.1] **A.** His symptoms imply occlusive disease above the common femoral level, confirmed by the absence of a femoral pulse.

[14.2] **A** and **B.** When tissue loss is noted, multilevel disease is usually present (in the aortoiliac and superficial femoral arteries).

[14.3] **D.** All patients require lifestyle modification, but the patient in question needs a complete multilevel revascularization.

CLINICAL PEARLS

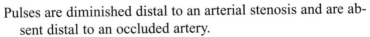

◈ Pulses are diminished distal to an arterial stenosis and are absent distal to an occluded artery.

◈ Claudication is extremely reproducible, with the same exertional load producing the same symptom complex.

◈ Rest pain is better called "metatarsalgia" in order to understand where the pain should be, making it different than pain in a foot with diabetic neuropathy.

REFERENCE

Rutherford RB, Baker JD, Ernst CB, et al. Recommended standards for reports dealing with lower extremity ischemia: revised version. J Vasc Surg 1997;26: 517–538.

A 22-year-old man presents to the hospital 1 hour after sustaining two stab wounds in an altercation. On examination, the patient appears intoxicated and grimaces during manipulation of the sites. His temperature is 36.8°C (98.2°F), pulse rate 86/min, blood pressure 128/80, and respiratory rate 22/min. A thorough physical examination reveals two stab wounds. One of the wounds is located at the anterior axillary line, 1 cm above the left costal margin, whereas the second wound is located 4 cm left of the umbilicus. There is no active bleeding from either wound site. The breath sounds are present and equal bilaterally. The abdomen is tender only in the vicinity of the injuries. The patient claims that the knife used in the attack was approximately 5 inches long.

 What is your next step?

 What are the potential injuries?

ANSWERS TO CASE 15: Penetrating Abdominal Trauma

Summary: A 22-year-old hemodynamically stable, intoxicated man presents with stab wounds to the left thoracoabdominal region and abdomen.

 Next step: Perform primary and secondary assessments focusing on the abdominal examination and obtain an upright chest radiograph (to assess for pneumothorax, hemothorax, and free intra-abdominal air).

 Potential injuries: Heart, lung, diaphragm, intra-abdominal injury.

Analysis

Objectives

1. Become familiar with the various possible approaches in the selective treatment of patients with a penetrating abdominal injury.
2. Become familiar with the benefits and potential limitations associated with the various diagnostic strategies for detecting intra-abdominal injuries.

Considerations

This patient has sustained penetrating thoracoabdominal and abdominal injuries. Initial attention should be directed to the primary survey, which includes assessment of the airway, breathing, and circulation (ABC's). These appear to be stable based on the scenario. For this patient the concerns include possible injury to the thoracic structures, diaphragm, and intra-abdominal structures. A reasonable approach for this asymptomatic patient with stab wounds to the left thoracoabdominal region and the abdomen includes an upright chest radiograph to rule out pneumothorax, hemothorax, and free air, with a study repeated in

6 hours if no abnormalities are seen initially. **A focused abdominal sonography for trauma (FAST) examination can then be performed to exclude pericardial effusion, which would indicate a cardiac injury.** The patient should then undergo diagnostic laparoscopy to determine if there is peritoneal penetration of the stab wound or if there is a diaphragm injury. **Any suspicion of a hollow viscus injury during laparoscopy should result in a celiotomy.**

APPROACH TO PENETRATING ABDOMINAL TRAUMA

Primary Survey

Patient treatment always begins with an evaluation and management of the airway, breathing, and circulation (the ABC's—a primary survey). Listening to the patient allows the examiner to determine the adequacy of the airway and brain perfusion and to make certain that there are no obvious neurologic deficits. **Breathing is evaluated by listening to the patient's breath sounds.** The finding of obvious decreased breath sounds on the left side is an indication for the placement of a chest tube. In addition to measuring vital signs, the examiner can evaluate the circulation by palpating the skin and observing the capillary refill. **Cool skin or a capillary refill greater than 2 seconds is an indication of shock.** The circulation evaluation includes an examination **for distended neck veins or muffled heart tones,** which are indications of **cardiac tamponade and require immediate treatment.**

A determination of the extent of disability is the equivalent of a rapid neurologic examination, and it includes assessing the pupillary response as well as the patient's response to verbal stimuli. The patient's clothes should be removed to look for evidence of other injuries. During the primary survey, an **upright chest radiograph** should be obtained. This chest radiograph is useful in the evaluation of **pneumothorax or hemothorax, the cardiac silhouette for evidence of cardiac injury and intra-abdominal free air** consistent with a hollow viscus injury. If the chest radiograph shows no abnormalities, it should be repeated at 4 to 6 hours to rule out a delayed pneumothorax. **FAST** should also be performed to rule out blood in the pericardium. The **sensitivity of FAST in detecting pericardial** blood has been shown to be

as high as 100%, but **its sensitivity in detecting abdominal injury approximates only 50%.**

Secondary Survey

Following the primary survey, a careful secondary survey should be performed to ascertain the extent of the patient's injuries. The most important part of the secondary survey in this patient is the abdominal examination. The presence of prominent physical findings such as **rigidity, guarding, or significant tenderness distant from the stab wounds is an indication for celiotomy.** It is important to note that the physical examination may not be reliable in patients with penetrating abdominal trauma, especially in those who are intoxicated.

Treatment Options

Patients with penetrating abdominal trauma have historically undergone mandatory surgical exploration, resulting in a high nontherapeutic celiotomy rate and a high complication rate. Currently, the practice of selective celiotomy has become widely accepted. This change in practice has resulted in alternative methods of evaluation, including admission to the hospital for serial abdominal examinations, local exploration of the wound followed by diagnostic peritoneal lavage (DPL), and abdominal computed tomography (CT) or exploratory laparoscopy.

Observation of asymptomatic patients with abdominal stab wounds for the development of positive physical findings results in a low nontherapeutic celiotomy rate. Patients who are observed require frequent evaluations for peritoneal findings or hemodynamic instability. Patients should be observed for a minimum of 24 to 48 hours. However, a policy of observing patients with stab wounds may result in a delay in the diagnosis of some injuries.

Local wound exploration of stab wounds permits a determination of fascial penetration. A sterile field is prepared around the stab wound, and the area is infiltrated with a local anesthetic. The stab wound is enlarged to permit adequate exploration, and the tract of the wound is followed. If the **anterior abdominal fascia has been penetrated, further evaluation is indicated.**

Diagnostic peritoneal lavage was designed to sample the intra-abdominal contents for blood, inflammation (white blood cell [WBC] count), or fecal matter. A catheter is placed in the abdomen utilizing the Seldinger (catheter over a guide wire) technique. The catheter is aspirated after placement to look for evidence of gross blood or fecal contents. If the aspiration results are negative, 1 liter of warmed normal saline is instilled into the abdomen and then removed by gravity. The criteria for a **positive DPL results in patients with blunt trauma** are well established and include **gross aspiration of 10 ml of blood, aspiration of fecal contents, or the presence of more than 100,000/mm^3 red blood cells (RBCs) or 500/mm^3 WBCs in the lavage fluid.**

Diagnostic Peritoneal Lavage Criteria

Although the criteria for grossly positive DPL results and the WBC count criteria (500 cells/mm^3) for penetrating are the same as for blunt trauma, the RBC count criteria have not been standardized. The published thresholds range from 1000/mm^3 to 100,000/mm^3. The use of low RBC count criteria results in sensitivities approaching 100%, but in nontherapeutic celiotomy rates as high as 30%. The use of higher erythrocyte thresholds is associated with a reduced sensitivity and a reduced nontherapeutic celiotomy rate. DPL is not a sensitive test for injuries to the diaphragm or retroperitoneal structures.

The use of **CT** has been described for the evaluation of penetrating torso injuries in hemodynamically normal patients. Oral, intravenous, and rectal contrast are used. Results from a CT scan are considered positive if there is evidence of peritoneal penetration, free intraperitoneal fluid or air, intraperitoneal extravasation of contrast material, or injury to an intraperitoneal organ. Abdominal CT imaging can be used to accurately follow the stab wound tract, allowing determination of the structures that are at risk for injury. Some solid organ injuries can be managed nonoperatively if a hollow viscus injury can be ruled out and the patient remains stable. CT scanning is noninvasive and specific for injury, but it has not been found to be sensitive in detecting diaphragm injuries.

Diagnostic laparoscopy is also an option in assessing patients with penetrating abdominal trauma. It is extremely useful in evaluating peritoneal penetration, solid organ injury, and diaphragm injury.

Laparoscopy has **not** been shown to be sensitive in detecting hollow viscus injury. **If there is any possibility of a hollow viscus injury based on the presence of peritoneal penetration and the trajectory of the stab wound tract, celiotomy should be performed.** Laparoscopy is unique in that it is accurate in the detection of diaphragm injuries and injuries that can be repaired using laparoscopic techniques. Laparoscopy obviates the need for a full celiotomy in approximately 50% of stable patients with abdominal stab wounds. The disadvantages of laparoscopy are its lack of sensitivity in detecting hollow viscus injuries and the requirement for an operative procedure.

Comprehension Questions

[15.1] A 25-year-old male sustains a stab wound to the abdomen just superior to the umbilicus. His skin is cool, and he is diaphoretic. His blood pressure is 74/40, and his pulse is 130/min. His abdomen is distended and diffusely tender. Which of the following management possibilities is most appropriate?

A. Abdominal CT scan
B. Laparoscopy
C. Celiotomy
D. Local wound exploration

[15.2] A 47-year-old male sustains a stab wound to the left upper quadrant of his abdomen. He complains of minimal pain. He is alert and hemodynamically normal, and the results from his abdominal examination show no abnormalities. Which of the following statements is true?

A. Abdominal CT is sensitive in the detection of diaphragm injuries.
B. The FAST examination reliably rules out intra-abdominal injury.
C. Local wound exploration revealing fascial penetration is an absolute indication for celiotomy.
D. The patient should be admitted for a 24- to 48-hour observation period.

[15.3] A 37-year-old female sustains a stab wound located at the anterior axillary line, 3 cm superior to the costal margin. The patient is alert and has normal mentation. Her blood pressure is 104/60, and her pulse is 110/min. What is the most appropriate next step?

    A. Listen to the patient's breath sounds.
    B. Obtain a chest radiograph.
    C. Perform a FAST examination.
    D. Examine her abdomen.

[15.4] A 56-year-old male has been stabbed in the right lower quadrant of his abdomen. He complains of pain at the wound site. His vital signs are normal, and the findings from his abdominal examination are normal. Local wound exploration reveals penetration of the anterior fascia, and DPL reveals 7000 RBCs/mm^3 and 750 WBCs/mm^3. What is the most appropriate next step?

    A. Repeat the DPL in 4 hours.
    B. Obtain an abdominal CT scan.
    C. Perform a laparoscopy.
    D. Perform a celiotomy.

Answers

[15.1] **C.** The patient has a life-threatening intra-abdominal hemorrhage, and after the ABC's and volume resuscitation, he needs immediate celiotomy.

[15.2] **D.** Asymptomatic stab wounds can be observed for the development of abdominal symptoms or hemodynamic instability. The sensitivity of the FAST examination is only 50%.

[15.3] **A.** The primary survey (ABC's) should be performed first.

[15.4] **D.** The DPL results are positive by WBC criteria, and hollow viscus injury is suspected. Celiotomy is the best method of excluding this type of injury

CLINICAL PEARLS

❖ The sensitivity of the FAST examination in detecting pericardial blood has been shown to be as high as 100%, but its sensitivity in detecting abdominal injury approximates 50%.

❖ An abdominal examination revealing prominent findings such as rigidity, guarding, or significant tenderness distant from the stab wounds is an indication for celiotomy.

❖ Selected patients who have sustained penetrating abdominal injury may be observed for a minimum of 24 to 48 hours.

❖ If the anterior abdominal fascia is penetrated by a wound, further evaluation is needed.

❖ Positive DPL results in blunt trauma patients include gross aspiration of 10 ml of blood, aspiration of fecal contents, or the presence of greater than 100,000 RBCs/mm^3 or 500 WBCs/mm^3 in the lavage fluid.

REFERENCES

Advanced trauma life support for doctors: instructor course manual, 6th ed. American College of Surgeons Committee on Trauma Staff. Chicago, IL, 1997:21–47.

Fabian TC, Croce MA. Abdominal trauma, including indications for celiotomy. In: Mattox KL, Feliciano DV, Moore EE, eds. Trauma, 4th ed. New York: McGraw-Hill, 2000:583–602.

A 37-year-old man is brought to the emergency center (EC) after being involved in a high-speed motor vehicle collision. The patient's vehicle crashed into a tree when he fell asleep at the wheel. The patient was restrained, his vehicle sustained severe front-end damage, and the air bags deployed in the vehicle. He was brought to the EC by paramedics. At the EC, his vital signs were blood pressure 110/80, pulse 110/min, respiration rate 28/min, Glasgow Coma Score (GCS) 14. The primary survey revealed a patent airway, diminished breath sounds on the left with exquisite chest wall tenderness, and subcutaneous emphysema. The heart sounds are normal and there is no jugular venous distension. The secondary survey revealed no abdominal tenderness, a stable pelvis, and no extremity abnormalities. A chest radiograph reveals several rib fractures on the left, a large pulmonary contusion, a left pneumothorax, and widening of the mediastinal structures.

◆ **What are the most likely diagnoses?**

◆ **How would you confirm the diagnosis?**

ANSWERS TO CASE 16: Chest Trauma (Blunt)

Summary: A 37-year-old man presents with multiple blunt chest injuries following a high-speed motor vehicle collision. In addition to injuries that have already been demonstrated by chest radiography, a major concern at this point is the possibility of thoracic aortic disruption.

◆ **Most likely diagnoses:** Blunt chest trauma with pulmonary contusion, pneumothorax, rib fractures, and possible thoracic aortic disruption.

◆ **Confirmation of diagnosis:** All of the diagnoses except for the aortic injury have been confirmed by chest radiography. The aortic injury can be diagnosed by angiography, computed tomography (CT) angiography, or transesophageal echocardiography.

Analysis

Objectives

1. Know the priorities in the treatment of patients with multiple blunt trauma.
2. Become familiar with the diagnosis and treatment of pneumothorax, pulmonary contusion, and thoracic aortic injury following blunt trauma.

Considerations

The initial assessment of the patient should begin with the airway, breathing, and circulation (ABC's), followed by the secondary survey. Simultaneously, intravenous lines should be placed, blood collected, and vital signs monitored. With the presence of diminished breath sounds, chest wall tenderness, and left-sided soft tissue crepitance, it would have been appropriate to place a left chest tube even without radiographic confirmation of left pneumothorax. Reassessment of the patient's respiratory status should be made and repeated chest radiographs

Table 16–1

CAUSES OF INSTABILITY AFTER BLUNT CHEST TRAUMA

INJURY	TREATMENT
Tension Pneumothorax	Tube thoracostomy Needle decompression
Hemothorax	Tube thoracostomy resuscitation Possible exploration, repair
Cardiac tamponade	Decompression (open, needle) Exploration repair
Cardiac contusion	Supportive care (inotropes, IABP?)
Air emboli	Exploration, repair
Injury to great vessels	Exploration, repair

IABP = intraaortic balloon pump

obtained immediately following chest tube placement. If the patient's respiratory status worsens or fails to improve dramatically, intubation should be considered to help improve cardiopulmonary stability while efforts are made to identify other potential life-threatening injuries. Once all the injuries have been identified (Table 16–1), they can be addressed according to their urgency.

APPROACH TO BLUNT CHEST TRAUMA

In the evaluation and treatment of patients with blunt chest trauma, it is critical to assess the magnitude of energy transfer that the accident has delivered to the injured victim. For instance, patients involved in a frontal impact collision with the deployment of air bags should be presumed to have absorbed a tremendous amount of kinetic energy to the chest wall and underlying structures. After the ABC's have been assessed, a secondary survey accomplished, and intravenous lines and blood studies performed, the patient should be examined for any change in clinical status (ie, mental status, vital signs, respiratory status). Often subtle changes forbode a looming catastrophe and require prompt reevaluation. As the assessment continues and injuries are identified, prioritizing attention depends on the severity and type of injury. A simple question to ask is "What will kill the patient **first?**" and address these issues first (Table 16–2).

The identification of **rib fractures,** especially fractures of the upper ribs (first and second), may indicate the presence of more severe associated injuries such as vascular injuries. The treatment of rib fractures is focused on management of the associated pain and the chest wall splinting that may lead to hypoventilation, atelectasis, and pneumonia. Therefore, adequate pain control may require the use of an epidural anesthetic.

Pneumothorax as identified by the chest radiograph results from disruption of the pleural surface. In general, simple traumatic pneumothorax may have been caused by a fractured rib penetrating the pleura or by direct injury to the pulmonary parenchyma. Proper insertion of a chest tube (tube thoracostomy) into the pleural space generally

Table 16–2

ASSESSMENT OF CASE #16'S INJURIES, DIAGNOSIS,
AND TREATMENT

INJURY	DIAGNOSIS	TREATMENT	COMMENT
Rib Fractures	PE, Chest x-ray, rib series	Conservative, pain management	Possible harbinger for other injuries, goal → pain control (epidural anesthesia) to prevent hypoventilation and associated pulmonary complications
Pneumothorax	PE, Chest x-ray	Tube thoracostomy	Should achieve full re-expansion Failure to re-expand or persistent air-leak → consider major tracheo-bronchial injury
Pulmonary contusion	Chest x-ray CT scan	Supportive care, Intubation	Ventilatory support on clinical grounds
Traumatic aortic rupture	Aortogram CT angiography TEE	Urgent repair	See Figure 16-2

PE = physical examination

results in reexpansion of the lung parenchyma. **If the lung fails to reexpand after chest tube placement and significant air leakage is noted, one should consider a major tracheobronchial injury.**

Pulmonary contusion results from hemorrhage into the alveolar and interstitial spaces. The clinical condition is determined by the severity of the injury and the extent of lung parenchyma involved. Severe pulmonary contusions may result in significant shunting and hypoxia. In general, supportive measures should be undertaken and the decision for ventilatory support made on clinical grounds. Because of capillary leakage, fluid restriction is usually advised but does not take precedence over adequate fluid resuscitation and oxygen delivery.

In the case of blunt chest trauma, **a widened mediastinum as revealed by a screening chest radiograph should raise a suspicion of traumatic rupture of the aorta (TRA)** (Figure 16–1). Although TRA is classically considered in the case of frontal impact (acceleration-deceleration) injuries, 25% of TRAs occur as a result of side impact

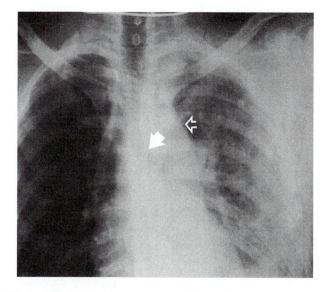

Figure 16–1. Traumatic rupture of the aorta. A widened mediastinum (open arrow) on the chest radiograph of a patient who had blunt trauma to the descending aorta. The left mainstem bronchus is depressed (solid arrow). (Reproduced, with permission, from Mattox KL, Feliciano DV, Moor EE. Trauma, 4th ed. New York: McGraw-Hill, 2000:562.)

collisions. The outcome with TRA is determined by whether the rupture is contained by the mediastinal pleura. Most patients with a free rupture into the pleural space die at the scene of the accident and never arrive at a hospital to receive medical attention. Thus, those who arrive

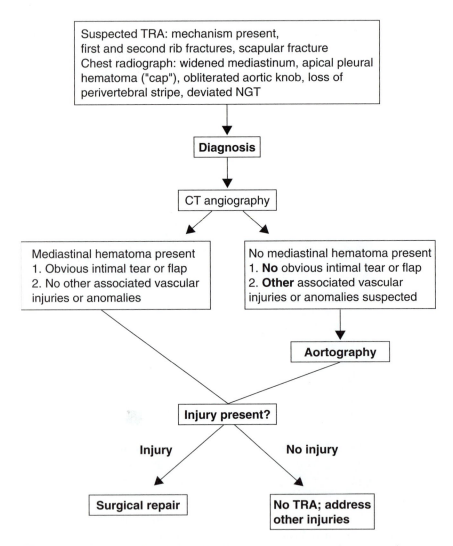

Figure 16–2.   An algorithm for the management of traumatic rupture of the aorta (TRA). NGT, nasogastric tube; CT, computed tomography.

for medical attention may need immediate diagnosis and treatment in order to prevent impending rupture. Debate exists as to the best tool for diagnosis. Although **the gold standard for the diagnosis of TRA remains an aortogram,** limitations in access (ie, a separate team is usually required to perform the test) and the invasiveness of the procedure have led to **CT angiography becoming more widely accepted for confirming the diagnosis of TRA.** Transesophageal echocardiography, not mentioned in the algorithm (see Figure 16–2), can be used for diagnosis but remains operator-dependent and is relatively invasive.

Comprehension Questions

[16.1] A 16-year-old man is brought into the ICU for multiple blunt trauma approximately 12 hours previously. His injuries included a femur fracture. He is noted to have a Po_2 of 60 mmHg despite the use of 100% oxygen by rebreather mask, and has become confused. The chest radiograph reveals clear lung fields and a normal cardiac size. Which of the following is the most likely diagnosis?

A. Pulmonary contusion
B. Fat embolism
C. Atelectasis
D. ICU psychosis

[16.2] A 43-year-old male is involved in a motorcycle accident in which his cycle slipped on wet pavement. He is brought into the hospital and noted to have multiple rib fractures, a tibial fracture, and significant contusions. The cardiac monitor reveals multiple premature atrial contractions. Which of the following is the most likely etiology for the cardiac arrhythmias?

A. Anxiety
B. Lower extremity fractures
C. Rib fractures
D. Blunt cardiac injury

[16.3] A radiologist evaluates a chest radiograph of a 19-year-old woman who was upended while riding her bicycle by a pickup truck. Which of the following findings is most likely to suggest a diagnosis of ruptured thoracic aorta?

A. A loss of aortic knob contour
B. Pneumomediastinum
C. Fracture of the sternum
D. Markedly enlarged cardiac silhouette

[16.4] Which of the following remains the gold standard in diagnosing TRA?

A. CT angiography
B. Magnetic resonance imaging
C. Chest radiograph
D. Aortogram

Answers

[16.1] **B.** Fat embolism syndrome is an exceedingly uncommon problem that may occur with major long bone fracture, and it can cause hypoxemia and CNS effects such as confusion or coma. Other findings include petechiae and retinal lesions.

[16.2] **D.** Blunt cardiac injuries may result in tachyarrhythmias or cardiac (pump) failure. Rib fractures are associated with pain, atelectesis, and pneumonia, but rarely with atrial arrhythmias.

[16.3] **A.** Chest radiographic findings consistent with thoracic aortic rupture include apical cap, deviated NG tube, obliteration of the aortic knob, and hemomediastinum (not pneumomediastinum).

[16.4] **D.** Aortography is considered the gold standard for diagnosis of TRA, although at many centers CT angiography is used.

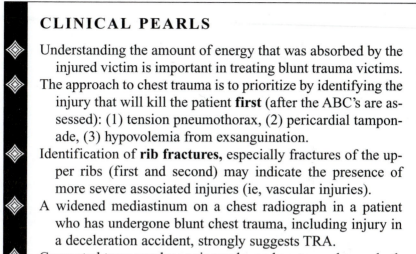

CLINICAL PEARLS

- Understanding the amount of energy that was absorbed by the injured victim is important in treating blunt trauma victims.
- The approach to chest trauma is to prioritize by identifying the injury that will kill the patient **first** (after the ABC's are assessed): (1) tension pneumothorax, (2) pericardial tamponade, (3) hypovolemia from exsanguination.
- Identification of **rib fractures,** especially fractures of the upper ribs (first and second) may indicate the presence of more severe associated injuries (ie, vascular injuries).
- A widened mediastinum on a chest radiograph in a patient who has undergone blunt chest trauma, including injury in a deceleration accident, strongly suggests TRA.
- Computed tomography angiography and aortography are both effective tests to confirm TRA.

REFERENCES

Estrera AL, Mattox KL, Wall MJ, Jr. Thoracic aortic injury. Semin Vasc Surg 2000;13:345–352.

Mattox KL, Wall MJ, LeMaire SA. Injury to the thoracic great vessels. In: Mattox KL, Feliciano DV, Moore EE, eds. Trauma, 4th ed. New York: McGraw-Hill, 2000:559–582.

A 20-year-old woman with abdominal pain is evaluated in the emergency department. She describes the gradual onset of pain 24 hours previously, and the pain has been persistent in its location in the lower abdomen. Shortly after the onset of pain, the patient developed nausea. She denies any diarrhea, dysuria, or previous abdominal symptoms. She had her last normal menstrual period 7 days ago, and she denies any abnormal patterns in her menses. The patient is sexually active with one partner. Her past medical and surgical history is unremarkable. She takes oral contraceptives and consumes alcohol socially. On physical examination, her temperature is 100.8°F (38.2°C) and her blood pressure, pulse, and respiration rate are normal. The cardiopulmonary examination is unremarkable. Her abdomen is soft, with tenderness to palpation in the right lower quadrant and suprapubic region. No peritoneal irritation or masses are detected. Her bowel sounds are hypoactive. The rectal examination reveals tenderness on the right side. Pelvic examination reveals no purulent discharge, however, there is tenderness in the right adnexa region. Laboratory studies reveal a white blood cell (WBC) count of 14,600/mm^3, normal hemoglobin and hematocrit values, and normal electrolyte and amylase levels. Urinalysis reveals concentrated urine with 3 to 5 red blood cells (RBCs per hpf), 5 to 10 WBCs per hpf, and negative results for leukocyte esterase. The results from a serum pregnancy test are negative.

◆ **What should be your next step?**

ANSWERS TO CASE 17: Abdominal Pain
(Right Lower Quadrant)

Summary: A 20 year-old woman has a 24-hour history of abdominal pain that is **atypical** for acute appendicitis. She has a low-grade fever and lower abdominal tenderness, with maximal tenderness in the right lower quadrant. Her laboratory tests are significant for leukocytosis, microscopic hematuria, and pyuria.

◆ **Next step:** Obtain a computed tomography (CT) scan of the abdomen and pelvis.

Analysis

Objectives

1.   Learn the pathophysiology of acute appendicitis.
2.   Learn the diagnostic approaches for patients with suspected acute appendicitis.

Considerations

The diagnosis of acute appendicitis is frequently made on the basis of clinical history, physical findings, and laboratory data. However, **when a patient presents with an atypical history and atypical physical and/or laboratory findings, it is important to determine whether the atypical presentation is due to another disease process or to atypical positioning of the diseased appendix.** Further diagnostic options (see Table 17–1) for an "atypical" patient include imaging studies (a CT scan, ultrasonography), clinical observation with serial laboratory evaluations, and diagnostic laparoscopy. The CT scan is selected in this case because it is sensitive for identifying inflammatory changes and thickening of the appendix. In a patient with fever, lower abdominal tenderness, and leukocytosis, these radiographic changes should be present if the findings are indeed caused by appendicitis. A factor that favors the use of a CT scan over ultrasonography in this case is that the

Table 17–1

DIAGNOSTIC OPTIONS FOR ACUTE APPENDICITIS*

	ADVANTAGES	DISADVANTAGES	RECOMMENDED USE
CT imaging	Identifies appendicitis changes or other pathology (~95% accuracy)	Limited sensitivity for early appendicitis and pelvic pathology	Inflammatory process not related to pelvic pathology
Ultrasonography	Greater sensitivity and specificity for gynecologic pathology than CT	Limited by body habitus, appendicitis signs less well defined	Suspected gynecologic pathology; young children
Clinical observation with serial laboratory studies	Allows the natural history of disease evolution	Limited application if localized pain, fever, and leukocytosis are already present	Possible early appendicitis and without localized signs
Diagnostic laparoscopy	Allows accurate assessment of pathology	Invasive; some morbidities	Inflammatory or pathology of uncertain source

*CT, computed tomography.

patient's history and examination results are not suggestive of pelvic pathology, which is more effectively evaluated by ultrasonography. For this patient, clinical observation with serial laboratory evaluation is not a good option because she already has localized abdominal pain, fever, and leukocytosis, and therefore continued observation for regression of these symptoms would lead to a delay in diagnosis. Diagnostic laparoscopy is an operative procedure with associated morbidity and is mainly indicated for patients with nonspecific clinical or radiographic evidence of inflammation or pathology that cannot be further delineated by additional imaging studies.

APPROACH TO SUSPECTED ACUTE APPENDICITIS

Definitions

Chronic or recurrent appendicitis: Occurs in 5% of patients with appendicitis and may result from antibiotic administration in patients with early acute appendicitis.

Interval appendectomy: Generally, this procedure is for the treatment of appendicitis complicated by abscess or phlegmon. The patient is treated initially with broad-spectrum antibiotic therapy and CT-guided drainage of the abscess to resolve the infectious process, followed by appendectomy after several weeks.

Mesenteric adenitis: An inflammatory condition occurring with a viral illness, resulting in painful lymphadenopathy in the small bowel mesentery. This process can be associated with right lower quadrant pain and tenderness and is especially common in children.

Clinical Approach

Pathogenesis and Clinical Presentation of Appendicitis   The appendix arises from the cecal diverticulum during embryonic development. During this process, it rotates from its posterior location toward the iliac fossa. Incomplete rotation occurs frequently, leading to variable appendiceal positioning and variations in clinical presentation. The development of appendicitis generally begins with luminal obstruction by a fecalith, lymphoid hyperplasia, or food matter. With this obstruction there is an increase in mucous secretion, venous and lymphatic congestion, and bacterial overgrowth (see Table 17–2). When unabated, this process leads to ischemic necrosis and perforation. **The classic history of acute appendicitis begins with vague pain in the periumbilical region, nausea, vomiting, and the urge to defecate;** these symptoms **are followed by localization of the pain in the right lower quadrant** associated **with localized peritonitis.** Approximately 20% of patients with acute appendicitis experience perforation within 24 hours of the onset of symptoms. Recognition of appendicitis can be delayed because of atypical presentations caused by retrocolic or pelvic locations. Similarly, antibiotic administration during the early course of appendicitis may alter the clinical course. **Only about 50% of patients with acute appendicitis show a classic presentation.**

Diagnosis   Patients with the classic presentation generally require only a thorough history and physical examination, a CBC with a differential count, urinalysis, and a pregnancy test (females only) for diagnosis. When patients with an atypical history, physical examination, or laboratory findings are encountered, selective application of diagnostic imaging is indicated to avoid delays in therapy and minimize the occurrence of nontherapeutic operations.

Table 17–2
CLINICAL-PATHOLOGIC CORRELATION

PATHOLOGIC CONDITION	CLINICAL SIGNS AND SYMPTOMS
Luminal obstruction	Poorly localized periumbilical pain, nausea, vomiting, and urge to defecate.
Inflammation	Location of pain depending on the position of the appendix; peritonitis is present only if the inflamed appendix or inflammatory changes involve the peritoneum.
Perforation	Transient improvement in pain but an increase in systemic toxicity.

Comprehension Questions

[17.1] Which of the following is the most appropriate management for a 19-year-old woman with a 2-day history of right lower quadrant pain and no fever? She has a tender right adnexal mass, a normal WBC count, negative findings from a pregnancy test, and normal urinalysis results.

A. CT of the abdomen and pelvis
B. Abdominal and pelvic ultrasonography
C. Diagnostic laparoscopy
D. Observation with serial laboratory studies

[17.2] A 24-year-old male complains of colicky intermittent umbilical and right lower quadrant abdominal pain of 24 hours duration. He complains of anorexia and nausea. His temperature is 98 F. Which of the following is the most likely diagnosis?

A. Acute appendicitis
B. Chronic appendicitis
C. Gastroenteritis
D. Acute pancreatitis

[17.3] An 18-year-old woman has a 1-day history of worsening lower abdominal pain, nausea and vomiting, and low-grade fever. Her temperature is 99°F, and she has mild lower abdominal tenderness and no rebound. She has possible right adnexal tenderness. Which of the following tests would most definitively differentiate pelvic inflammatory disease from acute appendicitis?

A. CT scan of the abdomen and pelvis
B. Magnetic resonance imaging of the abdomen and pelvis
C. Ultrasound examination of the pelvis
D. Laparoscopy

Answers

[17.1] **B.** For this patient with findings suggestive of pelvic pathology (an adnexal mass), ultrasonography is an accurate modality in defining the pathology.

[17.2] **C.** Intermittent pain is not typical for appendicitis. Acute pancreatitis typically presents as constant boring pain radiating to the back.

[17.3] **D.** Laparoscopy is the most accurate test to assess for acute pelvic inflammatory disease (an erythematous tube with purulent drainage from the fimbria) and to visualize the appendix.

CLINICAL PEARLS

◈ The options in assessing atypical presentations for appendicitis include imaging tests, clinical observation with a serial laboratory evaluation, and diagnostic laparoscopy.

◈ The classic history of acute appendicitis begins with vague pain in the periumbilical region, nausea, vomiting, and the urge to defecate; these symptoms are followed by localization of the pain in the right lower quadrant associated with localized peritonitis.

◈ Only about 50% of patients with acute appendicitis have the classic presentation.

◈ Ultrasonography is generally the best modality to assess pelvic pathology, whereas a CT scan is the best way to assess nongynecologic abdominal processes.

REFERENCES

Lally KP, Cox CS Jr, Andrassy RJ. Appendix. In: Townsend CM, Beauchamp RD, Evers BM, Mattox KL. Textbook of surgery: the biological basis of modern surgical practice. Philadelphia: Saunders, 2001:917–928.

Soybel DI. Appendix. In: Norton JA, Bollinger RR, Chang AE, Lowry SF, Mulvihill SJ, Pass HI, Thompson RW, eds. Surgery: basic science and clinical evidence. New York: Springer, 2001:647–666.

CASE 18

A 58-year-old woman complains of the sudden onset of right chest pain and shortness of breath 6 days following an uncomplicated left hemi-colectomy for adenocarcinoma of the descending colon. The patient has had an uncomplicated postoperative course until this time. During your evaluation, she appears anxious and is unable to remain comfortable. Her temperature is 37.9°C (100.2°F), pulse rate 105/min, blood pressure 138/80, and respiratory rate 32/min. She is receiving O_2 by nasal canula with an O_2 saturation of 96% by pulse oximetry. Despite this oxygen saturation, the patient continues to complain of difficulty breathing. There is no jugular venous distension. Her lungs are clear, with diminished breath sounds in both bases. Her cardiac examination reveals sinus tachycardia. Her abdomen is slightly tender and without distension, and the surgical incision is normal in appearance. Her legs reveal mild edema bilaterally and tenderness in the left calf. Laboratory evaluations reveal a white blood cell (WBC) count of 11,000/mm^3 with a normal differential, normal hemoglobin and hematocrit values, and a normal platelet count. The electrolyte levels are likewise normal. An arterial blood gas study reveals pH 7.45, P_{O_2} 73 mm Hg, P_{CO_2} 34 mmHg, and H_{CO_3} 24 mEq/L. A 12-lead electrocardiogram (ECG) reveals sinus tachycardia. The creatine kinase and troponin levels are within normal limits. A portable chest radiograph (CXR) demonstrates no infiltrates or effusions and minimal atelectasis in both lower lung fields.

◆ **What is the most likely diagnosis?**

◆ **What should be your next step?**

ANSWERS TO CASE 18: Venous Thromboembolic Disease

Summary: A 58-year-old woman has acute chest pain and dyspnea postoperatively. The results from cardiopulmonary and abdominal examinations are nonspecific. She has a minimally elevated leukocyte count and normal cardiac enzyme levels. Arterial blood gas studies indicate respiratory alkalosis and hypoxemia. The CXR and ECG show no obvious pathology.

◆ **Most likely diagnosis:** Pulmonary embolism (PE) is very likely with the sudden onset of chest pain and shortness of breath in a patient without pulmonary or cardiac pathology.

◆ **Next step:** Empiric systemic anticoagulation with confirmatory imaging pending.

Analysis

Objectives

1. Know the risk factors and causes of venous thromboembolic disease.
2. Know the applications and effectiveness of prophylactic measures for deep vein thrombosis (DVT).
3. Learn the diagnostic and therapeutic approaches for patients with suspected venous thromboembolism.

Considerations

The differential diagnosis for a 58-year-old woman with the sudden onset of chest pain and shortness of breath during the postoperative period includes cardiac ischemia, respiratory tract infection, acute lung injury, and PE. In this case, PE should be strongly considered based on the history of acute dyspnea and chest pain with a normal

WBC count, normal ECG and CXR results, and normal cardiac enzyme levels. As for most patients, making a definitive diagnosis of PE based on clinical criteria is difficult. However, this evaluation is vital in determining the level of clinical suspicion, which influences the diagnostic precision of subsequent imaging studies. In this case, the clinical picture indicates a high clinical probability of PE. The decision to **initiate systemic anticoagulation without a confirmed diagnosis of PE is justifiable based on a high clinical suspicion and the absence of contraindications to anticoagulation**. As one decides whether to initiate empirical treatment, it is important to bear in mind that **patients treated with early aggressive anticoagulation therapy are less likely to experience treatment failure or develop recurrences.**

APPROACH TO DEEP VENOUS THROMBOSIS AND PULMONARY EMBOLISM

Definitions

Venous duplex imaging: An accurate, noninvasive imaging modality combining ultrasonography and Doppler technology to assess the patency of veins and the presence of blood clot in veins; it is especially useful for the lower extremities.

Perfusion and ventilation (V/Q) scan: A radioisotope scan used to identify V/Q mismatches, which can indicate PE and other pulmonary conditions. Results must be interpreted based on coexisting pulmonary pathology and the clinical picture.

Computed tomography (CT) pulmonary angiography: A vascular contrast study involving CT imaging with a sensitivity for PE detection ranging widely from 64% to 93%; it is highly sensitive for PE involving the central pulmonary arteries but insensitive for subsegmental clots. Some advocate that it not be used as the initial imaging study and that it is perhaps best used with venous duplex or pelvic CT venography for better accuracy.

Pulmonary angiography: Considered the gold standard for the diagnosis of PE. It is accurate (approximately 96%) and carries

Table 18–1

APPROXIMATE DEEP VENOUS THROMBOSIS
PREVALENCE WITH AND WITHOUT PROPHYLAXIS

TREATMENT	GENERAL SURGERY (%)	TOTAL HIP REPLACEMENT (%)	TRAUMA (%)
No therapy	25	51	50–58
Low-dose heparin	8	31	44
Low-molecular-weight heparin	7	15	30; proximal deep vein thrombosis reduced to 6
Elastic stockings	9 (data include only low-risk patients)	22	No evidence available
Intermittent pneumatic compression device	10 (only low- to moderate-risk patients)	38	No evidence available

a false-negative rate of 0.6%, and especially has greater sensitivity than CT for subsegmental and chronic PE. The significant drawbacks are a major procedural complication rate of 1.3% and a mortality rate of 0.5%.

Thrombolytic therapy: Thrombolysis for PE has survival advantages in patients with massive PE, especially when it is associated with right heart dysfunction. Tissue plasminogen activator (TPA) is the most commonly used agent and may be given systemically or by catheter-directed infusion into the clot. Recent major surgery (such as within a 10-day period) and recent severe closed head injury are contraindications to therapy.

Pulmonary embolectomy: Surgical retrieval of clots in the pulmonary artery through a median sternotomy, requiring cardiopulmonary bypass. Major indication: massive PE with hemodynamic instability and hypoxia, where thrombolytic therapy is contraindicated. It is associated with 30% to 60% mortality.

Prophylaxis

The development of acute thromboembolic complications is presumed to be due to stasis, hypercoagulability, and vein wall injury that occur as the result of local and systemic effects of trauma and operative injuries, aging, and preexisting medical conditions. The incidence of deep vein thrombosis (DVT) in general surgery patients is estimated at about 25%, with most being asymptomatic. Major orthopedic surgery and major trauma are found to be associated with a significantly greater risk of this complication. Most patients with DVT have involvement of the tibial-level veins and may remain asymptomatic; however, involvement of the femoral and/or iliac veins dramatically increases the risk of PE and symptoms, such that about 30% to 50% of these patients may develop PE. All patients with identifiable risk factors should undergo prophylaxis against DVT/PE, which is effective in reducing the complication rate. In high-risk patients, prophylaxis is effective in reducing the occurrence of DVT/PE (Table 18–1).

Diagnosis

A suggested diagnostic approach is shown in Figure 18–1.

Treatment

In general, all patients with documented DVT and PE should undergo treatment with systemic anticoagulation therapy with heparin infusion, oral coumadin, or subcutaneous low-molecular-weight heparin. The duration of therapy for uncomplicated DVT is generally 3 months. Patients with PE and no identifiable hypercoagulability state should be treated for 6 months, and patients with documented hypercoagulability should be considered for life-long therapy (Table 18–2).

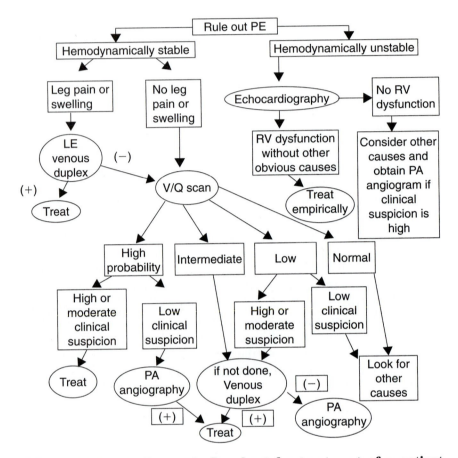

Figure 18–1. A diagnostic flowchart for treatment of a patient with suspected pulmonary embolism. (Adapted with modification from Shepard AD, Shin LH. Pulmonary thromboembolism. In: Cameron JL, ed. Current surgical therapy, 7th ed. St. Louis: Mosby-Year Book; 2001:1016.)

Table 18–2

DEEP VEIN THROMBOSIS TREATMENT AND EFFICACY

Unfractionated heparin	6% recurrence; 3% major bleeding; 1%–3% risk of heparin-induced thrombocytopenia
Low-molecular-weight heparin	3% recurrence; 1% major bleeding; associated with a lower risk of heparin-induced thrombocytopenia
Thrombolysis therapy	Indicated for iliofemoral deep vein thrombosis; contraindicated in recently postoperative patients or after recent head trauma

Comprehension Questions

[18.1] A 45-year-old diabetic male complains of pain and swelling in the right calf and thigh of 2 days' duration. Which of the following is the next appropriate step in the treatment of this patient?

   A. Begin systemic thrombolytic therapy.
   B. Perform a lower extremity venous duplex scan.
   C. Perform CT pulmonary angiography.
   D. Determine the D-dimer level. Perform pulmonary angiography if this level is elevated.

[18.2] Which of the following patients with confirmed femoral venous thromboses should not receive fractionated heparin therapy?

   A. A hemodynamically stable 80-year-old man with a documented PE
   B. A 20-year-old man who sustained a closed head injury 14 days ago
   C. A 23-year-old woman in her third trimester of pregnancy
   D. A 44-year-old woman with heparin-induced thrombocytopenia

[18.3] A 35-year-old male complains of dyspnea and left leg pain. He undergoes a V/Q scan, which is interpreted as being of low probability for PE. Which of the following is the most accurate statement?

A. The probability of PE is less than 1%.
B. The probability of PE is as high as 40%.
C. The next test should be a determination of the serum D-dimer level.
D. Pulmonary angiography should be performed to definitively rule out PE.

Answers

[18.1] **B.** Obtain a venous duplex scan of the legs. Systemic thrombolytic therapy is indicated only if patients have proven proximal DVT. D-dimer levels are elevated in 99.5% of all patients with DVT/PE, but this is also seen following trauma and surgery, and so the test is highly sensitive but nonspecific.

[18.2] **D.** Heparin-induced thrombocytopenia, which is usually an immunoglobin G–mediated reaction, is a contraindication to heparin therapy. Heparin does not cross the placenta and is not contraindicated during pregnancy. Generally, at 14 days following a closed head injury, there is no contraindication to anticoagulation.

[18.3] **B.** The probability of PE can be as high as 40% in a patient with a low-probability V/Q scan. The probability of PE in a patient with a low-probability V/Q scan and low clinical suspicion is about 4%. If the patient's V/Q scan indicates a low probability and the clinical suspicion is intermediate or uncertain, the risk for PE is approximately 16%. A venous duplex scan is indicated for further evaluation of intermediate- and high-risk patients.

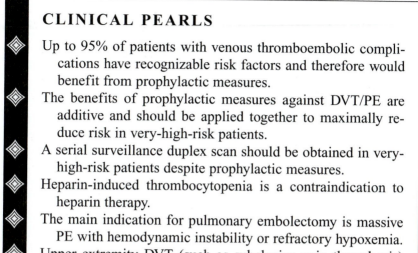

CLINICAL PEARLS

- Up to 95% of patients with venous thromboembolic complications have recognizable risk factors and therefore would benefit from prophylactic measures.
- The benefits of prophylactic measures against DVT/PE are additive and should be applied together to maximally reduce risk in very-high-risk patients.
- A serial surveillance duplex scan should be obtained in very-high-risk patients despite prophylactic measures.
- Heparin-induced thrombocytopenia is a contraindication to heparin therapy.
- The main indication for pulmonary embolectomy is massive PE with hemodynamic instability or refractory hypoxemia.
- Upper extremity DVT (such as subclavian vein thrombosis) carries a much higher PE risk than lower extremity DVT.

REFERENCES

Clagett GP, Anderson FA Jr, Geerts W, et al. Prevention of venous thromboembolism. Chest 1998;114:531S–560S.

Comerota AJ, Kagan SA. Venous disease. In: Townsend CM, Beauchamp RD, Evers BM, Mattox KL, eds. Textbook of surgery: the biologic basis of modern surgical practice, 16th ed. Philadelphia: Saunders, 2001;1418–1445.

A 65-year-old man presents with dyspnea on exertion and angina. The patient's current symptoms have been present for approximately 3 to 4 weeks. He denies any cough, weight loss, and gastrointestinal (GI) tract symptoms. His past medical history is significant for hypertension, stable angina, and colonic polyps that were removed 7 to 8 years ago by colonoscopy. The physical examination reveals a well-nourished African-American man who is in no acute distress. The findings from head and neck, cardiopulmonary, and neurologic examinations are unremarkable. Examination of the abdomen reveals an obese abdomen without tenderness or palpable masses. The rectal examination reveals no masses, a smooth and enlarged prostate, and strongly hemoccult-positive stool in the vault. The complete blood count reveals a normal white blood cell (WBC) count, hemoglobin 8.7 g/dL, hematocrit 29%, and mean cell volume 72 fL (normal 76 to 100 fL). The electrolyte levels and liver function studies are within normal limits. A 12-lead electrocardiogram reveals normal sinus rhythm and mild left ventricular hypertrophy. A chest radiograph reveals a normal cardiac silhouette, no pulmonary infiltrate, no pleural effusion, and no pulmonary mass.

◆ **What is the most likely mechanism causing this process?**

◆ **How would you confirm the diagnosis?**

ANSWERS TO CASE 19: Colorectal Cancer and Polyps

Summary: A 65-year-old man presenting with dyspnea on exertion and worsening angina pectoris due to anemia produced by occult GI tract bleeding.

◆ **Most likely mechanism:** Anemia due to occult GI tract bleeding.

◆ **Confirmation of diagnosis:** Esophagogastroduodenoscopy (EGD) to evaluate the upper GI tract and colonoscopy to evaluate for a possible colorectal source of bleeding.

ANALYSIS

Objectives

1. Be familiar with the clinical presentation and management of colorectal cancer.
2. Be familiar with the risk factors for and surveillance of high-risk patients.

Considerations

This patient presents with angina, dyspnea on exertion, microcytic anemia, and guiaic-positive stool. His presentation is strongly indicative of occult GI tract blood loss. **The lower GI tract is the most likely source of bleeding in patients who are not consuming aspirin or other nonsteroidal anti-inflammatory drugs.** In this case, the initial treatment should consist of transfusion to improve the patient's anemia, followed by endoscopic evaluation of the upper and lower GI tract with EGD and colonoscopy. If the source of the blood loss is not identified after these diagnostic procedures, evaluation of the small bowel for a blood loss source by contrast radiography should be performed. Given his previous history of **colonic polyps requiring endoscopic removal,** this man is at **risk for the development of polyps as well as colorectal cancer.** Thus, he should have been placed on a regular surveillance schedule 8 years ago, with repeated colonoscopy after 3 years. If negative results were obtained, he should have been placed on surveillance colonoscopy subsequently at 5-year intervals.

APPROACH TO COLORECTAL CANCER AND POLYPS

Definitions

Abdominoperineal resection: Resection of the rectosigmoid area for a low-lying rectal carcinoma. The procedure leaves the patient with a permanent colostomy.

Bowel preparation for elective colon surgery: A mechanical preparation consisting of a large volume of polyethylene glycol solution such as GoLYTELY or a smaller volume of phospho-soda *and* a broad-spectrum intravenous and/or oral nonabsorbable antibiotic. The goal is to decrease the bacterial count in the event of spillage of colonic contents.

Clinical Approach

Colorectal cancer is the fourth most common internal malignancy and the second most common cause of cancer death in the United States. (Lung cancer is the most common.) The average American has an approximately 5.5% to 6% lifetime risk of developing colorectal cancer. This cancer is predominantly a disease of the middle-aged and elderly population, with only 5% of cancers occurring in patients younger than 40 years of age. Roughly **70% of colorectal cancers initially develop as adenomatous polyps,** and through a series of mutations in protooncogenes and tumor suppressor genes, a malignant transformation occurs leading to the development of carcinoma. Based on the polypcarcinoma sequence of cancer development, it is possible to prevent cancer development by identifying and removing polyps prior to the development of invasive cancer. Patient surveillance can be accomplished by two effective approaches. Complete colonoscopy is effective as a screening tool; alternatively, flexible sigmoidoscopy with an air contrast barium enema has been shown to possess similar efficacy.

Clinical Presentation   The most common clinical presentations associated with colorectal carcinoma are chronic bowel habit changes and anemia (77% to 92%), obstruction (6% to 16%), and perforation (2% to 7%). Chronic bowel habit changes may be a change in the caliber of stools or diarrhea, which is more commonly seen with left-sided tumors and rectosigmoid tumors. Tumors of the right side are less likely to cause obstructive symptoms until late in the course of the disease, and in these cases patients typically present with symptoms related to anemia.

Cancer Staging   The TMN system and the Astler–Coller modification of the Duke classification are the most common staging systems used for colorectal carcinoma (Tables 19–1 and 19–2).

Treatment   Patients with colonic polyps can be treated with endoscopic resection. Endoscopic therapy is considered definitive when the

Table 19–1
TNM STAGING SYSTEM

STAGE	DEPTH	NODAL STATUS	DISTANT METASTASIS
Stage 1	T1, T2	N0	M0
Stage 2	T3, T4	N0	M0
Stage 3	Any T	N1, N2, N3	M0
Stage 4	Any T	Any N	M1

TX: Primary tumor cannot be assessed
T0:   No evidence of primary tumor
Tis: Carcinoma in situ
T1:   Tumor invasion into submucosa
T2:   Tumor invasion into muscularis propria
T3:   Tumor invasion through muscularis propria
T4a: Tumor perforation of visceral peritoneum
T4b: Tumor invasion of adjacent structure
NX: Regional lymph nodes cannot be assessed
N1:   1–3 regional lymph nodes
N2:   ≥4 regional lymph nodes involved
N3:   Regional lymph nodes involved along a major vascular structure
M0:   No distant metastatsis
M1:   Any distant metastatsis

Table 19–2
ASTLER–COLLER MODIFICATION OF THE
DUKE CLASSIFICATION

	TUMOR	NODES	DISTANT METASTASIS
A	Tis, T1, T2, T3	N0	M0
B	T4	N0	M0
C1	T1, T2, T3	N1, N2, N3	M0
C2	T4	N1, N2, N3	M0
D	Any T	Any N	M1

resection of the polyp is complete. **Cancer risks increase with larger polyps,** with the risk of carcinoma being approximately **1.3% for adenomatous polyps smaller than 1 cm, 9.5% for polyps 1 to 2 cm, and 46% for polyps larger than 2 cm.** Polypectomy alone is considered curative if the tumor has not penetrated the submucosa, whereas **submucosal penetration increases the likelihood of regional lymph node metastasis.** A patient with a reasonable life expectancy should undergo a **metastatic workup** including **chest radiography and abdomen and pelvic computed tomography (CT) scans prior to colonic resection to remove the involved colon as well as the regional lymph nodes (Figure 19–1).** Patients with invasive adenocarcinoma of the rectum (classically described as the lowest 15 cm of the GI tract) are not only at risk for metastasis but also at risk for local tumor recurrence because of the close proximity of the rectum to the surrounding structures. Following recovery from colon resection, patients with lymph node involvement (stage 3 disease) have a reduced possibility of tumor recurrence and improved survival when they are given adjuvant chemotherapy as either 5-fluorouracil (FU)/levamisole or 5-FU/ leucovorin. **The 5-year survival of patients by stage is as follows: stage 1, 76%; stage 2, 65%; stage 3, 42%; and stage 4, 16%.**

Adenocarcinoma of the Rectum

Approximately **30% of all colorectal carcinoma are located in the rectum.** Evaluation of patients for rectal carcinoma should include chest radiography and a CT scan of the abdomen and pelvis. In addition, endoscopic ultrasonography should be performed to determine the

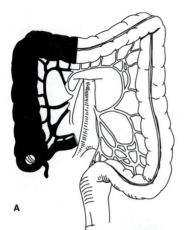

A

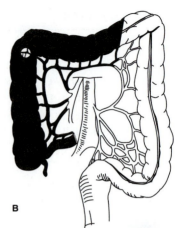

B

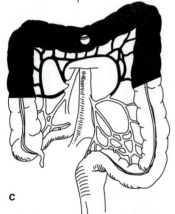

C

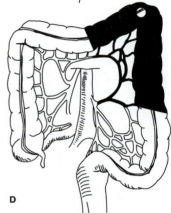

D

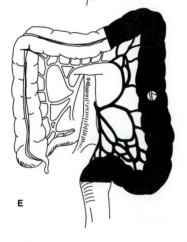

E

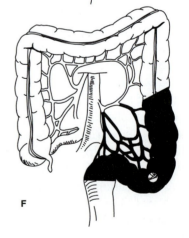

F

depth of tumor invasion and the status of the perirectal lymph nodes. The **surgical treatment** for most patients with **invasive rectal carcinoma** consists of **resection of the involved rectum with tumor-free margins.** For patients with **low-lying tumors in the rectum, abdominal perineal resection** is usually indicated. Patients with locally invasive rectal carcinoma experience a reduction in pelvic tumor recurrence when they complete a course of chemoradiation therapy prior to surgical resection (neoadjuvant therapy). **Neoadjuvant therapy appears to have additional benefits over postoperative chemoradiation therapy in rectal carcinoma in preventing local recurrence.** Patients with stage 3 rectal carcinoma who have not received neoadjuvant therapy may derive benefits from postoperative chemoradiation therapy.

Selected patients with localized rectal adenocarcinoma can be treated with localized transanal tumor excision. For maximal benefit, patients generally should have a tumor involving less than one-third of the rectal circumference, less than transmural involvement, a well to moderately differentiated histologic grade, and unaffected rectal lymph nodes.

Postoperative Follow-up

The incidence of **metachronous (subsequent) colorectal cancer is 1.1% to 4.7%.** It is not clear how often and by what means patients should be evaluated following the successful treatment of colorectal cancers. One such surveillance colonoscopy program advocates initial colonoscopy at 6 month intervals up to 1 year, followed by yearly colonoscopy for 2 years, and subsequently surveillance colonoscopy

---

Figure 19–1. Resection of colon cancer. (A) Right colectomy, (B) right hemicolectomy with division of middle colic pedicle, (C) transverse colectomy, (D) resection of splenic flexure sparing left colic artery, (E) left hemicolectomy, (F) sigmoid colectomy sparing left colic artery. (Reproduced, with permission, from Schwarz SI, Ellis H. Maingot's abdominal operations. New York: Appleton & Lange, 1989:1053, as modified in Niederhuber JE, ed. Fundamentals of surgery. NewYork: Appleton & Lange; 1998:322.)

every 3 years. In addition, patients should undergo a regular evaluation involving history and physical examinations and serial carcinoembryonic antigen measurements.

High-risk Patient Groups

Patients at high risk for colorectal cancer include those with familial adenomatous polyposis syndrome, familial cancer (first-degree relatives), familial nonpolyposis cancer syndrome, and a history of inflammatory bowel disease. Current recommendations include **colonoscopy with biopsies every 1 to 2 years for patients with a history of ulcerative colitis of more than 7 to 8 years' duration.** For patients with **familial nonpolyposis cancer syndrome, the initial colonoscopy** is recommended at **age 25,** followed by **yearly fecal occult blood testing and colonoscopy every 3 years (see Table 19–3).**

Table 19–3
RECOMMENDED SCREENING
AND SURVEILLANCE GUIDELINES*

Sporadic adenomatous polyposis
1. Complete colonoscopy and clearance of all polyps along with index polyp.
2. Repeat colonoscopy in 3 y (selectively—patients with tubular adenoma <1 cm may not require long-term follow-up).
3. If initial examination and clearance are suboptimal, initial follow-up colonoscopy should be at 1 y.

Familial adenomatous polyposis
1. Flexible sigmoidoscopy for all first-degree relatives of FAP, Gardner syndrome, and Turcot syndrome patients.
2. Screening colonoscopy should begin for known FAP patients at age 10–12 y and performed every 1–2 y until age 40, and then every 3 y thereafter.
3. Initial upper endoscopy at age 20 or at age of prophylactic colectomy.
   a. For mild duodenal disease, upper endoscopy every 2–3 y.
   b. For severe duodenal disease, upper endoscopy every 6 mo to 1 y.
4. Surveillance of all first-degree relative of FAP patient with abdominal CT for desmoid tumors.
5. Surveillance of first-degree relatives of Turcot syndrome patients with CT scan of the brain.

*FAP, familial adenomatous polyposis; CT, computed tomography.

Metastatic Disease

The presence of metastatic disease to the liver or lungs generally indicates the presence of disseminated disease. There are small subsets of patients who may develop isolated metastasis to these sites who can be appropriately treated by surgical resection.

Comprehension Questions

[19.1] Which of the following patients has the highest risk of developing colorectal cancer?

    A. A 45-year-old man whose younger brother has a history of colon cancer

    B. A 30-year-old woman with a BRCA-1 mutation

    C. A 55-year-old man with a 15-year history of ulcerative colitis

    D. A 50-year-old man with a history of resected adenomatous colonic polyps

    E. A 44-year-old male with familial adenomatous polyposis syndrome (polyposis coli)

[19.2] Which of the following is the most appropriate treatment for a 40-year-old man with a T3 N1 carcinoma of the cecum?

    A. Preoperative chemoradiation therapy followed by right hemicolectomy

    B. Right hemicolectomy and postoperative chemotherapy with 5-FU/levamisole

    C. Endoscopic removal of the tumor followed by chemoradiation therapy

    D. Right hemicolectomy and postoperative tamoxifen therapy

[19.3] Which of the following is the most appropriate follow-up for a 60-year-old man who underwent a colonoscopy and complete endoscopic removal of a 2-cm adenomatous polyp from the sigmoid colon?

A. Annual colonoscopy
B. Repeated colonoscopy at 3 years and, if the results are negative, repeated every 5 years
C. CT scan and repeated colonoscopy at 3 years and, if the results are negative, repeated every 5 years
D. Repeated colonoscopy every 2 years

Answers

[19.1] **E.** BRCA-1 does not confer an increased risk of colon cancer, whereas BRCA-2 does. The other conditions are associated with increased risks of developing colorectal cancer, but a patient with familial adenomatous polyposis syndrome (the colon is filled with thousands of polyps) has nearly a 100% risk of developing colon cancer.

[19.2] **B.** Right hemicolectomy with postoperative adjuvant chemotherapy using 5-FU/levamisole is indicated for this patient with stage 3 colon cancer. Radiation therapy is generally indicated for patients with rectal carcinoma. Tamoxifen therapy is not useful for colorectal carcinoma.

[19.3] **B.** The current recommendations for colonic polyp follow-up are as follows. Once the colon is cleared of polyps, repeated colonoscopy at 3 years and, if the results are negative, repeated colonoscopy every 5 years. A CT scan is not recommended for the follow-up of patients with polyps.

CLINICAL PEARLS

◈ Many of the symptoms associated with colorectal cancer are nonspecific, including postprandial bloating, distension, and constipation.

◈ Patients with familial adenomatous polyposis syndrome are at high risk for adenomas and adenocarcinomas of the duodenum in addition to colorectal cancers, and these patients require surveillance EGD.

◈ About 70% of colon cancers are thought to arise from adenomatous polyps. The larger the adenomatous polyp, the greater the risk of colon cancer.

◈ For rectal cancer, neoadjuvant chemotherapy seems to be helpful.

REFERENCES

Itkowitz SH, Kim YS. Colonic polyps and polyposis syndromes. In: Feldman M, Scharchmidt BF, Sleisenger MH, eds. Gastrointestinal and liver disease, 6th ed. Philadelphia. Saunders, 1998:1865–1905.

Welton ML, Varma MG, Amerhauser A. Colon, rectum, and anus. In Norton JA, Bollinger RR, Chang AE, Lowery SF, Mulvihill SJ, Pass HI, Thompson RW, eds. Surgery: basic science and clinical evidence. New York: Springer, 2001:667–762

CASE 20

A 33-year-old man presents for evaluation of swelling in his right thigh. He first noticed the swelling 8 to 10 weeks ago and attributed it to injuries incurred during long-distance running. The patient has no known medical problems. He is physically fit and runs approximately 3 to 5 miles daily. On examination, he is found to have a 6 × 5 cm, firm, non-tender mass in the anterior portion of the right thigh. There are no skin or motor/sensory changes in the right leg and no lymphadenopathy in the right groin. A radiograph of the thigh reveals no bony abnormalities.

◆ **What is the most likely diagnosis?**

◆ **How would you confirm the diagnosis?**

◆ **What is best therapy?**

ANSWERS TO CASE 20: Sarcoma (Soft Tissue)

Summary: A 33-year-old man presents with a large, nontender, soft tissue tumor that is highly suggestive of an extremity sarcoma.

◆ **Most likely diagnosis:** Soft tissue sarcoma (STS) should be highly suspected.

◆ **Confirmation of diagnosis:** A core needle biopsy of the mass should be obtained for tissue diagnosis.

◆ **Best therapy:** Surgical excision is the mainstay of therapy. Multimodality therapy, including radiation and chemotherapy delivered either preoperatively or postoperatively, may be indicated for selected high-grade, large STSs.

Analysis

Objectives

1. Become familiar with the presentation of extremity, truncal, and retroperitoneal sarcomas and the importance of obtaining tissue for early diagnosis and treatment.
2. Become familiar with the treatment options and outcome for patients with sarcomas.
3. Become familiar with the genetic conditions and risk factors associated with the development of sarcomas.

Considerations

The initial approach in this patient should include biopsy of the mass for pathologic diagnosis. The biopsy can be performed using a core needle or by open incision if a needle biopsy fails to obtain adequate tissue. **Excisional biopsy should never be attempted with lesions suspected to be STSs because of the difficulty in achieving ade-**

quate resection margins, which would compromise the definitive care of the patient. Young, healthy, active individuals with extremity STSs are frequently misdiagnosed as having a hematoma or a bruised muscle because sarcomas are infrequently encountered by physicians in most medical practices. Therefore, it is imperative to **consider STS whenever an unexplained soft tissue mass or swelling is identified** in an individual of any age. Certain clinical features in this case should further raise a **suspicion of STS,** including the **size of the lesion (6 × 5 cm), the absence of a specific event to account for a hematoma of this size, the firmness of the mass, and the absence of surrounding skin changes to suggest an inflammatory or infectious process.** As a rule, most patients with STS present without any regional lymphadenopathy or systemic symptoms such as weight loss, night sweats, or cachexia. Occasionally, STS may manifest as local pain, erythema, or tenderness over the mass and can be easily misdiagnosed as a soft tissue abscess; these symptoms are due to rapid tumor growth leading to partial necrosis of the STS.

APPROACH TO SARCOMAS

Sarcomas can be categorized as extremity, superficial truncal, and retroperitoneal. Extremity STSs are frequently diagnosed late, in part because of the failure of the patient to seek treatment and also because of misdiagnoses by physicians. The typical presentation is that of a new area of swelling in the arm or leg frequently thought to be a hematoma or bruised muscle and often noticed after trivial trauma to the area. It is important to note that trauma is not the cause of STS but rather is the event that brings attention to the mass itself. The differential diagnosis for a soft tissue mass include benign lipoma, which is much more common; however, STS should be suspected in any patient with a new fixed mass, a mass that is increasing in size, or a mass that is greater than 5 cm in diameter.

Approximately 50% of STS are found in the extremities, but the distribution can involve any site. Sarcomas arise from mesodermal tissue and can exist as one of many pathologic subtypes (eg, liposarcoma, fibrosarcoma, leiomyosarcoma, and malignant fibrohistiocytoma). The diagnosis of STS begins with development of a high index of suspicion based on the history and physical examination, followed by either a core biopsy or a fine-needle biopsy for diagnosis. **Patients with tumors of large size or high grade (highly mitotic) based on histologic study are at increased risk for pulmonary metastasis. These individuals should undergo CT imaging of the lung.** Staging of an extremity STS is based on size, grade, and superficial versus deep location. Table 20–1 outlines favorable and unfavorable characteristics of extremity and superficial trunk STSs. The staging for STS is still evolving. In general, sarcomas with three favorable signs are stage 0, those with two favorable signs are stage 1, those with one favorable and two unfavorable signs are stage 2, and those with three unfavorable signs are stage 3. All sarcomas with either lymph node or distant metastasis are considered stage 4. **Lymph node metastasis is rare in STS; however, when it occurs, patient survival is similar to that for individuals with distant metastasis. Distant metastasis occurs most commonly in the lungs.** Disease-specific survival (DSS) for patients with extremity STS varies depending on the site, histology, grade, and size. Basically, patients with low-grade tumors less than 5 cm have greater than a 90% 5-year DSS, whereas those with high-grade tumors greater than 5 cm have approximately a 50% 5-year DSS. Patients with stage 4 STSs have a 10% to 15% 5-year DSS. Nevertheless, when pulmonary metastases are amenable to complete resection, the 5-year DSS may be as high as 35%.

The **treatment of extremity STSs** has evolved substantially over the past several decades. Previously, amputation was the standard of care. However, a landmark prospective randomized study by the National Cancer Institute comparing limb-sparing surgery with radiation to am-

Table 20–1

CHARACTERISTICS OF EXTREMITY
SOFT TISSUE SARCOMAS

CHARACTERISTIC	FAVORABLE	UNFAVORABLE
Size	≤5 cm	>5 cm
Grade	Low	High
Depth	Superficial	Deep

putation found no survival benefits in performing amputations. **The current standard treatment is wide local excision, with all efforts made to obtain negative microscopic margins.** Complete resection of a muscle compartment results in greater functional loss and is generally unnecessary. Complete resection with a **2-cm gross margin** is reasonable to ensure negative microscopic margins. Patients with stage 0 disease rarely experience a recurrence or die of the disease, but the risk of local recurrence increases with the stage. Radiation therapy should be considered for stage 2 and 3 disease to reduce local recurrence. Generally, brachytherapy (radioactive catheters placed directly in the tumor resection bed) is given for high-grade tumors, and external beam therapy is given for larger, low-grade, and more deeply located tumors. Because brachytherapy catheters are placed intraoperatively, a tissue diagnosis should be obtained by core biopsy preoperatively whenever such therapy is considered.

Local recurrence of STS takes place despite resection with grossly clear margins. For this reason, every attempt should be made to obtain negative microscopic margins during the initial resection. With large tumors in deep locations, magnetic resonance imaging or CT imaging performed preoperatively can help to more clearly define the tumor's relationship to major structures. Patients with tumors encasing bone, major vessels, or nerves may be more appropriately treated with preoperative (neoadjuvant) chemoradiation to shrink the tumor to allow for limb-sparing surgery.

Postoperative Follow-up

Recommendations for follow-up after surgical resection currently are not standardized. A reasonable practice is to follow patients with a low risk for recurrence on a bi-yearly basis with a physical examination and on a yearly basis with a chest radiograph. Patients at high risk for recurrence are usually examined every 3 months, with chest radiographs obtained every 3 to 6 months indefinitely.

Retroperitoneal Sarcoma

Sarcomas arising from retroperitoneal structures tend to remain asymptomatic until they reach a large size. Most patients have late presentations, commonly with tumor involvement of contiguous structures. **Patients with high-grade and/or incompletely resected primary tumors have a substantial recurrence risk.** Unlike high-risk extremity STS, more likely to result in death because of recurrence at a distant site, **retroperitoneal sarcomas are much more likely to recur locally** and cause death as a result of local involvement. Lewis and colleagues evaluated 231 patients following the resection of retroperitoneal sarcomas and found 2- and 5-year survivals of 80% and 60%, respectively. It has been shown that **complete resection is best achieved during the initial surgery,** and the probability of complete resection is reduced with each subsequent operative attempt. Distant metastasis from retroperitoneal soft tissue, which infrequently occurs, often involves the liver and lungs. Postoperative follow-up for retroperitoneal sarcoma is not clearly defined. CT scans performed at 6-month intervals may be considered reasonable.

Genetic and Environmental Predisposition to Sarcomas

Both physical and genetic factors can predispose to the development of sarcomas. Physical factors include prior radiation, lymphedema, and chemical exposure (including prior chemotherapy). The genetic predisposing factors are listed in Table 20–2. Patients with neurofibromatosis are prone to develop sarcomas arising from nerve structures, as well as paragangliomas and pheochromocytomas. The development of retinoblastoma in patients with the Li–Fraumeni syndrome (an autosomal dominant disorder with predisposition to the early onset of many types of cancers) has been genetically linked to mutations in *Rb-1* and

Table 20–2
GENETIC PREDISPOSITION ASSOCIATED
WITH SARCOMAS

Neurofibromatosis
Li–Fraumeni syndrome
Retinoblastoma
Familial polyposis coli

p-53 genes, respectively. Whereas patients with the Li–Fraumeni syndrome have been shown to have an increased risk for several cancers, those with retinoblastoma are prone to develop osteosarcomas. Patients with familial polyposis coli have an increased risk of developing desmoid tumors, which are generally considered benign tumors with a predilection for local recurrence following excision.

Comprehension Questions

[20.1] A 35-year-old man notices a firm, nontender, 10-cm mass in his thigh after falling off a ladder. What is the most appropriate first step following a history and a physical examination?

A. Observation to see if it changes over the next month
B. Core needle biopsy followed by a CT scan of the extremity
C. Immediate resection with wide margins
D. Ultrasonography of the mass

[20.2] A 41-year old woman underwent excision of what was thought to be a superficial lipoma of the upper extremity. Findings from pathology studies subsequently revealed a 3-cm, low-grade sarcoma with positive histologic margins. Which of the following treatments is most appropriate?

A. Follow-up physical examination in 6 months
B. External beam radiation
C. Chemotherapy
D. Reexcision to obtain negative margins

[20.3] What is the most common site of metastasis of extremity sarcoma?

A. Lymph nodes
B. Liver
C. Lung
D. Bone

[20.4] A 54-year-old woman is seen in a follow-up after resection of a large retroperitoneal sarcoma. Which of the following locations is the most likely site of recurrence?

A. Peritoneal or retroperitoneal space
B. Liver
C. Lung
D. Recurrence is unlikely following complete resection.

[20.5] Which of the following is *not* considered an independent risk factor for the recurrence of retroperitoneal sarcoma?

A. High grade
B. Incomplete resection
C. Resection for recurrence
D. Being less than 50 years of age

Answers

[20.1] **B.** The finding of a **nontender** mass is inconsistent with a soft tissue injury despite the history of a fall; therefore a core biopsy is indicated.

[20.2] **D.** Surgical resection to achieve negative margins is the best treatment in this case.

[20.3] **C.** The lungs are the most common site of metastasis for extremity STS.

[20.4] **A.** Local and regional recurrence is the most likely cause of treatment failure for retroperitoneal sarcomas.

[20.5] **D.** Age is not a risk factor for retroperitoneal sarcoma recurrence.

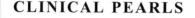

CLINICAL PEARLS

◈ Features of an extremity mass that are suggestive of sarcoma include the size of the lesion (>5 cm), the absence of a specific event to account for a hematoma, firmness of the mass, and the absence of surrounding skin changes suggesting an inflammatory or infectious process.

◈ The diagnosis of STS begins with a high suspicion based on the history and physical examination, followed by performance of a diagnostic core biopsy or fine-needle biopsy.

◈ The current standard therapy for sarcomas is wide local excision with all efforts made to obtain negative microscopic margins, followed by radiation therapy in high-risk patients.

◈ Prior radiation or chemotherapy and genetic factors such as neurofibromatosis are risk factors for STS.

REFERENCES

Brennan MF, Lewis JJ, eds. Diagnosis and management of soft tissue sarcoma. London: Martin Dunitz, 2002.

Lewis JJ, Leung D, Woodruff JM, Brennan MF. Retroperitoneal soft tissue sarcoma: analysis of 500 patients treated and followed at a single institution. Ann Surg 1998;228:355–365.

Pisters PWT, Leung DHY, Woodruff J, et al. Analysis of prognostic factors in 1041 patients with localized soft tissue sarcoma of the extremities. J Clin Oncol 1996;14:1679–1689.

Rosenberg SA, Kent H, Costa J, et al. Prospective randomized evaluation of the role of limb-sparing surgery, radiation therapy, and chemoimmunotherapy in the treatment of adult soft-tissue sarcoma. Surgery, 1978;84:62–69.

CASE 21

A 23-year-old female medical student presents for the evaluation of an asymptomatic neck mass that was found during a practice head and neck examination performed by a fellow medical student. The student is otherwise healthy and denies any previous medical problems. Evaluation of her neck reveals a 4-cm discrete, nontender, firm mass in the right inferior pole of the right lobe. The remainder of the thyroid is normal. No other abnormalities are noted during the rest of her physical examination. The patient denies any family history of thyroid disease or other endocrinopathies. She denies any unusual exposure to ionizing radiation. Thyroid function studies are obtained and reveal normal serum thyrotropin (TSH) and thyroxine (T$_4$) levels.

◆ **What is your next step?**

ANSWERS TO CASE 21: Thyroid Mass

Summary: A 23-year-old medical student presents for the evaluation of an asymptomatic 4-cm, discrete, nontender, firm mass in the inferior pole of the right lobe of the thyroid gland. She denies any previous medical problems, a prior history of head or neck irradiation, or a family history of thyroid cancer or other endocrinopathies. Her serum TSH level is normal.

◆ **Next step:** Fine-needle aspiration for a cytologic assessment for malignancy.

Analysis

Objectives

1. Know the approach to evaluate thyroid nodules, especially concerning cancer risks.
2. To review the diagnostic evaluation of a patient with a thyroid nodule.
3. To identify the indications for surgical treatment of a thyroid nodule.

APPROACH TO THYROID NODULES

Definitions

Multiple endocrine neoplasia (MEN) 2 syndrome: An autosomal dominant syndrome with medullary thyroid carcinoma, pheochromocytoma, and parathyroid hyperplasia or adenomas.

Follicular adenoma: Benign thyroid nodules noted to be fairly common in adults; they usually take up radioactive iodine.

Papillary thyroid carcinoma: The most common type of thyroid carcinoma, usually well-differentiated.

Medullary carcinoma: A type of thyroid cancer occurring sporadically or in familial clusters (MEN); they usually do not take up radioactive iodine.

Clinical Approach

A patient with a thyroid nodule should be questioned about symptoms of hyper- or hypothyroidism, compressive symptoms such as dyspnea, coughing or choking spells, dysphagia or hoarseness, and a prior history of head or neck irradiation. Patients should also be asked about a family history of thyroid cancer, hyperparathyroidism, or pheochromocytoma. Symptoms of hyper- or hypothyroidism may be present in patients with thyroiditis. Symptoms of hyperthyroidism are also seen in patients with benign functioning follicular adenomas. The presence of **compressive symptoms,** which occur from thyroid enlargement and impingement on **adjacent structures, most notably the trachea, esophagus, and recurrent laryngeal nerve are indications for surgery.** A patient with a **solitary thyroid nodule and a prior history of low-dose head or neck irradiation** has a **40% risk of carcinoma.** A **family history of thyroid cancer** should increase the physician's suspicion of carcinoma in a patient with a thyroid nodule. Twenty percent to 30% of medullary thyroid cancers occur as part of a familial syndrome; the most notable are MEN 2A and MEN 2B (Table 21–1). Five percent of papillary cancers are familial.

On physical examination, the size and character of the thyroid nodule should be noted. The thyroid gland should be examined for other nodules, and the neck for associated cervical lymphadenopathy and the position of the trachea. The **presence of associated adenopathy should increase suspicion of malignancy.**

The primary challenge in the management of a thyroid nodule is selecting for surgery those patients with a high risk for cancer and avoiding operations in patients with benign disease. **Currently, fine-needle aspiration biopsy (FNAB) is the initial and most important step in the diagnostic evaluation of a dominant thyroid nodule.** Management of nodular thyroid disease is dependent on the results from the FNAB (Figure 21–1). Patients with a malignant FNAB are treated with thyroidectomy. A cytologic diagnosis of malignancy is very reliable

Table 21–1

MULTIPLE ENDOCRINE NEOPLASIA

Multiple endocrine neoplasia 2A
  Medullary thyroid cancer
  Pheochromocytoma
  Hyperparathyroidism
  Lichen planus amyloidosis
  Hirschsprung disease
Multiple endocrine neoplasia 2B
  Medullary thyroid cancer
  Pheochromocytoma
  Marfanoid habitus
  Mucosal neuromas
  Ganglioneuromatosis of the gastrointestinal tract

---

with only a 1% to 2% incidence of false-positive results. Patients with benign FNAB results are followed with a yearly physical examination of the neck and a serum TSH level test. Thyroidectomy is reserved for progressive nodule enlargement or compressive symptoms. The incidence of false-negative FNAB results is approximately 2% to 5%.

A cellular FNAB result refers to a specimen with cytologic features consistent with either a follicular or a Hürthle cell neoplasm. A follicular or Hürthle cell carcinoma cannot be distinguished from a follicular or Hürthle cell adenoma using cytologic criteria alone. A diagnosis of follicular or Hürthle cell carcinoma is based on the presence of capsular or vascular invasion as observed in a tissue sample. For patients with a cellular FNAB, the results of a serum TSH level test are reviewed. A solitary nodule in a patient with a normal or an increased serum TSH level is almost always hypofunctioning, whereas in approximately 90% of patients with a hyperfunctioning nodule, the serum TSH level is low. **Clinically significant carcinoma occurs in less than 1% of patients with hyperfunctioning nodules compared to 10% to 20% of patients with hypofunctioning nodules.** As a result, iodine-123 thyroid scintigraphy is recommended for patients with a cellular FNAB when the serum TSH level is low. **Thyroidectomy** is recommended for patients with a **cellular FNAB when the serum TSH level is normal or high or when a hypofunctioning nodule** is demonstrated

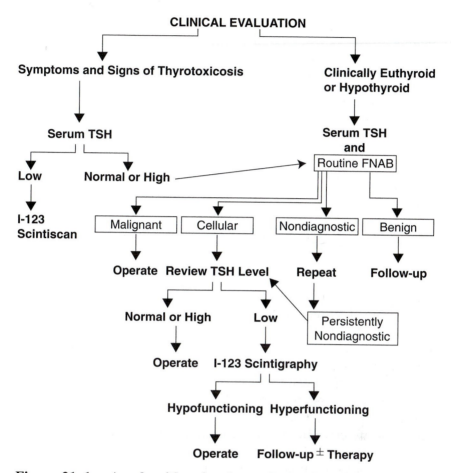

Figure 21–1.   An algorithm for the evaluation of patients with a dominant thyroid nodule. (Reproduced, with permission, from McHenry CR, Slusarczyk SJ, Askari AT, et al. Refined use of scintigraphy in the evaluation of nodular thyroid disease. Surgery 1998; 124:660.)

on thyroid scintigraphy. Patients with a solitary hypofunctioning nodule and a cellular FNAB have been reported to have a 20% to 30% incidence of carcinoma.

In patients with nondiagnostic FNAB results, the biopsy should be repeated because an adequate specimen is obtained with a repeated biopsy in more than 50% of patients. For patients with **persistently nondiagnostic FNAB results, an operation is recommended when the serum TSH level is normal or high,** and iodine-123 scintigraphy is performed in patients with a low serum TSH level. **Surgery is recommended for patients with persistently nondiagnostic FNAB results and a hypofunctioning nodule.** A 9% incidence of carcinoma has been reported in this subset of patients.

Comprehension Questions

[21.1] In which of the following situations would the results of thyroid scintigraphy most likely impact treatment?

A. FNAB results consistent with a malignant neoplasm
B. FNAB results consistent with a benign neoplasm
C. FNAB results consistent with a follicular neoplasm
D. Prior history of head or neck irradiation

[21.2] A 40-year-old woman presents with a single thyroid nodule. Which of the following situations would be associated with the highest risk of malignancy?

A. A prior history of head or neck irradiation
B. Hyperfunction of the nodule seen on thyroid scintigraphy
C. Hypofunctioning of the nodule seen on scintigraphy (cold nodule)
D. History of Graves disease

[21.3] In which of the following situations is thyroidectomy the best choice for treatment of a thyroid nodule?

A. Initial nondiagnostic FNAB results
B. Hypothyroidism
C. A mother who had papillary carcinoma
D. FNAB results consistent with a benign neoplasm when compressive symptoms are present

[21.4] Which of the following procedures should be performed routinely in a patient with a thyroid nodule who is clinically euthyroid?

A. FNAB and determination of a screening serum TSH level
B. Measurement of radioiodine uptake and thyroid scintiscanning
C. Measure of serum T_4, triiodothyronine (T_3), and TSH levels
D. Ultrasound examination of the thyroid gland to distinguish a solid from a cystic nodule

Answers

[21.1] **C.** Radionuclide scanning can determine the function of the nodule. With a fine-needle aspirate showing a follicular pattern, a "cold" hypofunctioning pattern is associated with a significant risk of cancer, whereas a "warm or hot" functioning pattern is associated with a low (1% risk) of cancer.

[21.2] **A.** A history of head and neck irradiation greatly increases the risk of a thyroid nodule being malignant.

[21.3] **D.** Compressive symptoms are life-threatening, and urgent surgical intervention is considered the best therapy.

[21.4] **A.** FNAB and a TSH level test for the assessment of thyroid function are the two most important initial tests for evaluating a thyroid nodule.

CLINICAL PEARLS

◆ Currently, FNAB is the initial and most important step in the diagnostic evaluation of a dominant thyroid nodule.

◆ Thyroid enlargement and impingement on adjacent structures, most notably the trachea, esophagus, and recurrent laryngeal nerve, are indications for surgery.

◆ A patient with a prior history of neck irradiation or a family history consistent with MEN syndromes has a high risk of thyroid cancer.

◆ A nonfunctioning "cold" thyroid nodule has significantly more risk for cancer than a "hot" functioning nodule.

REFERENCES

McHenry CR. Goiter and nontoxic benign thyroid conditions. In: Bland KI, ed. The practice of general surgery. Philadelphia: Saunders, 2002:1041–1048.

McHenry CR, Slusarczyk S, Ascari AT, Lange RL, Smith CM, Nekl K, Murphy TA. Refined use of scintigraphy in the evaluation of nodular thyroid disease. Surgery 1998;124:656–662.

Mittendorf EA, McHenry CR. Follow-up evaluation and clinical course of patients with benign nodular thyroid disease. Am Surg 1999;65(8):653–658.

A 33-year-old man presents with a sudden onset of left chest pain and shortness of breath that occurred while he was working in his yard. The patient denies any trauma to his chest and any cough or other respiratory symptoms prior to the onset of pain. His past medical history is unremarkable. He takes no medications. He consumes one pack of cigarettes a day and two to three beers a day. On physical examination he appears anxious. His temperature is normal, his pulse rate 110/min, his blood pressure 124/80, and his respiratory rate 28/min. The pulmonary examination reveals diminished breath sounds on the left and normal breath sounds on the right. A cardiac examination demonstrates no murmurs or gallops. Results from the abdominal and extremity examinations are unremarkable. The laboratory examination reveals a normal complete blood count and normal serum electrolyte levels. The chest radiograph shows a 50% left pneumothorax, without effusion or pulmonary lesions.

◆ **What is your next step?**

◆ **What are the risk factors for this condition?**

ANSWERS TO CASE 22: Pneumothorax (Spontaneous)

Summary: An otherwise healthy 33-year-old man presents with a large primary spontaneous pneumothorax.

◆ **Next step:** Perform either tube thoracostomy or needle aspiration to allow reexpansion of the left lung.

◆ **Risk factors for this condition:** Primary spontaneous pneumothorax is due to the rupture of subpleural blebs. Secondary spontaneous pneumothorax may be caused by bullous emphysematous disease, cystic fibrosis, primary and secondary cancers, and necrotizing infections with organisms such as *Pneumocystis carinii.*

Analysis

Objectives

1. Be able to define primary and secondary spontaneous pneumothorax.
2. Be able to outline treatment and diagnostic strategies for patients presenting with spontaneous pneumothorax.

Considerations

The patient is a young male, the type of individual most likely to develop spontaneous pneumothorax. The most common cause is the rupture of a subpleural bleb. This patient does not have any risk factors for secondary causes of spontaneous pneumothorax such as malignancy, tuberculosis, or chronic obstructive pulmonary disease. The best management would be insertion of a chest tube or needle aspiration to allow for reexpansion of the lung.

APPROACH TO SPONTANEOUS PNEUMOTHORAX

Definitions

Pneumothorax: Condition whereby air enters the pleural space, thus preventing expansion of the lung parenchyma.

Tension pneumothorax: Caused by a flap-valve effect such that air enters the pleural space but cannot exit until the pleural pressure is so great that it prevents blood from entering the chest.

Open pneumothorax: Injury to the full thickness of the chest wall such that the negative intrapleural pressure results in air being sucked directly though the chest wall defect, preventing air from being taken in through the trachea; it requires a mechanical covering over the chest wound.

Flail chest: Injury to multiple ribs leading to a paradoxical inward movement of the affected chest region on inspiratory effort, resulting in little air movement. This condition is best treated with endotracheal intubation and positive pressure ventilation.

Tube thoracostomy: Placement of a catheter (chest tube) into the pleural space to evacuate air, blood, or fluid to permit better ventilation.

Clinical Approach

The initial management of pneumothorax requires reexpansion of the lung. This often requires tube thoracostomy, but thoracentesis or pleural catheter drainage can be attempted for smaller pneumothoraces (<30% of the width of the hemithorax). Small, asymptomatic pneumothoraces (<15% of the width of the hemithorax) can be initially observed with serial chest radiographs. If the pneumothorax does not improve or the patient develops symptoms (chest pain, dyspnea), tube thoracostomy will be required.

Spontaneous pneumothorax can be classified as either primary or secondary. **Primary pneumothorax is usually caused by the rupture of subpleural pulmonary blebs.** This condition is more commonly observed in young males (15 to 35 years old) without other risk factors for

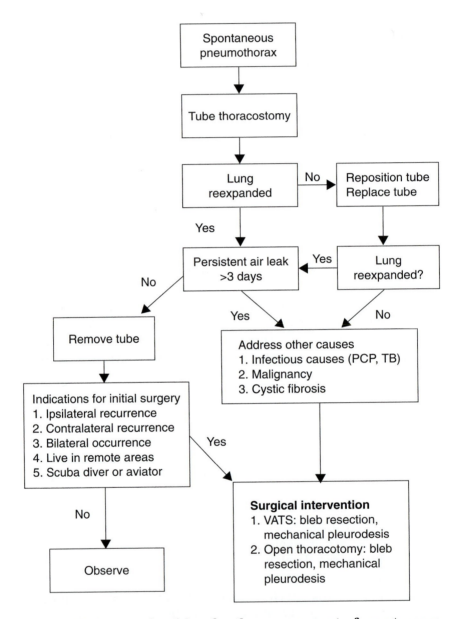

Figure 22–1. An algorithm for the management of spontaneous pneumothorax. PCP, Pneumocystis carinii pneumonia; TB, tuberculosis; VATS, video-assisted thoracoscopy.

spontaneous pneumothorax. **Secondary spontaneous pneumothorax** results from an **acquired process** and is most commonly seen in **older patients with chronic obstructive pulmonary disease.** These patients may present with severe respiratory difficulty due to the already present diffuse lung disease. Other reasons for secondary spontaneous pneumothorax include malignancy, infection (tuberculosis, *P. carinii*), catamenial, asthma, and cystic fibrosis. For management of these problems see Figure 22–1.

Chest tube management is sufficient treatment for most cases of spontaneous pneumothorax, with 15% to 20% requiring surgical intervention. Surgery is indicated for first-time spontaneous pneumothorax when there is persistent air leakage (>3 to 5 days), when the lung fails to reexpand, in patients who are at high risk for recurrence (bilateral pneumothoraces, a previous history of contralateral pneumothorax, significant bullous disease on radiographs), in patients who have limited access to medical care (those living in remote areas), and in patients whose occupation produces an increased risk (scuba divers, pilots).

The recurrence rate for spontaneous pneumothorax is 30% after the first occurrence, 50% after the second, and 80% after the third. Therefore, **immediate surgical intervention is indicated after the second recurrence.**

Comprehension Questions

[22.1] Which of the following is a risk factor for the development of spontaneous pneumothorax?

    A. Female gender
    B. Age 55–70 years
    C. Tall, thin physique
    D. History of tuberculosis

[22.2] Which of the following factors is most predictive of the recurrence of pneumothorax?

    A. Patient's occupation
    B. Location of blebs

C. Presence of chronic obstructive pulmonary disease

D. Number of previous episodes of pneumothorax

[22.3] A 33-year-old woman who underwent multiple enterotomies for penetrating abdominal trauma has a subclavian central line placed and subsequently develops "air hunger." Which of the following is the most likely etiology?

A. Acute psychosis

B. Panic disorder

C. Hemothorax

D. Pneumothorax

E. Pulmonary embolism

Answers

[22.1] **C.** Spontaneous pneumothorax occurs more commonly in young males who are thin and tall, and in smokers.

[22.2] **D.** The number of prior episodes of pneumothorax is more predictive of a recurrence, with an 80% recurrence rate after three previous episodes.

[22.3] **D.** A fairly common complication of the placement of central venous catheters is pneumothorax.

CLINICAL PEARLS

◈ Although most cases of pneumothorax can be managed with a tube thoracostomy, aggressive surgical intervention is indicated for cases where there is a high risk of recurrence.

◈ The general therapeutic goal is to address the underlying problem (blebs, infection, etc) and to achieve pleural apposition (reexpansion of the lung).

◈ Failure to achieve pleural apposition or persistent air leakage requires surgical intervention.

REFERENCES

Abolnik IZ, Lossos IS, Gillis D, Breuer R. Primary spontaneous pneumothorax in men. Am J Med Sci 1993;305:297.

DeVries WC, Wolfe WG. The management of spontaneous pneumothorax and emphysema. Surg Clin North Am 1980;60:851.

Dines DE, Clagett OT, Payne SW. Spontaneous pneumothorax in emphysema. Mayo Clin Proc 1970;45:481.

A 38-year-old man fell 15 feet from a ladder while trying to rescue a cat. During the evaluation at the hospital, he was found to have a closed fracture of the right femur, a fracture of the right radius and ulna, and soft tissue contusions and abrasions. The patient underwent open reduction and internal fixation of his femur and external fixation of his forearm without apparent complications. On postinjury day 2, he began to complain of difficulty in breathing. On physical examination, his temperature is found to be 38.4°C (101°F), pulse rate 120/min, blood pressure 148/86, respiratory rate 34/min, and Glasgow Coma Score 15. The patient appears anxious and complains of difficulty breathing but is without chest pain. Auscultation of the chest reveals diminished breath sounds bilaterally with scattered rhonchi. The results of a cardiac examination are unremarkable. The abdomen is nondistended and nontender. Examination of the extremities reveals postinjury soft tissue swelling. Laboratory studies reveal the following: white blood cell (WBC) count 16,000/mm^3, hemoglobin 10.8 g/dL, platelet count 185,000/mm^3. Arterial blood gas studies reveal pH 7.4, Pao$_2$ 55 mm Hg, Paco$_2$ 40 mmHg, and HCO$_3$ 24 mEq/L. A chest radiograph (CXR) reveals bilateral nonsegmental infiltrates and no effusion or pneumothorax.

◆ **What are your next steps?**

◆ **What is the most likely diagnosis?**

ANSWERS TO CASE 23: Postoperative Acute Respiratory Insufficiency

Summary: A previously healthy young man develops acute respiratory insufficiency after being injured in a fall and undergoing operative repair of traumatic orthopedic injuries.

◆ **Next steps:** Administration of supplemental oxygen and transfer to the intensive care unit for closer observation and possible mechanical ventilation if the patient's condition does not improve or deteriorates.

◆ **Diagnosis:** Acute respiratory insufficiency due to acute lung injury (ALI).

Analysis

Objectives

Learn the presentations and differential diagnosis of acute respiratory insufficiency surgical patients.

1. Learn the pathophysiology of ALI.
2. Be familiar with the types of invasive and noninvasive modes of pulmonary support.

Considerations

The timing of the development of respiratory insufficiency is relatively early for pulmonary embolism (PE) but within the expected time frame for ALI. The patient's pulmonary examination reveals diminished breath sounds and scattered rhonchi, nonspecific findings compatible with ALI. The CXR reveals bilateral nonsegmental infiltrates, and an arterial blood gas study shows moderate hypoxemia. Typically, PE presents with a relatively normal CXR. By strict definition, ALI requires the respiratory insufficiency to be acute in onset, associated with a Pao_2:Fio_2 value less than 300, bilateral infiltrates, and a pulmonary capillary wedge pressure of less than 18 mm Hg. Although many features of this case suggest a diagnosis of ALI, other potential diagnoses must be considered and excluded, including aspiration pneumonitis, atypical pneumonia, atelectasis, and PE. During the initial evaluation of any patient with acute respiratory insufficiency, it is important to consider the diagnosis, but the primary consideration should be to determine the most appropriate level of respiratory support. For this patient, it is important to remember that even though he does not appear to require immediate mechanical ventilatory support, his oxygenation and pulmonary compliance defects may progress and cause further respiratory embarrassment.

APPROACH TO ACUTE RESPIRATORY INSUFFICIENCY

Definitions

Aspiration: Spillage of gastric contents into the bronchial tree causing direct injury to the airways, which can progress to a chemical burn or pneumonitis (especially when pH <3) and predispose to bacterial pneumonia. When the aspirated gastric contents contain particulate matter, bronchoscopy may be helpful in clearing the airway. Half of affected patients develop subsequent pneumonia not prevented by empirical antibiotics.

Pneumonia: Pulmonary infection due to impairment of the lung's defense mechanisms. Incisional pain frequently affects the patient's ability to clear airway mucus, leading to small airway obstruction and ineffective bacteria clearance. Most commonly, nosocomial organisms are those that colonize patients during hospitalization.

Pulmonary embolism: A major source of morbidity and mortality in surgical patients. The prophylaxis, diagnosis, and treatment of PE are continuous concerns for the surgeon. Bed rest, cancer, and trauma increase the risk of deep vein thrombosis (DVT) and PE occurrence. PE may be clinically silent or symptomatic. In high-risk surgical patients, the risk of developing a clinically significant PE is 2% to 3%, and the risk of developing a fatal PE approaches 1%. The clinical hallmarks include acute onset hypoxia associated with anxiety leading to tachypnea and hypocarbia without significant CXR abnormalities.

Lung contusion: Blunt trauma to the chest is a common cause of pulmonary dysfunction resulting from direct parenchymal injury and impaired chest wall function. An injured chest wall leads to impaired breathing mechanics that can range from splinting secondary to a rib fracture to the severe impairment of a flail chest. The morbidity from lung contusion is attributed to direct parenchymal injury and bronchoalveolar hemorrhage, causing V/Q mismatch leading to hypoxia. This condition is worsened by chest wall injury pain, leading to atelectasis in the uninvolved lung.

Acute respiratory distress syndrome (ARDS): The most severe form of ALI ($Pao_2:Fio_2 < 200$), this condition encompasses a spectrum of lung injuries characterized by increasing hypoxia and decreased lung compliance. Initially, an injury to the pulmonary endothelial cells leads to an intense inflammatory response. Inhomogeneous involvement of the lung occurs, with interstitial and alveolar edema, loss of type II pneumocytes, surfactant depletion, intra-alveolar hemorrhage, hyaline membrane deposition, and eventual fibrosis. These changes manifest clinically as severe hypoxia, decreased lung compliance, and the increased dead space ventilation.

Atelectasis: The collapse of alveolar units in patients who undergo general anesthesia, which causes a reduction in functional residual capacity that is further reduced because of incisional pain. The subsegmental atelectasis may progress to obstruction and inflammation, leading to larger airway obstruction and segmental collapse. Most patients have only a low-grade fever and mild respiratory insufficiency.

Cardiogenic pulmonary edema: Myocardial dysfunction most frequently resulting from ischemia can produce left ventricular dysfunction, fluid overload, and pulmonary interstitial edema. The increase in the amount of interstitial water compresses the fragile bronchovascular structures, thereby increasing the V/Q mismatch and resulting in hypoxia.

Clinical Approach

Patient Assessment   In treating patients with acute respiratory insufficiency, the first priority is to assess and stabilize the airway, breathing, and circulation (ABC's). Patients with lethargy and diminished mentation may benefit from immediate endotracheal intubation to protect against aspiration. The assessment of each patient should be directed toward the immediate status as well as toward the anticipated future status of the patient's ventilation and oxygenation. The adequacy of oxygenation is evaluated by pulse oximetry or Pao_2 measurement by arterial blood gas (ABG) studies. The **inability to maintain a Pao_2 of 60 mmHg or an oxygen saturation of less than 91% with a supplemental nonrebreathing O_2 mask are indicative of a significant alveolar-arterial (A-a) gradient and intubation and mechanical ventilation may be needed.** Hypoxemia frequently causes agitation and confusion, and an uncooperative patient can contribute to delays in diagnosis. The adequacy of ventilation is generally assessed by observing the patient's respiratory efforts and subjective symptoms, and quantified by the measurement of $Paco_2$ by ABG analysis. It is important to bear in mind that ventilation assessment requires the use of all these data should not be made on the basis of a blood gas value alone.

Pathophysiology of Acute Lung Injury   Acute lung injury encompasses a spectrum of lung disease from mild forms to severe lung injury or ARDS. The inciting event can be a direct or indirect pulmonary insult (Figure 23–1). The resultant cascade of events includes both cellular and humoral components that produce an inhomogeneous injury. The inflammatory response involves activated polymorphonucleocytes that generate oxygen radicals, cytokines, lipid mediators, and nitric oxide. The complement, kinin, coagulation, and fibrinolytic systems are also involved. Endothelial damage ensues with an increase in microvascular permeability leading to the accumulation of extravascular lung water. This soon results in diminished lung volume and decreased lung compliance. Lung compliance is further hampered due to the sloughing of type I pneumocytes and a decrease in surfactant production by type II pneumocytes. The process continues, further aggravating interstitial edema, alveolar collapse, and lung consolidation. In the

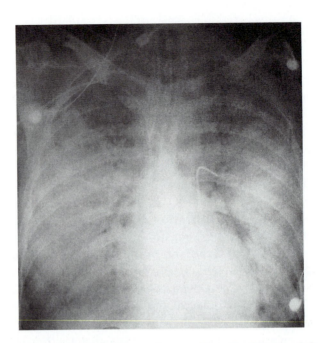

Figure 23–1.   A chest radiograph revealing the bilateral dense pulmonary infiltrates typical of acute respiratory disease syndrome. (Reproduced, with permission, from Mattox KL, Feliciano DV, Moore EE, eds. Trauma, 4th ed. New York: McGraw-Hill, 2000:526.)

pathogenesis, inflammatory cells and fluid are sequestered within the lungs, leading to a decrease in pulmonary compliance and an increase in the work of breathing. During the prodromal phase of ALI, the patient may simply complain of difficulty in catching his breath, leading to tachypnea. **Ventilation is reflected by the $Paco_2$, but the patient's appearance, respiratory rate, and respiratory efforts are equally important endpoints.** Hypercapnia is not associated with anxiety or agitation; therefore patients with an altered level of consciousness should have $Paco_2$ (by ABG) or end-tidal CO_2 (by capnography) monitoring to assess ventilation.

Noninvasive Pulmonary Support   Patients with acute postoperative respiratory insufficiency can be provided with supplemental oxygen and noninvasive respiratory support, including a continuous positive airway pressure mask (useful for atelectasis) and chest physiotherapy, including bronchodilators and mucolytic agents (useful for atelectasis, pneumonia, and reactive airway disease). Patients with a significant A-a gradient may benefit from mechanical ventilator support for oxygenation.

Mechanical Ventilation Modes

Conventional Ventilation   Conventional ventilation or positive pressure ventilation fills the lungs via supra-atmospheric pressure applied through an endotracheal tube to the airways. This creates a positive transpulmonary pressure that ensures inflation of the lungs. Exhalation is passive and occurs after release of the positive pressure. The major settings are volume- and pressure-controlled, where the tidal volume delivery is based on either volume- or pressure-limiting settings.

High-frequency Ventilation   High-frequency ventilation also utilizes an endotracheal tube to facilitate gas exchange; however, high-frequency ventilation delivers very small tidal volumes, on the order of 1 mL/kg body weight at a very high rate, about 100 to 400 breaths per minute. Although this mode has an important role in the treatment of respiratory insufficiency in neonates, it has not had the same success in adults.

Liquid Ventilation   The theoretical advantage of liquid ventilation lies in its ability to reduce the amount of energy necessary to overcome surface tension at the gas–liquid interface of alveoli. Because diseased lungs have less surfactant, liquid ventilation can improve lung compliance. Studies are needed to document the clinical benefits of this ventilation mode.

Extracorporeal Life Support   Cardiopulmonary bypass or extracorporeal life support uses a heart-lung machine to take over pulmonary and/or cardiac function. If cardiac function is adequate, a venovenous circuit can be used to remove carbon dioxide and oxygenate the blood.

As in the case of high-frequency ventilation, the early success achieved in neonates has not been duplicated in adult populations.

Comprehension Questions

[23.1] A 57-year-old woman develops an acute onset of respiratory distress 7 days following colectomy for adenocarcinoma of the colon. She had been doing well up until this time. The physical examination reveals diminished breath sounds at the lung bases. The CXR reveals atelectasis of the left lower lobe segment. Which of the following is the *most appropriate* treatment at this time?

    A. Provide supplemental oxygen and begin chest physiotherapy.

    B. Provide supplemental oxygen and initiate chest physiotherapy and antibiotic therapy.

    C. Begin antibiotic therapy and immediate bronchoscopy to open up the lungs.

    D. Provide supplemental oxygen, obtain venous duplex scans of the lower extremities and a lung V/Q scan, and consider starting heparin therapy.

[23.2] Diagnostic bronchoscopy is most appropriate in which of the following patients?

    A. A 33-year-old man with right lower lobe hospital-acquired pneumonia

    B. A 40-year-old man with AIDS who develops fever, acute respiratory distress, and bilateral pulmonary infiltrates

    C. A 66-year-old man with dementia who develops a right upper lobe infiltrate following an episode of aspiration

    D. A 30-year-old man who develops ARDS associated with fever and a loculated right pleural effusion

[23.3] A 34-year-old woman is hospitalized for septic shock due to toxic shock syndrome. She is treated with intravenous nafcillin, and is noted to have hypoxemia. A chest radiograph reveals diffuse infiltrates in bilateral lung fields. Which of the following would most likely differentiate ARDS from cardiogenic pulmonary edema?

A. Pulmonary artery catheter readings
B. Serum colloid osmotic pressure
C. Urinary electrolytes and partial excretion of sodium
D. Ventilation-perfusion scan

Answers

[23.1] **D.** Provide supplemental O_2, perform a workup for PE, and consider empirical treatment. This patient develops a sudden onset of respiratory distress 7 days postoperatively. The clinical presentation is highly suggestive of PE. The diagnosis of atelectasis as the primary cause of this patient's clinical picture should not be readily accepted until PE can be ruled out.

[23.2] **B.** Diagnostic bronchoscopy and bronchoalveolar lavage are indicated in an immunocompromised individual with new-onset fever and bilateral pulmonary infiltrates.

[23.3] **A.** The pulmonary capillary wedge pressure (PCWP) approximates the left ventricular end-diastolic pressure. A low-normal pulmonary artery wedge pressure (<18 mm Hg) supports leaky capillaries (ARDS) as the etiology, whereas a high PCWP suggests a hydrostatic mechanism, cardiogenic pulmomary edema.

REFERENCES

Artigas A, Bernard GR, Carlet J, Dreyfuss D, Gattinoni L, Hudson L, Lamy M, Marini JJ, Matthay MA, Pinsky MR, Spragg R, Suter PM. The American-European Consensus Conference on ARDS. Part 2: ventilatory, pharmacologic, supportive therapy, study design strategies, and issues related to recovery and remodeling–acute respiratory distress syndrome. Am J Respir Crit Care Med 1998;157:1332–1347.

Bernard GR, Artigas A, Brigham KL, Carlet J, Falke K, Hudson L, Lamy M, Legall JR, Morris A, Spragg R, and the Consensus Committee. The American-European Consensus Conference on ARDS. Definitions, mechanisms, relevant outcomes, and clinical trial coordination. Am J Respir Crit Care Med 1994;149:818–824.

Shapiro BA, Peruzzi WT. Changing practices in ventilator management: a review of the literature and suggested clinical correlations. Surgery 1995;117(2):121–133.

Following recovery from an exploratory laparotomy and repair of a colon injury caused by a gunshot wound to the abdomen, a 24-year-old man developed an infection in the superior portion of his wound that required local wound care. He was discharged from the hospital on postoperative day 10 and has returned about 2 weeks later for a follow-up visit to the outpatient clinic. The patient indicates that he has been doing well except for fluid drainage from his open midline abdominal wound. On physical examination, his temperature is 37.5°C (99.5°F), pulse rate 70/min, blood pressure 130/80, and respiratory rate 18/min. The results of his cardiopulmonary examinations are within normal limits. Examination of the abdomen reveals a small amount of serosanguinous fluid from the superior aspect of his surgical incision. There is no redness, swelling, or tenderness around the incision. A 4-cm fascia defect in the superior aspect of the wound is present without signs of evisceration.

◆ **What are the complications associated with this condition?**

◆ **What are the risk factors for this condition?**

◆ **What is the best treatment?**

**ANSWERS TO CASE 24: Fascial Dehiscence and
Incisional Hernia**

Summary: A 24-year-old man presents with stable abdominal wound
dehiscence 3 weeks following exploratory laparotomy for the treatment
of traumatic injuries.

 Complications: Abdominal fascia dehiscence can lead to
abdominal evisceration, the development of enterocutaneous
fistulas, and the subsequent formation of incisional hernias.

 Risk factors: Contributing factors include technical failure of
surgical techniques or anesthetic relaxation. The occurrence of a
deep wound infection is contributory. Finally, patient factors
include old age, diabetes mellitus, malnutrition, and perioperative
pulmonary disease.

 Best treatment: Local wound care, followed by elective repair of
the fascia defect (incisional hernia) at a later time.

Analysis

Objectives

1. Recognize the contributing factors and preventive measures for
   wound dehiscence and incisional hernias.
2. Become familiar with the treatment of wound dehiscence and
   incisional hernias.

Considerations

Disruption of the fascia following an abdominal operation is referred to
as fascial dehiscence. **Two factors guide the management of fascia
dehiscence found in the early postoperative period: (1) stability of
the intra-abdominal contents, and (2) the presence or absence of
ongoing infection.** In this patient's case, the dehiscence appears stable

and without risk of evisceration. This opinion is based on the appearance of the wound and the time of occurrence 3 weeks after the initial surgery when fibrous scar formation should be sufficient to prevent abdominal evisceration. With the absence of symptoms, fever, and local infection, it is unlikely that an ongoing infectious process exists; however, the complete evaluation should include a leukocyte count with a differential. The treatment of stable wound dehiscence consists of local wound care. The patient needs to be advised that an incisional hernia will eventually develop and will require repair at a later time. **Early reoperation is indicated for patients at risk for evisceration enterocutaneous fistula, or uncontrolled sepsis.**

APPROACH TO FASCIAL DEHISCENCE AND INCISIONAL HERNIAS

Definitions

Fascia dehiscence: The disruption of fascia closure within days of an operation; this complication may occur with or without evisceration.

Evisceration: The presence of abdominal viscera (bowel or omentum) protruding through a fascial dehiscence or traumatic injury.

Enterocutaneous fistula: A direct communication between the small bowel lumen and a skin opening. It can be the primary process leading to wound dehiscence, but this complication frequently develops from wound dehiscence and direct trauma to the underlying bowel. It can be a devastating complication leading to septic and metabolic derangements, long-term disability, and mortality.

Incisional hernia: Delayed development of a fascia defect due to inadequate healing. For some patients this condition can remain undetectable for as long as 5 years after the operation.

Physiology of Wound Healing

Fascial dehiscence and incisional hernias generally develop as a result of inadequate healing of the fascia closure after surgery. **The phases of wound healing are the inflammatory, proliferation, and remodeling**

Table 24–1
PHASES OF WOUND HEALING

Inflammatory phase	Begins immediately and ends within a few days. Inflammatory cells function in sterilizing the wound and secreting growth factors stimulating fibroblasts and keratinocytes in the wound repair process.
Proliferation phase	Deposition of the fibrin-fibrinogen matrix and collagen, resulting in formation of the wound matrix and an increase in wound strength.
Remodeling phase	Capillary regression leads to a less vascularized wound, and with collagen cross-linking there is a gradual increase in wound tensile strength.

phases (Table 24–1). Numerous environmental and host factors can affect the wound-healing process (Table 24–2). An understanding of the temporal occurrence and clinical implications of wound-healing events helps with the appropriate management of these complications (Figure 24–1).

Table 24–2
CLINICAL FACTORS AFFECTING WOUND HEALING

Infections	Lead to delays in fibroblast proliferation, wound matrix synthesis, and deposition.
Nutrition	Vitamin C deficiency leads to inadequate collagen production. Vitamin A deficiency leads to impaired fibroplasias, collagen synthesis, cross-linking, and epithelialization. Vitamin B6 deficiency causes impaired collagen cross-linking.
Oxygenation	Collagen synthesis is augmented with oxygen supplementation.
Corticosteroids	Reduce wound inflammation, collagen synthesis, and contraction.
Diabetes mellitus	Association with microvascular occlusive disease leading to poor wound perfusion; impair keratinocyte growth factor and platelet-derived growth factor functions in the wound.

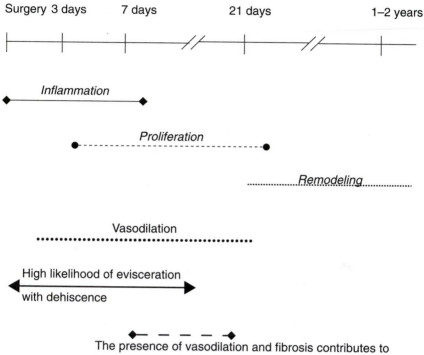

Surgery 3 days   7 days   21 days   1–2 years

Inflammation

Proliferation

Remodeling

Vasodilation

High likelihood of evisceration
with dehiscence

The presence of vasodilation and fibrosis contributes to
increased technical difficulty in reoperation during this time.

Figure 24–1.   Temporal relationships of wound repair and implications in management. (Modified, with permission, from Norton JA, Bollinger RR, Chang AE, et al, eds. Surgery: basic science and clinical evidence. New York: Springer, 2001:221-239.)

Clinical Approach

About 2% to 20% of patients who undergo abdominal surgery develop fascial defects, with the incidence increased fourfold in patients with wound infections. Factors contributing to dehiscence and hernia formation include the patient factors listed in Table 24–2, the technical characteristics listed in Table 24–3, and environmental factors such as tobacco smoking, which causes a decrease in collagen strength. It is generally believed that a significant proportion of fascial defects arise as a result of technical problems.

Table 24–3

TECHNICAL FACTORS RELATED TO ABDOMINAL
CLOSURE FAILURE

Inadequate tissue incorporation
Inappropriate sutures
Excessive tension
Inadequate patient relaxation
Inappropriate suture placement

Management   Fascial defects may be seen early in the postoperative course as drainage of serous or serosanguinous fluid from an otherwise normal wound, or as development of a soft tissue mass beneath the incision. The discovery of significant fluid drainage from an abdominal incision should alarm the examiner to the possibility of fascia dehiscence. When this occurs in the early postoperative period, the initial management consists of opening of the skin incision and meticulously inspecting the wound and fascia. Depending on the precise timing and circumstances, the treatment may require an immediate return to the operating room for repair or initial local wound care with delayed repair of the hernia. **Immediate surgery is indicated for evisceration, impending evisceration, bowel exposure with a concern for enterocutaneous fistula formation, and untreated intra-abdominal infections.** Factors favoring delayed management include a stable dehiscence with no exposed bowel and the risk of a "hostile" abdominal environment associated with reoperation at this time.

Incisional Hernia Repair   Unlike the repair of a groin hernia, the repair of an incisional hernia is associated with a high wound infection rate (7% to 20%) and a high recurrence rate (20% to 50%). Contributing to a poor outcome are the coexisting conditions that may have originally led to development of the hernia (wound infection, patient factors, and fascia weakness). Primary repair of an incisional hernia is performed infrequently because of the high rate of recurrence; therefore, whenever feasible, incisional hernias should be repaired with the placement of prosthetic material. Repair can be performed by an open or a laparoscopic approach, and there is currently no convincing evidence indicating a clear advantage for either repair technique.

Comprehension Questions

[24.1] Which of the following conditions has been shown to have detrimental effects on wound healing?

    A. Obesity
    B. Hyperthyroidism
    C. C-reactive protein deficiency
    D. Diabetes mellitus

[24.2] Five days following abdominal surgery, a patient is noted to have 30 to 40 ml of serosanguinous fluid draining from her midline laparotomy wound. Which of the following is the most appropriate management?

    A. Reinforce the wound dressing and reassure the patient that it is a wound seroma that will resolve spontaneously
    B. Initiate antibiotic therapy
    C. Perform an immediate laparotomy
    D. Open the wound to evaluate the fascia

[24.3] A 36-year-old nursing student undergoes a laparotomy for appendicitis and asks about the possibility of incisional hernia formation. Which one of the following statements is a *true* statement regarding incisional hernias?

    A. The incidence may reach upward of 20% in infected wounds.
    B. Repairs are generally associated with less than 2% recurrence.
    C. Primary repair is associated with less infection and a lower recurrence rate.
    D. Formation of a hernia is nearly always recognized within 3 months after surgery.

Answers

[24.1] **D.** Diabetes mellitus is associated with poor wound healing.

[24.2] **D.** The drainage of a large amount of serosanguinous fluid is highly suggestive of fascia dehiscence; therefore direct evaluation of the fascia should be performed.

[24.3] **A.** The incidence of incisional hernia may approach 20% in infected wounds. Up to 20% to 50% of repairs may eventually fail. Primary repairs are seldom performed because of the high rate of hernia recurrence.

CLINICAL PEARLS

◆ The tensile strength of uncomplicated wounds steadily increases for about 8 weeks, when it reaches 75% to 80% of that of normal tissue; thereafter the wound continues to strengthen, but the strength never reaches that of uninjured tissue.

◆ The use of braided, nonabsorbable suture material is associated with the entrapment of infected debris within the suture material and may lead to an increased number of infections. Therefore, this type of suture material should be avoided in the closing of an infected abdomen.

◆ The 4:1 ratio refers to the optimal ratio of suture length to wound length that is required so that an adequate amount of tissue is incorporated into the fascia closure.

◆ Reclosure of a previously healed fascial incision is associated with lower strength of healing and increased wound breakdown.

REFERENCES

Gilbert AI, Graham MF, Voigt WJ. Incisional, epigastric, and umbilical hernias. In: Cameron JL, ed. Current surgical therapy, 7th ed. St. Louis: Mosby-Year Book, 2001:661–616.

Lorenz HP, Longaker MT. Wounds: biology, pathology, and management. In: Norton JA, Bollinger RR, Chang AE, Lowery SF, Mulvihill SJ, Pass HI, Thompson RW, eds. Surgery: basic science and clinical evidence. New York: Springer, 2001:221–239.

A 58-year-old man underwent an emergency laparotomy with sigmoid colectomy and colostomy for a perforated diverticulitis 7 days previously. Since the operation, the patient has had intermittent fevers to 39.0°C (102.2°F). He has been unable to eat since the surgery because of persistent abdominal distension. His indwelling urinary catheter was removed 2 days ago, and the patient denies any urinary symptoms. On examination, his temperature is 38.8°C (101.8°F), pulse rate 102/min, and blood pressure 130/80. His skin is warm and moist. The lung examination reveals normal breath sounds in both lung fields, and his heart rate is regular without murmurs. His abdomen is distended and tender throughout, and the surgical incision is open without any evidence of infection. His current medications include maintenance intravenous fluids, morphine sulfate, and intravenous cefoxitin and metronidazole. A complete blood count reveals a white blood (WBC) count of 20,500/mm^3.

 What is the most likely diagnosis?

 What is the next step?

ANSWERS TO CASE 25: Postoperative Fever (Intra-abdominal Infection)

Summary: A 58-year-old man has fever and ileus following sigmoid re-section and colostomy for a perforated diverticulum. His physical ex-amination does not reveal infection of the respiratory or urinary system or of the surgical site.

◆ **Most Likely Diagnosis:** Intra-abdominal infection.

◆ **Next step:** A thorough fever workup including an abdominal and a pelvic computed tomography (CT) scan.

Analysis

Objectives

1. Recognize the sources of fever in postoperative patients and be-come familiar with strategies for fever evaluation.
2. Understand the principles of diagnosis and treatment of intra-abdominal infections.
3. Understand the pathogenesis of intra-abdominal infections.

Considerations

Persistent fever following definitive operative therapy for an intra-abdominal infection suggests the persistence of infection or the devel-opment of another infectious process. It is important to bear in mind that a hospitalized patient may have various sources of fever, including nosocomial infections and noninfectious causes. The possibility of uri-nary, respiratory, and blood-borne infections should be assessed with urinalysis, chest radiography, and blood cultures. A CT scan of the ab-domen and pelvis is a useful diagnostic modality for intra-abdominal infections and is indicated in this setting. When identified, abscesses can be drained percutaneously under CT guidance (Figure 25–1). In-flammatory changes without abscesses are suggestive of persistent sec-

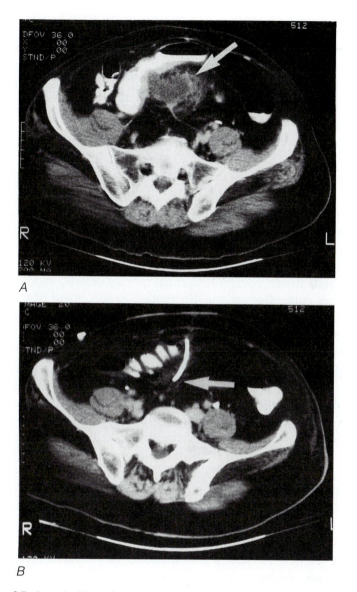

Figure 25–1.   A diverticular abscess noted by arrow (A) and then evacuated by computed tomography–guided percutaneous drainage (B). (Reproduced, with permission, from Schwarz SI, Shires GT, Spencer FC, et al, eds. Principles of surgery, 7th ed. New York: McGraw-Hill, 1999:1041.)

ondary peritonitis. Persistent secondary peritonitis may also be due to inappropriate or inadequate antimicrobial therapy; in these cases, treatment consists of extending the course of therapy or modifying the antimicrobial regimen.

APPROACH TO FEVER AND INTRA-ABDOMINAL INFECTION

Definitions

Postoperative fever: Fever is arbitrarily defined by most clinicians as oral temperature higher than 38.0° to 38.5°C (100.4° to 101.3°F).

Surgical site infections: Infections involving the skin and subcutaneous tissue, which are divided into superficial and deep categories depending on whether there is involvement of the fascia. CT imaging can be helpful when a deep surgical space infection is suspected.

Superficial surgical site infections: Infectious processes above the fascia constitute superficial infections. These are treated primarily by wound exploration and drainage of the infected material, although systemic antibiotic therapy may be needed when there is extensive surrounding cellulitis (>2 cm from the incision margins) or if the patient is immunocompromised.

Deep surgical site infections: Infectious processes involving the fascia. The presence of deep surgical site infection mandates an evaluation for possible deep surgical space infection. A CT scan should be considered if deep surgical space infection is suspected.

Deep surgical space infections: Also referred to as intra-abdominal infections in the setting of postoperative abdominal surgery, they include secondary peritonitis, tertiary peritonitis, and intra-abdominal abscesses.

Secondary microbial peritonitis: Spillage of endogenous microbes into the peritoneal cavity following viscera perforation. The persistence of this infection is affected by microbial inoculum volume, the inhibitory and synergistic effects of the polymicrobial environment, and host response. Recurrent infections may result from insufficient antimicrobial therapy or inadequate control of the infectious source.

Tertiary microbial peritonitis: This condition occurs in patients who fail to recover from intra-abdominal infections despite surgical and/or antimicrobial therapy because of diminished host peritoneal response. Frequently, low virulence or opportunistic pathogens such as *Staphylococcus epidermidis, Enterococcus faecalis,* and *Candida* species are identified.

Intra-abdominal abscess: A defined intraperitoneal collection of inflammatory fluid and microbes resulting from a host compartmentalizing process in which fibrin deposition, omental containment, and ileus of the small bowel localize the infectious material. This response produces loculated, infected inflammatory fluid that cannot be eliminated by the host translymphatic clearance process.

Preemptive antibiotic therapy: Administration of antibiotics when a large microbial inoculum is thought to have occurred, such as with a perforated diverticulum with significant peritoneal spillage. Therapy should be directed toward gram-negative aerobes and anaerobes. The optimal therapeutic duration and endpoints are controversial.

Clinical Approach

Fever that occurs in a hospitalized surgical patient can have a number of causes. These include infections related to the original disease process, such as secondary peritonitis, intra-abdominal abscess, and wound infection. In addition, many hospital-acquired (nosocomial) infections can also occur, including urinary tract infection, pneumonia, bacteremia, intravenous catheter infection, and antibiotic-associated colitis. Noninfectious etiologies include systemic inflammatory response syndrome, endocrinopathies (adrenal insufficiency, thyrotoxicosis), drug reactions, and transfusion reactions. Generally, **a febrile postoperative patient who has had abdominal surgery for an infectious process is presumed to have an intra-abdominal infectious complication until proven otherwise.**

Pathophysiology of Intra-abdominal Infections   Perforation of the gastrointestinal tract results in microbial spillage into the peritoneal cavity.

The severity of peritoneal contamination is related to the location of the perforation that determines the concentration and diversity of endogenous microbes (ie, colon contents with 10^{11} to 10^{14} of aerobic and anaerobic microbes per gram of contents versus stomach contents containing 10^2 to 10^3 aerobic microbes per gram of contents). A number of adaptive host responses occur following the inoculation of bacteria into the peritoneal cavity; these include peritoneal macrophage and polymorphonucleocyte (PMN) recruitment and the development of ileus and fibropurulent peritonitis to localize the spillage. Normal peritoneal activity includes translymphatic clearance of sequestered microbes and inflammatory cells, leading to the resolution of peritonitis. Several factors influence the resolution or progression of secondary peritonitis: (1) the size of the microbial inoculum, (2) the timing of diagnosis and treatment, (3) the inhibitory, synergistic, or cumulative effects of microbes on the growth of other microbes, and (4) the status of the host peritoneal defenses.

The goals in the management of secondary peritonitis are directed toward eliminating the source of microbial spillage (an appendectomy for a perforated appendix or closure of a perforated duodenal ulcer) and early initiation of preemptive antibiotic therapy. With appropriate therapy, secondary peritonitis resolves in the majority of the patients; however, approximately 15% to 30% of individuals develop complications with recurrent secondary peritonitis, tertiary peritonitis, or intra-abdominal abscesses. Factors contributing to the recurrence of secondary peritonitis include inappropriate and/or insufficient antimicrobial therapy and inadequate source control. Tertiary peritonitis, which is primarily due to a failure of the host immune response, is treated with additional antimicrobial therapy and optimization of the host condition. **Patients with suspected deep surgical space infections following abdominal surgery should undergo CT imaging to search for intra-abdominal abscesses.** When identified, abscesses can be treated by percutaneous drainage. Patients with ongoing gastrointestinal tract spillage or abscesses that are inaccessible by percutaneous drainage should undergo open surgical drainage to control the primary source of infection. Initial systemic antibiotic therapy for the treatment of secondary peritonitis should be directed toward anaerobes and gram-negative aerobes, and this can be accomplished with a single broad-spectrum agent or combination therapy (Table 25–1).

Table 25–1
ANTIMICROBIAL THERAPY
FOR INTRA-ABDOMINAL INFECTIONS

Standard dual-agent therapy
    Aminoglycoside plus metronidazole or clindamycin
    This regimen should be used with extreme caution for older patients and those with renal insufficiency; aminoglycoside peak and trough levels should be monitored closely with prolonged use in most if not all patients.
Nonstandard dual-agent therapy
    1. Second- or third-generation cephalosporin plus metronidazole or clindamycin
       For example, cefotetan, cefoxitin, ceftriaxone, cefotaxime, cefepime
    2. Fluoroquinolone plus metronidazole or clindamycin
       Ciprofloxacin, levofloxacin, gatifloxacin
Single-agent therapy
    1. For treatment of mild or moderate infections (eg, perforated appendix in otherwise healthy individuals)
       Cefoxitin, cefotetan, ceftriaxone, ampicillin–sulbactam
    3. For treatment of severe infections or infections in immunocompromised hosts
       Imipenem–cilastatin, meropenin, pipercillin–tazobactam, ticarcillin–cluvulanate

Comprehension Questions

[25.1] A 66-year-old woman undergoes exploratory laparotomy for suspected appendicitis. A ruptured appendix with purulent drainage into the peritoneal cavity is noted. Which of the following statements is most correct regarding this patient's condition?

    A. The resulting infection is a difficult problem to resolve even with appropriate surgical and antimicrobial therapy.

    B. The most common organisms involved are *Candida* and *Pseudomonas* species.

    C. Treatment can be effectively accomplished with the use of first-generation cephalosporins.

    D. Persistent secondary peritonitis may result because of inappropriate antibiotics selection or insufficient duration of therapy.

[25.2] Which of the following is most accurate regarding patients who develop fever during the postoperative period?

    A. They should receive broad-spectrum antibiotics until the fever resolves.

    B. They require no specific therapy because fever is a physiologic response to surgical stress.

    C. A thorough search for the fever source is required. Presumptive antibiotics should be given if the patient exhibits physiologic signs of sepsis or if the patient is immunocompromised.

    D. The patients should undergo an immediate reoperation.

[25.3] A 39-year-old male undergoes ileal resection and bowel anastomosis because of a perforation due to Crohn disease. Following surgery, he has persistent fever and abdominal pain despite the administration of intravenous cefoxitin and gentamicin. A CT scan reveals a 4 × 5 cm heterogeneous fluid collection in the pelvis. Which of the following is the best therapy for this patient?

    A. Add vancomycin to the regimen

    B. Add fluconazole to the regimen

    C. Administer a thrombolytic to dissolve the pelvic hematoma

    D. Percutaneous drainage of the fluid collection

Answers

[25.1] **D.** Inappropriate selection of and insufficient duration of antimicrobial therapy are the major causes of persistent secondary peritonitis. Gram-negative and anaerobic bacteria are the most commonly involved bacteria.

[25.2] **C.** Routine antimicrobial therapy is not indicated for all febrile postoperative patients; however, patients with a poor physiologic reserve and a compromised immune system should be treated with broad-spectrum presumptive antimicrobial therapy prior to definitive diagnosis of the fever source.

[25.3] **D.** This patient likely has an abscess, which is best treated by percutaneous drainage with CT guidance.

CLINICAL PEARLS

❖ Prolonged dysfunction of the gastrointestinal tract following gastrointestinal surgery frequently indicates the presence of intra-abdominal infectious complications, whereas the prompt return of gastrointestinal function following surgery generally indicates the absence of intra-abdominal infections.

❖ Atelectasis is the most common cause of fever in a patient during the first 24 hours following surgery.

❖ With the availability of many effective antibiotics against gram-negative organisms, aminoglycosides are rarely used as first-line therapy.

❖ The colon has a very large number of bacteria (10^{11} to 10^{14} of aerobic and anaerobic microbes per gram of contents) versus the stomach (containing 10^2 to 10^3 aerobic microbes per gram of contents).

❖ Computed tomography imaging is often helpful in identifying intra-abdominal abscesses.

REFERENCES

Barie PS. Perioperative management. In: Norton JA, Bollinger RR, Chang RR, Lowry SF, Mulvihill SJ, Pass HI, Thompson RW, eds. Surgery: basic science and clinical evidence. New York: Springer, 2001:363–395.

Dunn DL: Diagnosis and treatment of infection. In: Norton JA, Bollinger RR, Chang AE, Lowry SF, Mulvihill SJ, Pass HI, Thompson RW, eds. Surgery: basic science and clinical evidence. New York: Springer, 2001:193–219.

O'Grady NP, Barie PS, Bartlett JG, et al: Practice guidelines for evaluating new fever in critically adult patients. Clin Infect Dis 1998;26:1042–1059.

A 22-year-old man presents to the emergency department complaining of headache, palpitations, chest tightness, and nausea that have been occurring intermittently over the past 2 months. He takes no medications and has no significant past medical or family medical history. He appears anxious and diaphoretic. His temperature is 37.2°C (100.0°F), heart rate 112/min, blood pressure 210/102, and respiratory rate 20/min. Immediately following a change from a supine to an upright position, his pulse rate increases to 130/min and his blood pressure drops to 160/86. He has a fine tremor in both hands. The results of the rest of his physical examination are unremarkable. The findings from serum electrolytes studies and a complete blood count are normal. A 12-lead electrocardiogram reveals left ventricular hypertrophy.

◆ **What is the most likely explanation for the patient's signs and symptoms?**

◆ **How would you confirm the diagnosis?**

ANSWERS TO CASE 26: Pheochromocytoma

Summary: A 22-year-old man presents with severe hypertension with orthostatic changes, anxiety, diaphoresis, and tremor, which are signs and symptoms compatible with pheochromocytoma.

◆ **Explanation:** Pheochromocytoma causing excessive catecholamine production.

◆ **Confirm diagnosis:** Documentation of elevated urinary or serum catecholamine levels.

Analysis

Objectives

1. Become familiar with the clinical presentation of a patient with pheochromocytoma.
2. Describe the laboratory studies used for confirming the diagnosis of pheochromocytoma and the imaging modalities used for localizing a pheochromocytoma.
3. Be able to outline a diagnostic plan for pre-, intra-, and postoperative treatment of a patient with a pheochromocytoma.

Considerations

A history of chest pain, palpitation, nausea, and diaphoresis are not specific for pheochromocytoma; however, the presence of these symptoms in a patient with **profound hypertension and severe orthostatic changes are highly suggestive of pheochromocytoma.** The diagnosis can be confirmed by measuring the **serum-free metanephrine levels. A computed tomography (CT) scan of the abdomen should be performed to localize the tumor. All patients require thorough preparation prior to any operative intervention.**

APPROACH TO PHEOCHROMOCYTOMA

Pheochromocytoma is a tumor that most commonly arises from the chromaffin cells of the adrenal medulla and secretes catecholamines. **Pheochromocytoma is known as the "10% tumor" because 10% are bilateral, extra-adrenal, multiple, malignant, or familial.** The hallmark clinical manifestation of pheochromocytoma is **hypertension** that can be either paroxysmal or sustained. **Headache, palpitations, and profuse sweating** are other common manifestations. Anxiety and abdominal pain may also occur.

The diagnosis of pheochromocytoma usually requires a demonstration of excess catecholamine production by one of two methods: **a 24-hour urine collection to test for metanephrine, normetanephrine, and vanillylmandelic acid (VMA) and/or measurement of plasma-free metanephrine levels.** Measurements of plasma-free metanephrine levels have a sensitivity of 99% and a specificity of 89% and as a result have been advocated by some as the initial biochemical test for the diagnosis of pheochromocytoma.

Imaging and Localization

Once a pheochromocytoma has been diagnosed by biochemical studies, tumor localization is the next step. Preoperative imaging studies are also important to exclude multiple, bilateral, or extraadrenal pheochromocytomas. Abdominal CT imaging and magnetic resonance imaging (MRI) have at least 95% sensitivity in detecting an adrenal pheochromocytoma. A pheochromocytoma usually appears bright on a T_2 weighted magnetic resonance image. Both CT imaging and MRI have a specificity of as low as 50% in some studies related to the high frequency of adrenal masses that are not pheochromocytomas. **An iodine-131 *m*-iodobenzylguanidine (MIBG) scan is usually obtained for confirmation of pheochromocytoma because of its superior specificity of 90% to 100%.** Positron emission tomography (PET) imaging can be used when conventional imaging studies cannot localize the tumor.

Patient Preoperative Preparation

A preoperative chest radiograph should be obtained for all patients because the lung is one of the most common sites for metastasis. An electrocardiogram and an echocardiogram are frequently useful, as chronic catecholamine excess may cause cardiomyopathy. **Preoperative blood pressure control is essential to minimize the risk of a hypertensive crisis.** The preferred method is to administer an alpha-adrenergic blocking agent 1 to 2 weeks before surgery. This allows for relaxation of the constricted vascular tree and correction of the reduced plasma volume, which helps to prevent the hypotension that can often occur following tumor removal. A beta-adrenergic blocking agent is added to oppose the reflex tachycardia associated with alpha blockade. In general, **administration of a beta-blocking agent should not be started without prior alpha blockade because this may precipitate a hypertensive crisis related to unopposed alpha-receptor stimulation.**

Traditionally, phenoxybenzamine has been the preferred alpha-adrenergic antagonist. α-Methyl-*p*-tyrosine, which is often used in combination with phenoxybenzamine, competitively inhibits tyrosine hydroxylase, the rate-limiting enzyme in catecholamine synthesis. Newer, selective alpha-1-blocking agents have also been used with good results.

Surgical Concerns

The intraoperative management is critical because of **the danger of large fluctuations in blood pressure, heart rate, and fluid balance.** Usually, continuous blood pressure monitoring is accomplished with an arterial line, and central venous and Foley catheters are inserted for volume assessment and intravenous fluid replacement. An intravenous nitroprusside continuous infusion is often administered for the control of hypertension, and a short-acting beta-blocker, such as esmolol, is used to control any tachycardia. Adrenalectomy can be accomplished either laparoscopically or through an open technique. **Acute hypotension may occur following excision of a pheochromocytoma related to sudden diffuse vasodilatation.** Continuous intravenous neosynephrine is used when the blood pressure fails to respond to fluid administration.

Postoperatively, a normotensive state is achieved in approximately 90% of patients following tumor excision.

Follow-up

Because **histopathologic studies cannot always identify whether a tumor is benign or malignant,** all patients are followed for life. In general, **plasma-free metanephrine levels** are measured 1 month after surgery and at yearly intervals thereafter.

Comprehension Questions

[26.1] Which of the following tests is *best* for excluding the possibility of a pheochromocytoma?

A. CT imaging
B. MRI
C. Plasma catecholamine levels
D. Plasma-free metanephrine levels

[26.2] Which of the following imaging studies has the *highest specificity* when used to confirm the presence of a pheochromocytoma?

A. CT imaging
B. MRI
C. MIBG imaging
D. PET

[26.3] A 22-year-old male is diagnosed as having a pheochromocytoma and is being prepared for adrenalectomy. Which of the following is most important in the preoperative preparation of this patient?

A. Fluid restriction to avoid exacerbation of hypertension
B. Selective beta-agonist therapy to avoid tachycardia

    C. Selective alpha-receptor antagonist for control of hypertension

    D. Cortisol hydroxylase inhibitor for control of heart rate, anxiety, and blood pressure

[26.4] Which of the following statements regarding adrenalectomy for a pheochromocytoma is most correct?

    A. It results in blood pressure improvement, but it is rare that the blood pressure normalizes.

    B. It corrects hypertension only in patients with benign disease.

    C. It may lead to profound intraoperative hypotension.

    D. It should be reserved for patients with hypertension refractory to drug therapy

Answers

[26.1] **D.** Plasma-free metanephrine measurement is 99% sensitive for pheochromocytoma, and so it may be the most effective as a screening test.

[26.2] **C.** An MIBG scan is highly specific in confirming pheochromocytoma.

[26.3] **C.** Due to the catecholamine excess, patients with pheochromocytoma are generally volume depleted, so fluid restriction is not indicated. Beta adrenergic blockade (not agonist) is used after alpha-blockade is achieved. Finally, a tyrosine hydroxylase inhibitor may be used to control the blood pressure.

[26.4] **C.** Excision of a pheochromocytoma may result in immediate intraoperative hypotension.

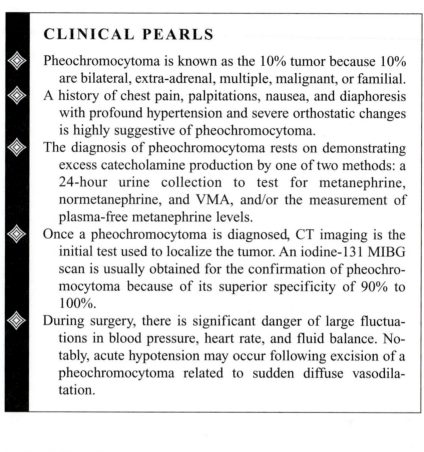

CLINICAL PEARLS

◆ Pheochromocytoma is known as the 10% tumor because 10% are bilateral, extra-adrenal, multiple, malignant, or familial.

◆ A history of chest pain, palpitations, nausea, and diaphoresis with profound hypertension and severe orthostatic changes is highly suggestive of pheochromocytoma.

◆ The diagnosis of pheochromocytoma rests on demonstrating excess catecholamine production by one of two methods: a 24-hour urine collection to test for metanephrine, normetanephrine, and VMA, and/or the measurement of plasma-free metanephrine levels.

◆ Once a pheochromocytoma is diagnosed, CT imaging is the initial test used to localize the tumor. An iodine-131 MIBG scan is usually obtained for the confirmation of pheochromocytoma because of its superior specificity of 90% to 100%.

◆ During surgery, there is significant danger of large fluctuations in blood pressure, heart rate, and fluid balance. Notably, acute hypotension may occur following excision of a pheochromocytoma related to sudden diffuse vasodilatation.

REFERENCES

Graham DJ, McHenry CR. Diagnosis of tumors of the adrenal glands. Hospital Physician. General Surgery Board Review Manual 2001;7(2):1–12.

Graham DJ, McHenry CR. Management of tumors of the adrenal gland. Hospital Physician. General Surgery Board Review Manual 2001;7(3)1–12.

A 52-year-old woman presented with atrial fibrillation and an acute abdomen 8 days ago. She was taken to the operating room for exploratory laparotomy after the initial evaluation suggested the perforation of a hollow viscus. During the operation she was discovered to have a superior mesentery artery (SMA) embolism. She required resection of the infarcted bowel and a jejunal-colonic anastomosis was performed. On postoperative day 8, the patient was provided with enteral nutritional support with a polymeric formula diet through a nasogastric feeding tube. After the initiation of tube feeding, she began to produce a large amount of liquid stools. During the initial evaluation, the results of her physical examination are unremarkable except for postoperative changes. Her stool sample was analyzed and found negative for fecal leukocytes and *Clostridium difficile.*

◆ **What is the most likely diagnosis?**

◆ **What is the best therapy?**

ANSWERS TO CASE 27: Short Bowel Syndrome

Summary: A 52-year-old patient required right colon and extensive small bowel resection after an embolus was found in her SMA 8 days previously. She now has severe diarrhea with stool negative for fecal leukocytes or *C. difficile* toxin.

◆ **Diagnosis:** Malabsorption and diarrhea due to short bowel syndrome.

◆ **Best therapy:** Bowel rest and parenteral nutrition until bowel adaptation occurs.

Analysis

Objectives

1. Be familiar with the different routes of enteral nutritional support.
2. Know the advantages and disadvantages of enteral and parenteral nutrition.
3. Be familiar with small bowel adaptations following massive resection and the options for short- and long-term management of short gut syndrome.

Considerations

A patient presents with postenteral feeding diarrhea after a massive small bowel resection. The SMA supplies blood to most of the small bowel and proximal colon. Because an SMA embolus typically lodges in the distal artery, it causes necrosis of the right colon, ileum, and distal jejunum. In this case, the absence of fecal leukocytes and *C. difficile* toxin makes an infectious cause of the diarrhea unlikely. Her surgical history and negative laboratory test results indicate malabsorption due to short bowel syndrome.

APPROACH TO SHORT BOWEL SYNDROME
AND MALNUTRITION

Pathophysiology

Short bowel syndrome, which results from either extensive bowel resection or a functional defect such as radiation enteritis or severe inflammatory bowel disease, is characterized by diarrhea, dehydration,
electrolyte disturbance, malabsorption, and progressive malnutrition.
The ileum and jejunum of the small intestine are the most important organs in dietary nutrient digestion and absorption. Nutrients are digested
in the small intestinal lumen and absorbed by intestinal epithelia lining
along the lumen. The normal small bowel length is approximately 300
to 500 cm. **An individual with less than 200 cm of small bowel** (or
approximately one-third of the normal intestinal length) **may develop
diarrhea and malabsorption problems.** The pathophysiologic consequences of short bowel syndrome depend on the extent and site of
bowel loss and the adaptation of the remaining bowel. The **most common causes of short bowel syndrome are Crohn disease and mesenteric infarction in adults, and necrotizing enterocolitis and small
bowel volvulus in infants.**
    After an extensive small bowel resection, the remaining intestine un-
dergoes both structural and functional adaptations. Structural changes
include an increase in villous height, mucosal surface area, bowel luminal circumference, and wall thickness; functionally, there is usually
an increase in nutrient absorption and a decrease in diarrhea and malabsorption. The adaptive process begins within 12 to 24 hours and continues for 1 to 2 years. The degree of intestinal adaptation depends on
many variables including the length and site of intestinal loss, the functional status of the remaining bowel, and the time that has elapsed since
the insult. Intestinal failure associated with short bowel syndrome may
be temporary or permanent.

Treatment

Nutritional Support Nutritional support, the cornerstone of short
bowel syndrome management, is utilized to meet caloric requirements

and to promote gut adaptation to allow patients to survive on an oral diet.

Routes of nutritional support: (1) Enteral feeding via mouth, nasogastric or nasojejunal tube, gastrostomy, or jejunostomy; (2) total parenteral nutrition; (3) a combination of both.

Enteral nutrition: The advantages of enteral nutrition are that it is more physiologic, is more economical, and promotes intestinal mucosal hyperplasia and gut adaptation. The disadvantage is that it requires enough healthy intestine to absorb sufficient nutrients.

Parenteral nutrition: The advantages of parenteral nutrition are that it provides sufficient nutrition to support growth and development in children and weight gain and positive nitrogen balance in adults regardless of the length of the bowel. The disadvantages of parenteral nutrition include intestinal atrophy, intravenous line sepsis, high cost, high morbidity and mortality (liver dysfunction), and poor quality of life. The initial decision between enteral and parenteral nutrition is based on whether the patient is able to maintain a healthy nutritional status via enteral feeding alone. With patients receiving only parenteral nutrition, a period of transition is usually needed before full enteral feedings are tolerated. Specific intestinal nutrients, such as the amino acids ornithine and glutamine, triglycerides, and soluble and short-chain fatty acids, are important in promoting adaptation.

Medical Therapy The restriction of oral intake or the use of medications that reduce gastrointestinal motility, such as loperamide and codeine phosphate, are helpful. Other agents that decrease gastric secretion, such as proton pump inhibitors (PPIs) and octreotide, can be used to treat patients with a high output from ostomy sites, severe diarrhea, or malabsorption.

Surgical Therapy Surgical intervention may be useful in carefully selected patients with either temporary or permanent short bowel syndrome. Small bowel transplantation holds potential future promise. A recent study noted that transplant recipients had a 1-year overall survival of 69%, with three-quarters of the survivors not requiring total parenteral nutrition (TPN). Other operative procedures, utilized with the goal of promoting absorption and/or delaying intestinal emptying, include lengthening of the intestine, implantation of artificial intestinal valves, and the use of reversed intestinal segments or a recirculating loop.

Comprehension Questions

[27.1] A 2-month-old preterm baby is noted by a neonatologist to have probable short bowel syndrome. Which of the following is the most likely cause?

    A. Crohn disease
    B. Hirschsprung disease
    C. Necrotizing enterocolitis
    D. Radiation enteritis

[27.2] A 40-year-old man underwent massive bowel resection (from the ligament of Treitz to the midtransverse colon) secondary to SMA thrombosis. Which of the following therapies is most appropriate?

    A. Oral diet
    B. Feeding gastrostomy
    C. Short-term TPN and progressive advance to an oral diet
    D. Small bowel transplantation

[27.3] A 50-year-old woman has undergone multiple small bowel re-sections for severe Crohn disease. She notices weight loss and disturbances in electrolyte levels while on an oral diet. Which of the following therapies is most appropriate?

    A. Complete bowel rest and long-term TPN
    B. Small bowel transplantation.
    C. Continued limited oral diet with short-term TPN support and progress toward a total oral diet.
    D. Continued observation and no intervention at this time.

Answers

[27.1] **C.** Necrotizing enterocolitis is the most common cause of short bowel syndrome in an infant of this age, particularly a preterm infant.

[27.2] **D.** The loss of the entire absorptive surface of the bowel in this patient is incompatible with enteral nutritional tolerance because there is no ileum or jejunum left. Therefore, small bowel transplantation is an appropriate consideration.

[27.3] **C.** Initial TPN and a subsequent slow reintroduction of enteral feeding are appropriate for this patient to allow for adaptive changes in the intestine.

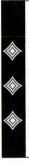

CLINICAL PEARLS

Individuals with less than 200 cm (one-third) of small bowel are at risk for diarrhea and malabsorption.

The most common causes of short bowel syndrome in adults are Crohn disease and mesenteric infarction.

Selected patients with short bowel syndrome may be candidates for small bowel transplantation.

REFERENCES

Platell CFE, Coster J, McCauley RD, Hall JC. The management of patients with the short bowel syndrome. World J Gastroenterol 2002;8(1):113–120.

Wilmore DW, Byrne TA, Persinger RL. Short bowel syndrome: new therapeutic approaches. Curr Probl Surg 1997;34(5):391–444.

A 43-year-old woman presents with a sudden onset of abdominal pain. She denies previous abdominal complaints. Her systolic blood pressure is 88 mm Hg on evaluation and becomes stable at 120 mmHg after the infusion of 2 L of intravenous fluid. The abdominal examination demonstrates no peritoneal signs, her bowel sounds are hypoactive, and there is mild right upper quadrant tenderness. The hematocrit value is 22%. A computed tomography (CT) scan is performed and demonstrates free intra-abdominal blood and a 5-cm solid mass in the right hepatic lobe with evidence of recent bleeding into the mass. By history, the patient denies recent trauma, weight loss, a change in bowel habits, hematemesis, or hematochezia. The only medication she takes is an oral contraceptive agent, which she has been using without problems for about 20 years.

◆ **What are your next steps?**

◆ **What is the most likely diagnosis?**

ANSWERS TO CASE 28: Liver Tumor

Summary: A 43-year old woman who uses an oral contraceptive presents with acute abdominal pain, hypotension, anemia, and recent intra-abdominal hemorrhage. CT imaging shows a right hepatic tumor.

 Next steps: Hemodynamic monitoring and admission to the intensive care unit with serial hematocrit determinations are indicated. Once the patient is stable, the etiology of the liver mass should be sought.

 Most likely diagnosis: Hepatic adenoma with hemorrhage.

Analysis

Objectives

1. Develop a differential diagnosis for hepatic masses based on patient characteristics and risk factors.
2. Know the pertinent differences in the management of primary and secondary liver masses.
3. Understand the natural history and imaging characteristics of liver tumors to avoid unnecessary investigations and operations.

Considerations

Most patients with liver tumors are asymptomatic or may have only vague symptoms. This patient's dramatic presentation is unusual when compared to that of all patients with liver tumors but represents a classic presentation of hepatic adenoma complicated by hemorrhage. This type of tumor was quite uncommon prior to the introduction of oral contraceptives, but this disease process is now recognized as being associated with exposure to estrogenic compounds. Benign focal liver masses are present in 9% to 10% of the general population, and most of these individuals are asymptomatic and can be treated with observation. Hepatic adenoma is an exception to this rule. Because of the propensity of these tumors to produce symptoms, cause hemorrhage, and undergo malignant transformation, most patients with hepatic adenomas should be advised to undergo tumor resection. Hepatic adenomas are hormonally stimulated; therefore, some patients with small, asymptomatic adenomas can be initially treated with cessation of the use of oral contraceptives and close surveillance at 3- to 6-month intervals.

APPROACH TO HEPATIC TUMORS

Definitions

Primary liver tumor: A tumor originating from liver tissue and derived from hepatocyte, bile duct epithelial, or mesenchymal tissue. This tumor may be benign, have a potential for malignant transformation, or be frankly malignant in nature.

Secondary liver tumor: A tumor that arises from tissue outside the liver and spreads to the liver by a metastatic process. This tumor is by definition malignant.

Benign tumor: A tumor that does not have the biologic ability to spread via the lymphatic or vascular system. This type of tumor may cause significant symptoms or may be locally aggressive.

Malignant tumor: A tumor with the potential to spread by either a lymphatic or a hematogenous route.

Focal nodular hyperplasia (FNH):   The second most common benign liver tumor, which is usually found in reproductive-age women. Most FNH is asymptomatic and is discovered incidentally. FNH is a truly benign tumor without malignant potential. Some FNH may be difficult to distinguish from adenomas on the basis of radiographic criteria, and has a characteristic "central scar" pattern on a CT scan. Biopsy may be needed if the tumor cannot be differentiated from hepatic adenoma. Surgery is indicated when malignancy cannot be excluded and when FNH produces severe symptoms.

Hemangioma: The most common benign liver tumor. This lesion may produce vague abdominal pain but frequently is asymptomatic. **Spontaneous rupture is rare.** The diagnosis may be made on the basis of contrast CT imaging, magnetic resonance imaging, or tagged red blood cell scan findings. **Biopsy is contraindicated because it may result in life-threatening hemorrhage.** Indications for surgery are severe symptoms, inability to rule out the possibility of malignancy, and rupture.

Clinical Approach

Liver tumors may be found incidentally or during the evaluation of nonspecific abdominal symptoms; however, more frequently, they are identified in patients at risk for primary or secondary liver tumors (eg, a patient with cirrhosis or with a history of advanced breast carcinoma who develops upper abdominal pain). The approach to a hepatic mass in a patient begins with a thorough history and physical examination, imaging studies, measurement of serum tumor markers, and in some cases tissue biopsy. **The primary goals of the evaluation** are to determine whether the lesion in question is **a primary versus a secondary liver tumor, characterize the nature of the tumor, and define the location and local extent of the mass.**

Imaging Liver Tumors   Selection of the imaging modality is perhaps the most crucial aspect of the evaluation. Proper selection of imaging studies may help establish the diagnosis of many liver tumors, thus avoiding unnecessary biopsies and/or operations for some patients. Although liver tumors are readily visualized by ultrasonography and CT scans, these images generally provide insufficient information for patient treatment. CT with angioportography, magnetic resonance imaging (MRI), angiography, and laparoscopic ultrasonography are the modalities available for the further characterization of liver tumors. The imaging selection criteria for primary and secondary liver tumors are listed in Table 28–1.

Secondary Liver Tumors   The liver is a frequent site of malignant metastasis, most commonly involving colorectal carcinoma. Listed below are the characteristics associated with secondary liver tumors.

1. Resection of a primary tumor with known metastatic potential within the previous 5 years (eg, a history of stage III adenocarcinoma 2 years previously).

Table 28-1

IMAGING MODALITIES FOR LIVER TUMORS

MODALITY	HEMANGIOMA	FOCAL HYPERPLASIA	ADENOMA	HEPATOCELLULAR CARCINOMA	METASTATIC ADENOCARCINOMA
Computed tomography angioportography	High sensitivity and specificity, early contrast enhancement with peripheral outlining of tumor	Low specificity (central scar is characteristic finding)	Low specificity	Low specificity	High sensitivity and specificity, gold standard
Magnetic resonance imaging	High sensitivity and specificity	Low specificity (central scar is characteristic finding)	Low specificity	Low specificity	High sensitivity and specificity
Angiography	Gold standard test with high sensitivity and specificity, but invasive	High sensitivity and specificity, but invasive	Low specificity	Low specificity	Infrequently used
Laparoscopic ultrasound	Poor	Poor	Helpful when combined with laparoscopic biopsy	Gold standard test	Highly sensitive when combined with laparoscopic biopsy
Biopsy	Contraindicated because of high risk for bleeding	Rarely useful	Helpful	Mandatory	Mandatory

2. Current signs and symptoms of an untreated primary tumor with known metastatic potential (eg, a large left breast mass and multiple hepatic lesions in a 74-year-old woman).
3. Miliary or diffuse distribution of hepatic lesions.
4. Significant elevation of tumor marker levels (>10-fold) in the setting of a new liver mass.

When a secondary liver tumor of unknown primary origin is identified, an investigation to identify the primary malignancy should be undertaken. Important in this evaluation are the history and physical examination. Weight loss, a history of new narrow-caliber stools, and a rectal examination with hemocult-positive results should prompt further gastrointestinal tract evaluation. A history of long-time smoking in an elderly male with hematemesis and a new hilar mass seen on chest radiography should prompt further evaluation of the respiratory tract, including a cytologic examination of the sputum, bronchoscopy, and subsequent CT-guided biopsy. The search for the primary tumor is important not only in treating the primary site but also in considering treatment of the liver metastasis. Although the presence of liver metastasis frequently indicates an advanced tumor stage and may preclude the possibility of cure, certain tumor types and distribution in carefully selected patients are amenable to curative resection or ablative therapy. Liver transplantation has no role in the treatment of patients with secondary liver tumors.

Primary Liver Tumors   Tumor markers are invaluable tools in the evaluation of both secondary and primary liver masses. Although the specificity of most tumor markers for a given primary cancer is not high, these assays are sensitive in most cases and are an important part of the workup for liver masses. Table 28–2 lists some of the primary tumor markers that are helpful in the diagnosis of liver masses.

Many liver tumors are either cancerous or have significant premalignant potential or significant morbidity such as bleeding or the production of abdominal pain. For this reason, early surgical consultation is recommended to facilitate the appropriate workup and diagnosis. When appropriate imaging studies are unable to verify the lesion as a tumor without malignant potential, biopsy of the mass or masses may be needed to determine the tumor type and subsequent therapy. Liver

Table 28–2
TUMOR MARKERS POTENTIALLY USEFUL FOR
IDENTIFYING THE ORIGIN OF SECONDARY
LIVER TUMORS

TUMOR MARKER*	TYPE OF CANCER
CEA	Colon cancer
AFP	Hepatocellular carcinoma
CA 19-9	Pancreatic cancer
CA 125	Ovarian cancer
β-hCG	Testicular cancer
PSA	Prostate cancer
CA 50	Pancreatic cancer
Neuron-specific enolase	Small cell lung cancer
CA 15-3	Breast cancer
Ferritin	Hepatocellular carcinoma

*CEA, carcinoembryonic antigen; AFP, α-fetoprotein; CA 19-9, carbohydrate antigen 19-9; CA 125, carbohydrate antigen 125; β-hCG, β-human chorionic gonadotropin; PSA, prostate-specific antigen; CA 50, carbohydrate antigen 50; CA 15-3, carbohydrate antigen 15-3.

resection is both safe and in many cases may provide either a cure or long-term survival benefits. **The cornerstone of workup for a liver mass is the development of an appropriate differential diagnosis based on history and physical examination, and appropriate imaging to facilitate diagnosis.**

Comprehension Questions

[28.1] A 30-year-old woman is noted to have a hepatic mass on laparoscopy for a sterilization procedure. She undergoes a liver biopsy which reveals focal nodular hyperplasia. Which of the following is the most correct statement regarding this condition?

A. These tumors have malignant potential over 10-20 years
B. Surgical excision is often the best therapy
C. Angiography has high sensitivity and specificity for the diagnosis of this tumor
D. Oral contraceptive use is a risk factor

[28.2] A 65-year-old man is found to have a 6-cm mass of his liver on sonography of his gall bladder. He has a history of hepatitis B surface antigen present on serology, but his liver transaminase levels are within normal limits. Which of the following is the most appropriate therapy for this patient?

A. Superior mesenteric artery embolization procedure
B. Surgical resection
C. Intravenous interferon therapy
D. Prolonged antibiotic therapy for probable amebic abscess

[28.3] A 75-year-old icteric woman is noted to have multiple lesions in her liver which on CT imaging is suspicious for metastatic cancer. Which of the following is the most likely source of the primary cancer?

A. Stomach
B. Lung
C. Colon
D. Cervix

Answers

[28.1] **C.** Focal nodular hyperplasia is the second most common hepatic tumor. It is not associated with oral contraceptive use, and is usually asymptomatic. It has no malignant potential, and rarely needs biopsy for diagnosis since angiography is an excellent diagnostic tool for this disorder.

[28.2] **B.** This patient is at risk for hepatocellular carcinoma since he has a large hepatic mass and a likely chronic hepatitis B infection (surface antigen positive). Surgical resection is the best therapy for early stage disease and the only hope for cure in this condition. Interferon therapy is used for hepatitis C disease.

[28.3] **C.** The colon is the most common primary site when metastatic disease is found in the liver.

CLINICAL PEARLS

◈ Hemangiomas are the most common benign tumors of the liver and are usually asymptomatic.

◈ Hepatic adenomas are associated with estrogen use and should be excised because of the risk of hemorrhage or malignant transformation.

◈ The most common metastatic disease to the liver is colorectal cancer.

◈ Because of the risk of hemorrhage, hepatic hemangiomas should be ruled out prior to needle biopsy.

REFERENCES

Blumgart LH, Fong Y. Surgery of the liver and biliary tract, 3rd ed. Philadelphia: Saunders, 2000.
Dutta S, Warren RS. Benign liver tumors. In: Cameron JL. Current surgical therapy, 6th ed. St. Louis: Mosby-Year Book, 1998:331–346.

A 62-year-old man presents to the emergency department with a 1-week history of left lower quadrant abdominal pain and diarrhea. He complains of increased pain, nausea, vomiting, and fever. He has had two prior episodes of similar left lower quadrant pain that resolved with antibiotic treatment alone. He has no cardiac or pulmonary risk factors. On examination, his blood pressure is 140/80, heart rate 110/min, and temperature 101.5°F. His abdomen is soft and mildly distended, with left lower quadrant tenderness to palpation. He does not have evidence of generalized peritonitis. His white blood cell (WBC) count is 20,000/mm³.

 What is the most likely diagnosis?

 How would you confirm the diagnosis?

 What are the complications associated with this disease process?

ANSWERS TO CASE 29: Diverticulitis

Summary: A 62-year-old man presents with signs and symptoms compatible with recurrent sigmoid diverticulitis.

◆ **Most likely diagnosis:** Acute sigmoid diverticulitis with an abscess.

◆ **Confirmation of diagnosis:** Computed tomography (CT) imaging demonstrating sigmoid diverticula, colonic wall thickening, and mesenteric fat stranding.

◆ **Associated complications:** Perforation, abscess formation, bowel obstruction, and development of fistulas.

Analysis

Objectives

1. Be able to explain the etiology of diverticular disease and the pathophysiology of diverticulitis.
2. Be able to discuss the workup and management of diverticulitis and its complications.

Considerations

This patient's clinical history of left lower quadrant pain and fever are suggestive of acute sigmoid diverticulitis. Although he has no evidence of generalized peritonitis, the presence of fever, leukocytosis, and tachycardia are of concern. **A CT scan in this case is very helpful in assessing for complications of diverticulitis, particularly an abscess.** Small mesenteric abscesses associated with diverticulitis usually resolve with antibiotic therapy alone, whereas large abscesses may require CT-guided drainage in addition to antibiotic therapy. If the patient fails to improve clinically after 72 hours with nonoperative treatment, surgical intervention is usually warranted. Over the long term, the risk of recurrence is high given the patient's prior history; therefore, elective surgical resection with primary anastomosis is recommended even if the current bout of infection is successfully treated with conservative measures.

APPROACH TO DIVERTICULITIS

Definitions

Diverticulosis: Outpouchings of the colon that do not contain all layers of the colon wall, most commonly in the sigmoid colon in Western societies. Right-sided or cecal diverticulosis tends to occur in Asian populations.

Diverticulitis: Inflammation of a diverticulum caused by obstruction of the neck of the diverticulum and microperforation.

Clinical Approach

The diagnosis of diverticulitis can often be made clinically based on history and a physical examination. However, when the diagnosis is uncertain, when there are signs of systemic toxicity, or when there is a lack of improvement, further diagnostic studies are indicated. An abdominal CT scan is the radiologic examination of choice. A barium enema is generally deferred because of concerns for intraperitoneal leakage of barium, and colonoscopy should be used with caution. However, after the acute episode is resolved, these tests can be used to document the presence of diverticulosis or fistulas and to assess for other pathologic conditions such as malignancies.

Uncomplicated Diverticulitis Simple or uncomplicated diverticulitis can usually be managed nonoperatively. Mild cases of diverticulitis can be treated on an outpatient basis, but otherwise patients should be hospitalized for hydration, treatment with intravenous antibiotics, bowel rest, and observation. After the clinical resolution of acute diverticulitis, patients with their first episode who are older than age 50 years and who are not immunocompromised do not require further treatment.

However, patients who are **immunocompromised tend be unresponsive to medical treatment alone and usually require surgical intervention.** Patients who have had two or more episodes of diverticulitis should undergo elective resection. Because of an increased risk of complications and a more aggressive course, surgical resection may be indicated in patients less than 40 years old with their first episode of diverticulitis.

Complicated Diverticulitis   **Complicated diverticulitis typically requires surgical management.** Perforated diverticulitis with peritonitis should be treated with surgical exploration. If the patient is hemody-

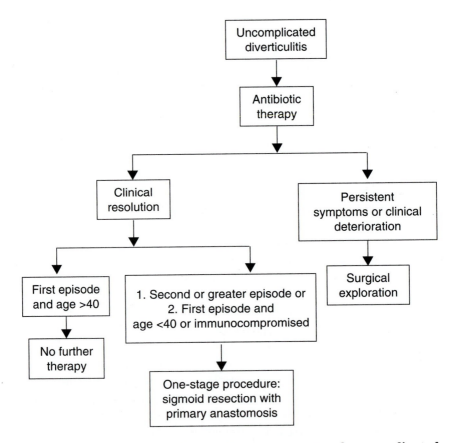

Figure 29–1. An algorithm for the management of uncomplicated diverticulitis.

namically unstable or fecal peritonitis is present, surgical resection, colostomy, and closure of the rectal stump (Hartmann procedure) are recommended. Reanastomosis should then be performed at a later date. In the absence of significant contamination, primary anastomosis can be performed with or without proximal diversion.

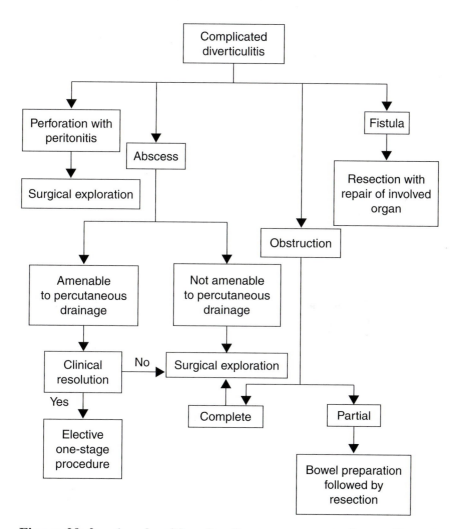

Figure 29–2. An algorithm for the management of complicated diverticulitis–early complications.

Perforation that results in localized fluid collection or a diverticular abscess can be initially managed with nonoperative therapy in the absence of peritoneal signs or systemic toxicity. Typically, mesenteric abscesses are treated with antibiotic therapy, and pelvic abscesses can be initially managed with percutaneous drainage. An elective one-stage procedure should then be performed at a later date. Intestinal obstruction can occur either at the time that acute diverticulitis occurs secondary to inflammation or at a later date because of a stricture. If the patient has a partial bowel obstruction, resection with anastomosis may be feasible after bowel preparation. However, patients with complete bowel obstruction should undergo urgent surgical intervention.

Diverticular fistulas can occur between the sigmoid colon and the bladder, vagina, skin, or another loop of bowel. A barium enema, a CT scan, and sigmoidoscopy can be used to attempt to visualize a fistula. Cystoscopy or a vaginal speculum examination can be utilized to demonstrate a colovesical or a colovaginal fistula, respectively. **Treatment consists of resection of the sigmoid colon, excision of the fistulous tract, and repair or resection of the other involved organ.** See Figures 29–1 and 29–2 for management schemes.

Comprehension Questions

[29.1]   A 57-year-old man presents to his primary care physician with left-sided abdominal pain of 5 days' duration, nausea, vomiting, and diarrhea. He is unable to maintain his oral intake at home. On presentation, he has mild tenderness to palpation in the left lower quadrant without peritoneal signs. His WBC count is 14,000/mm^3. He has never had a similar episode in the past. What is the appropriate treatment for this patient?

A. Hospitalize for bowel rest, administration of intravenous fluids and antibiotics, and close observation

B. Prescribe a course of outpatient antibiotics with appropriate follow-up

C. Obtain an emergent barium enema to diagnose diverticulitis

D. Consult the surgery department regarding future elective sigmoid resection

[29.2] A 61-year-old woman presents to the emergency room with left-sided abdominal pain of 10 days' duration. She has had constipation and states that her last bowel movement was 2 days ago. She also complains of fever to 102°F and nausea and vomiting. On examination, she is diffusely tender to palpation. Plain films demonstrate dilated loops of small bowel and a paucity of gas in the rectum. Her WBC count is 26,000/mm^3. What is the appropriate next step in the treatment of this patient?

A. Barium enema to confirm the diagnosis of diverticulitis
B. Urgent sigmoidoscopy to evaluate for diverticulitis versus colonic neoplasm
C. Urgent surgical exploration
D. Admission for nasogastric decompression and administration of intravenous antibiotics

[29.3] A 59-year-old woman presents to her primary care physician with complaints of pneumaturia or air in the urine and recurrent urinary tract infections. She has a prior history of diverticulitis occurring 6 months ago. Which of the following is an appropriate next step?

A. Order a CT scan of the abdomen to look for a colovesical fistula.
B. Schedule the patient for cystoscopy to look for a fistula opening.
C. Order a barium enema to demonstrate a possible fistula.
D. All of the above.

[29.4] Which of the following is the most common cause of gastrointestinal tract fistulas?

A. Peptic ulcer disease
B. Inadvertent enterotomy
C. Crohn disease
D. Ulcerative colitis
E. Diverticulitis

Answers

[29.1] **A.** The patient clinically has diverticulitis and is unable to maintain oral hydration. He should be admitted to the hospital. Surgery is not indicated at this point for a patient his age with his first episode of uncomplicated diverticulitis.

[29.2] **C.** The patient clinically has evidence of a complete bowel obstruction, and the tenderness and leukocytosis are worrisome. Surgical exploration is therefore warranted. A barium enema and colonoscopy are contraindicated in this situation.

[29.3] **D.** All of the listed tests can be used to confirm the diagnosis of a colovesical fistula and to localize the fistulous tract.

[29.4] **E.** The most common cause of gastrointestinal tract fistulas is diverticulitis, usually causing a colovesical (colon-to-bladder) fistula. Air or stool in the urine or frequent urinary tract infections are typical.

CLINICAL PEARLS

◆ Computed tomography imaging is often helpful in identifying and guiding percutaneous drainage of abscesses related to diverticulitis.

◆ Diverticulitis is the most common cause of gastrointestinal tract fistulas.

◆ Surgical intervention for uncomplicated diverticulitis is appropriate for patients with multiple episodes and possibly for the first episode in a young patient.

◆ Complicated diverticulitis such as perforation or fistula is usually treated surgically.

REFERENCE

Knol JA. Colonic diverticular disease. In: Bell RH, Rikkers LF, Mulholland MW, eds. Digestive tract surgery: a text and atlas. Philadelphia: Lippincott-Raven, 1996:1363–1386.

During a routine physical examination, a family physician identifies an asymptomatic pulsatile abdominal mass in a 62-year-old man. The ultrasound evaluation that followed demonstrated a 4.2-cm aneurysm in the infrarenal aorta. This patient is subsequently referred to you for evaluation and further treatment. His past medical history is significant for hypertension and stable angina. He has a history of smoking 40 packs of cigarettes per year. His current medications include aspirin, a beta-blocker, and nitrates. The patient describes himself as an active individual who is retired and plays 18 holes of golf twice a week. On examination, the carotid pulses and upper extremity pulses are found to be normal. The abdomen is nontender with a prominent aortic pulsation. Pulses in the femoral and popliteal regions are easily palpated and appear more prominent than usual.

◆ **What are the complications associated with this disease process?**

◆ **What is the best treatment?**

ANSWERS TO CASE 30: Abdominal Aortic Aneurysm

Summary: A 62-year-old reasonably healthy man presents with an asymptomatic 4.2-cm abdominal aortic aneurysm (AAA).

◆ **Complications:** Rupture, thrombosis, distal embolism, and other peripheral aneurysms.

◆ **Best treatment:** The best treatment for this patient is debatable. The risk of complications from the aneurysm must be weighed against the risk of surgical or endovascular intervention.

Analysis

Objectives

1. Be familiar with the presentation, evaluation, treatment, and follow-up of patients with aneurysms.
2. Be familiar with the risks and outcomes associated with elective open aneurysm repair, elective endovascular repair, and the repair of ruptured aneurysms.

Considerations

A relatively healthy 62-year-old man presenting with a 4.2-cm AAA can be observed with serial examinations and repeated ultrasonography or undergo elective aneurysm repair. The risks and benefits of the options must be discussed with the patient. If the patient wishes to undergo elective repair, a thorough evaluation to assess other comorbidities should to be undertaken.

APPROACH TO ABDOMINAL AORTIC ANEURYSM

More than 95% of AAAs develop as complications of atherosclerosis, and more than 90% are infrarenal in location. Many are found asymptomatically, but some can cause distal emboli or pain. Others are found in association with other peripheral (ie, popliteal and femoral) aneurysms. The majority of AAA are detected asymptomatically. AAA is a disease where size matters. Because of the relationship between AAA size and the risk of rupture, the maximal diameter is an important discriminant in assessment and management. The law of Laplace (wall tension is proportional to the square of the radius and the inverse of wall thickness) provides the physics behind the pathophysiology of AAA rupture. **Once an AAA reaches 5 cm in diameter, the risk of rupture is 25% over 5 years.** At 6 cm it rises to 40% over 5 years, and at 7 cm it exceeds 60% over 5 years.

Repair of a ruptured AAA can be attempted in only half of patients, as the others never reach the hospital alive. Even today, 40% to 60% of patients with a ruptured AAA do not survive emergency surgery. As good-risk patients have a mortality rate of 1% to 3% when undergoing elective surgery, the **usual criterion for recommending repair is when an AAA reaches 5 cm.** However, as AAAs arise in patients with atherosclerosis, there is a significant association with other risks and comorbidities that can complicate repair. **Cardiac complications remain the most common cause of perioperative morbidity and mortality.**

Abdominal aortic aneurysms found on routine examination should have their size confirmed by an imaging study. Ultrasound is inexpensive and safe but not as reproducible over time. Computed tomography (CT) scanning requires radiation exposure but can give enough information to assess suitability for endovascular aneurysm repair (EVAR) or conventional open surgery. Arteriography cannot diagnose an AAA as it only delineates the lumen of a vessel. However, a preoperative angiogram helps in operative planning for both EVAR and open repairs. Open repair has withstood the test of time and remains the standard of care. However, patients with a higher risk for open repair complications (severe coronary artery disease, chronic obstructive pulmonary disease, obesity, malignancy, adhesions, and others) can be offered protection from rupture with EVAR. One must realize that EVAR currently has a risk of rupture of 0.7% to 1.0% per year (according to the Eurostar Registry). In addition, because of technical issues in EVAR, following EVAR the patient requires intensive imaging follow-up every 3 to 6 months. Because of associated risk profiles, the ultimate perioperative patient mortality for EVAR is still in the 2% to 3% range. **The actual recommendation for EVAR versus open AAA repair should be made by a trained vascular specialist well versed in both techniques.**

For a patient who presents with AAA rupture (back pain, hypotension, and a pulsatile epigastric mass), operative open repair is the most available and most potentially life-saving therapy. If AAA rupture is clinically suspected, the patient should undergo emergent operative repair. There is no role for radiologic imaging if the clinical impression is a ruptured AAA—the delay involved in obtaining imaging is too risky for the patient as compared to a potentially negative exploration.

Comprehension Questions

[30.1] What is considered appropriate surveillance for a patient with a small, asymptomatic AAA?

    A. Observation with yearly ultrasound
    B. Observation with a yearly CT scan
    C. Ultrasound of the femoral and popliteal arteries
    D. All of the above

[30.2] Which of the following conditions does *not* indicate the need for operative repair in the patient described at the beginning of the case?

    A. Presenting 11 months later with an AAA that is 5.5 cm in size
    B. Unexplained back pain in a 4.2-cm aneurysm and normotensive.
    C. Bilateral embolization to all his toes.
    D. Presenting 3 years later with shock and severe abdominal pain.
    E. The AAA is 4.3 cm on ultrasound 2 years later

Answers

[30.1] **D.** All of the listed choices are part of a conservative protocol for the follow-up of patients with AAA. The choice of ultrasound or computed tomography for the imaging depends on which is more available in one's practice environment.

[30.2] **E.** The patient in D is presenting with a rupture. The patient in B is the most controversial candidate for operative repair, however, if a complete workup cannot find another cause of back pain, then the AAA must be implicated and strong recommendations for repair should be made.

CLINICAL PEARLS

◈ Patient diagnosed with an AAA should have a thorough pulse examination to look for associated aneurysms in the periphery and/or concomitant occlusive disease.

◈ Abdominal aortic aneurysms are palpated in the epigastrium, and iliac aneurysms in the infraumbilical position.

◈ In general, AAA exceeding 5 cm should undergo elective repair because of the risk of rupture.

◈ In the case of a suspected rupture, negative laparotomy findings are much better than delay in control of the AAA in the operating room.

REFERENCES

Shermerhorn ML, Cronenwett JL. Abdominal aortic aneurysm. In: Cameron JL, ed. Current surgical therapy, 7th ed. St. Louis: Mosby-Year Book, 2001:807–812.

Vallabhaneni SR, Harris PL. Lessons learned from the EUROSTAR registry on endovascular repair of abdominal aortic aneurysm repair. Eur J Radiol 2001; 39(1):34–41.

A 45-year-old woman is admitted to the general surgical ward after an elective cholecystectomy. Eight hours later, a nurse notes the following vital signs: heart rate 130/min, respiratory rate 24/min, blood pressure 90/74, temperature 36.8°C (98.2°F), and 91% O_2 saturation with a 6-L/min nasal cannula. The physical examination reveals a mildly distended, nontender abdomen. The patient is confused and agitated. The skin turgor is poor. Only 50 mL of urine output has been recorded over the last 4 hours. Hemoglobin obtained at the onset of hypotension was 11.5 g/dL (compared to an immediate postoperative hemoglobin of 13.1 g/dL).

◆ **What is the most likely diagnosis?**

◆ **What should be the next step in treatment?**

ANSWERS TO CASE 31: Hemorrhagic Shock

Summary: A 45-year-old woman presents with postoperative hypotension probably due to hemorrhagic shock.

◆ **Most likely diagnosis:** Hemorrhagic shock secondary to postoperative bleeding.

◆ **Next steps:** Blood transfusion and a return to the operating room for surgical control of the bleeding.

Analysis

Objectives

1. Recognize the presence of hemorrhagic shock and understand the principles of early treatment.
2. Describe the causes of postoperative hypotension.
3. Understand the indications for invasive monitoring and relate the findings associated with various states of shock.

Considerations

Hypotension is not uncommonly seen in patients who undergo major surgery. Although most postoperative hypotension is benign in nature, a cause of greater concern (such as postoperative bleeding) should be assumed until proven otherwise. This requires clinical judgment and assessments at the patient's bedside. **In patients with acute and active bleeding, the hemoglobin level may not drop proportionately to the blood loss** because enough time has not elapsed for equilibration in the absence of rapid fluid resuscitation. In other words, **patients with active bleeding may have a relatively normal hemoglobin level on initial evaluation.** For the patient described above, other possible causes of hypotension include hypovolemia from third-space fluid loss, a reaction to medication (eg, narcotics and anesthetic agents), and cardiopulmonary complications unrelated to surgery (Table 31–1). An-

Table 31–1
CAUSES OF POSTOPERATIVE HYPOTENSION

Postoperative bleeding
Intravascular volume depletion due to third-space losses
Myocardial infarction
Pulmonary embolus
Cardiac arrhythmia
Sepsis
Medications (opioids, sedatives, antihypertensive medications, others)
Anaphylactic shock
Mechanical (cardiac tamponade, tension pneumothorax)
Adrenal insufficiency

other point to keep in mind in evaluating hypotensive patients is that younger individuals with a greater physiologic reserve can tolerate relatively larger amounts of blood loss prior to showing overt signs of shock. This patient has presented with clear physiologic signs of shock associated with a drop in the hemoglobin level, which strongly suggests hemorrhage; the treatment for this condition is resuscitation and reoperation.

APPROACH TO HEMORRHAGIC SHOCK

An initial evaluation of postoperative hypotension should include a review of the pertinent history and a physical examination, recent vital signs and urine output, all administered medications, and a focused examination for signs of bleeding. The physical examination signs may be subtle in postoperative patients: the abdomen may not be distended, and the operative site may not be tender because of postoperative narcotic administration. Patients without signs of cardiac failure should initially receive an intravenous fluid bolus of isotonic crystalloid.

Patients who initially respond to fluid therapy but subsequently experience a drop in arterial blood pressure after fluid resuscitation should be assumed to have ongoing bleeding. This type of clinical response is an indication for a blood transfusion. In addition to **strongly considering** a return to the operating room, these patients

Table 31–2

HEMODYNAMIC VARIABLES IN DIFFERENT SHOCK STATES

SHOCK STATE	CARDIAC INDEX	SYSTEMIC VASCULAR RESISTANCE	PULMONARY CAPILLARY WEDGE PRESSURE	PRIME MOVER*
Normal	2.4–3.0 L/min-m²	800–1200 dyne·s or dyne-sec/cm⁵	8–12 mmHg	Not applicable
Distributive (sepsis, neurogenic, anaphylaxis)	Elevated	Decreased (due to decreased vascular tone)	Low to normal	Decreased vascular tone
Cardiogenic (myocardial infarction, cardiomyopathy)	Decreased	Increased	Increased	Decreased cardiac contractility
Hypovolemic (hemorrhage, dehydration)	Decreased (because of decreased volume)	Increased (to attempt to maintain blood pressure)	Decreased	Decreased preload
Obstructive (tamponade, tension pneumothorax, pulmonary embolus)	Decreased	Increased	Normal to increased flow	Obstruction of blood flow

*The prime mover is the initial pathophysiologic change; this change then causes compensatory changes in other variables.

Table 31–3

HELPFUL ENDPOINTS OF ADEQUATE RESUSCITATION

Clinical variables
   Mentation
   Heart rate
   Skin turgor
   Blood pressure
   Urine output 50 mL/h
   Appropriate response to therapeutic interventions
Laboratory studies: normal lactate/acid base status
Invasive measures: pulmonary artery catheter measurement of carbon monoxide,
diffusing capacity of oxygen, pulmonary capacity wedge pressure

should be evaluated for coagulopathy with international normalized ratio, partial thromboplastin time, and platelet count measurements.

Most patients with postoperative hypotension can be evaluated and treated by an astute clinician at the bedside using clinical measures of perfusion status. An elevated **lactate level** suggests a global deficit in oxygen delivery and requires further attempts to correct this problem. The placement of a **pulmonary artery catheter** may be considered when the cause of postoperative hypotension remains uncertain or when there is no response to initial therapeutic interventions or a persistent elevation in lactate levels. Measurements from the pulmonary artery catheter can help establish the diagnosis and assist in directing fluid resuscitation (see Tables 31–2 and 31–3).

Comprehension Questions

[31.1] A 31-year-old male in the intensive care unit (ICU) has had a pulmonary artery catheter placed because of persistent hypotension after multiple blunt trauma. Initial readings include a cardiac index of 4.1 L/min-m^2, systemic vascular resistance of 420 dyne-s/cm^5, and pulmonary capillary wedge pressure (PCWP) of 12 mm Hg. Which of the following conditions is most likely?

A. Myocardial infarction
B. Neurogenic shock
C. Severe diarrhea leading to intravascular depletion
D. Simple pneumothorax

[31.2] A 65-year-old man is noted to have a blood pressure of 90/62 mmHg on the evening after an uncomplicated small bowel resection of obstruction. His heart rate is 110/min, and respiratory rate 24/min, temperature 37.4°C (99.3°F), urine output only 15 cc over two hours, and oxygen saturation by pulse oximetry is 95%. His preoperative hemoglobin level was 12.6 g/dL. Which of the following statements is most accurate regarding this patient?

A. A hemoglobin level performed in the recovery room after surgery of 12.4 g/dL is good evidence against active hemorrhage.
B. Intravenous furosemide (lasix) should be administered.
C. This patient is most likely affected by anxiety and a mild anxiolytic and careful observation should be initiated.
D. Initial therapy should be intravenous cystalloid fluid bolus.

[31.3] A 56-year-old woman is admitted to the ICU for ventilator management after an abdominal aortic aneurysm repair. The patient is noted to have a urine output of 20 cc over 3 hours. Her blood pressure is 100/55 mmHg, HR 110/min and Temp 35.6°C (96.1°F). Her serum tropinin levels are noted to be elevated. Which of the following is the most likely diagnosis?

A. Intraabdominal hemorrhage
B. Renal insufficiency
C. Myocardial infarction
D. Post-surgical hypothermia

[31.4] A 34-year-old woman has an acutely ruptured ectopic pregnancy with an estimated 1500- ml hemoperitoneum. Which of the following parameters is most likely to be abnormal?

A. PO$_2$ level
B. Central venous pressure
C. Hemoglobin level
D. Platelet count

Answers

[31.1] **B.** Neurogenic shock is hypotension caused by an imbalance between the vasodilatory and vasoconstrictive influences of the arterioles and venules. This patient has a normal filling pressure (PCWP 12 mmHg), a normal cardiac index, and low peripheral vascular resistance reflective of the venous dilation.

[31.2] **D.** This patient has hypotension, tachycardia, tachypnea, and low urine output following surgery. These are indicators of volume depletion. A normal hemoglobin level acutely does not accurately reflect volume status.

[31.3] **C.** Serum troponin elevation is highly suggestive of myocardial infarction. A 12-lead EKG and echocardiography are often performed as adjunctive studies.

[31.4] **B.** The hemoglobin and hematocrit values are not acutely affected, but the central venous pressure that reflects volume in the right heart will be low.

CLINICAL PEARLS

◈ Do not be falsely reassured by a normal hemoglobin value in hypotensive surgical patients: They bleed whole blood!

◈ Clinical measures of perfusion status are adequate in most patients for determination of the adequacy of resuscitation.

◈ A pulmonary artery catheter should be considered if one is unsure why a patient is hypotensive, if a patient does not respond appropriately to initial fluid therapy, or when the lactate level is persistently elevated.

◈ Young people with a good cardiac reserve and patients on beta-blockers may not exhibit the expected tachycardia response to hemorrhage until late in the course of shock.

REFERENCES

Fundamental critical care support course text, 2nd ed. Anaheim, CA: Society of Critical Care Medicine, 1998.

Irwin RS, Cerra FB, Rippe JM, eds. Intensive care medicine, 4th ed. Philadelphia: Lippincott-Raven, 1998.

Marino P. The ICU book, 2nd ed. Philadelphia: Lippincott Williams & Wilkins, 1997.

A 26-year-old man is seen in the emergency center for abdominal pain that began after returning home from a party where he consumed pizza and eight beers. The pain is constant, located in the upper part of his abdomen, and radiates to his back. Approximately 3 to 4 hours after onset of the pain, the patient vomited a large amount of undigested food, but the emesis did not resolve his pain. His past medical history is unremarkable, and he consumes alcohol only during the weekends when he attends parties with his friends. On examination, the patient appears uncomfortable. His temperature is 38.8°C (101.8°F), heart rate 110/min, blood pressure 110/60, and respiratory rate 28/min. The abdomen is distended and tender to palpation in the epigastric and periumbilical areas. Laboratory studies reveal a white blood cell (WBC) count of 18,000/mm^3, hemoglobin 17 g/dL, hematocrit 47%, glucose 210 mg/dL, total bilirubin 3.2 mg/dL, AST 380 U/L, ALT 435 U/L, lactose dehydrogenase (LDH) 300 U/L, serum amylase 6800 IU/L. Arterial blood gas studies (room air) reveal pH 7.38, PaCO$_2$ 33 mmHg, PaO$_2$ 68 mm Hg, HCO$_3$ 21 mEq/L. Chest radiography reveals the presence of a small pleural effusion.

◆ **What is the most likely diagnosis?**

◆ **What are your next steps?**

◆ **What are complications associated with this disease process?**

ANSWERS TO CASE 32: Pancreatitis (Acute)

Summary: A 26-year-old man presents with acute nausea and vomiting and abdominal pain radiating to the back following binge drinking. The clinical presentation of fever, leukocytosis, hemoconcentration, and hypoxemia suggests severe acute pancreatitis.

◆ **Most likely diagnosis:** Acute pancreatitis.

◆ **Next steps:** Resuscitative measures including administration of supplemental oxygen and intravenous fluids.

◆ **Complications of the disease:** Acute pancreatitis can cause local complications including hemorrhage, necrosis, fluid collection, and infection. Pancreatitis may also lead to systemic complications such as pulmonary, cardiac, and renal dysfunction.

Analysis

Objectives

1. Be familiar with the diagnosis and initial treatment of patients with acute pancreatitis.
2. Recognize the value and limitations of clinical prognosticators and computed tomography (CT) scans in evaluating patients with acute pancreatitis.
3. Understand the diagnosis and management of the regional and systemic complications of acute pancreatitis.

Considerations

This patient, with a history of alcohol consumption and the sudden onset of abdominal and back pain, likely has acute alcoholic pancreatitis. This diagnosis is further supported by findings from the patient's physical examination and the elevated serum amylase level. The amylase level itself does not correlate with the severity of the disease; however,

his fever, tachypnea, and hyperdynamic state are due to the systemic inflammation related to acute pancreatitis. The presence of three of the
Ranson criteria (WBC, LDH, and AST measurements) and radiographic evidence of pleural effusion indicate a severe process. Based
on these initial findings, close monitoring of the patient's cardiopulmonary status in an intensive care unit and a CT scan of his
abdomen to assess the pancreas for evidence of necrosis may be
appropriate.

APPROACH TO ACUTE PANCREATITIS

Definitions

Infected pancreatic necrosis: An infectious complication with
    necrotic pancreas and peripancreatic tissue, which is due to sec-
    ondary infection by bowel-derived microorganisms within the
    first few weeks of onset. Antibiotic prophylaxis may be beneficial
    in preventing this complication, and operative debridement is
    usually indicated in managing this process.
Pancreatic abscess: Secondary infection of the pancreas and peri-
    pancreatic fluid collection. This condition is recognized by the ac-
    cumulation of thick, purulent fluid and infected debris. Surgical
    drainage is generally indicated in treating this condition.
Infected pancreatic pseudocyst: Usually a late process that oc-
    curs several weeks or months after the onset of severe pancreati-
    tis. This process can be adequately treated by percutaneous or op-
    erative drainage.

Clinical Approach

In the United States the most common etiologies of acute pancreatitis
are gallstones and alcohol consumption. Acute pancreatitis should be
diagnosed early because it may alter the management of the disease.
The diagnosis is based on the history and typical clinical presentation
of severe epigastric pain that radiates to the back, nausea, vomiting, and
fever. Serum amylase and lipase levels confirm the diagnosis in patients with the aforementioned symptoms, but by themselves are not diagnostic because they can be elevated in other pathologic conditions.

The severity of acute pancreatitis ranges from mild and self-limited (85% of cases) to severe and complicated (15% of cases). Mild pancreatitis is characterized by edema of the pancreas and rarely proceeds to necrosis or infection. Severe pancreatitis is characterized by necrosis of the pancreas and may be complicated by infection in approximately 50% of cases. Furthermore, severe pancreatitis is associated with increased microvascular permeability, leading to large volume losses of intravascular fluid into the tissues, thereby decreasing perfusion of the lungs, kidneys, and other organs. **The most important element in preventing multiple-organ failure is fluid resuscitation and intensive monitoring.** Recently, much investigation has focused on the systemic inflammatory response syndrome and multiple-organ failure during pancreatitis.

Prognostic Criteria   Several prognostic systems have been developed to differentiate between mild and severe pancreatitis. The most widely used system is the Ranson criteria (Table 32–1), which include five parameters determined at the time of admission and six parameters determined during the subsequent 48 hours. The Ranson criteria attempt to reflect the severity of the retroperitoneal inflammatory process, and the original purpose was to help predict patient outcome. **Patients with three or more Ranson criteria have more severe disease and an in-**

Table 32–1
RANSON CRITERIA

ON ADMISSION	SUBSEQUENT 48 HOURS
White blood cell count $>16,000/mm^3$	Hematocrit fall of 10%
Glucose >200 mg/dL	Calcium <8 mg/dL
Age >55 y	Serum urea nitrogen increase of 5 mg/dL
Aspartate aminotransferase >250 U/L	Fluid requirement of >6 L
Lactate dehydrogenase >350 U/L	Base excess of >4 mEq/L
	Po_2 <60 mmHg

creased risk of complications and death; however, with the recent improvements in patient care, the high mortality rates identified by the investigators are no longer applicable. Although helpful in the diagnosis, serum amylase and lipase levels do not correlate with the severity of pancreatitis. Other prognostic systems such as APACHE II and C-reactive protein levels have similar sensitivity and specificity compared to the Ranson criteria.

Computed Tomography Imaging of the Abdomen   **Contrast-enhanced CT imaging of the pancreas should be performed when the diagnosis of pancreatitis is in question.** In addition, patients who do not improve clinically in 3 to 5 days or who have severe pancreatitis based on the Ranson score should undergo contrast-enhanced CT scanning of the pancreas to determine the presence of necrosis. Two or more extra-pancreatic fluid collections or necrosis (nonenhancement) of more than 50% of the pancreas indicates severe disease and an increased risk of complications. **Necrotizing pancreatitis is complicated by infection approximately 50% of the time, and prophylactic antibiotics should be administered when necrosis is confirmed by a CT scan.** Severe pancreatitis can lead to other complications such as hemorrhage and splenic vein thrombosis. Pancreatic abscesses and pseudocyst formation are other possible complications of acute pancreatitis.

The diagnosis of acute pancreatitis is initially a presumptive one. Patients presenting with acute abdominal symptoms require careful clinical, biochemical, and radiologic evaluations to exclude other intra-abdominal processes such as bowel obstruction, perforated viscus, and mesenteric ischemia. It is also important to determine the severity of the disease. The presence or absence of gallstones should be determined as early as possible, usually with ultrasonography. **Patients with gallstone pancreatitis require cholecystectomy once the pancreatitis has resolved.**

Treatment   The **initial treatment of acute pancreatitis is nonoperative and focuses on fluid resuscitation, maintenance of ventilation, adequate oxygenation, and renal perfusion.** Patients with severe pancreatitis should be monitored in an intensive care unit. **Gastric decompression** is indicated for patients with nausea and vomiting. Approximately **85% of patients improve** with these supportive measures. In the 15% of patients who do not improve within 3 to 5 days, a **contrast-enhanced CT scan** of the pancreas should be obtained to determine the presence of **pancreatic necrosis.** Broad-spectrum antibiotics against enteric pathogens are indicated in treating necrotizing pancreatitis. One very effective **antibiotic in penetrating** the pancreatic tissue is imipenem/cilastatin. Aggressive nutritional support and proper electrolyte replacement are also important in the successful management of patients with severe pancreatitis.

Percutaneous needle aspiration of fluid collections or necrotic areas found on CT imaging can be performed to identify the presence of infection and guide therapeutic decisions about the need for drainage. When infected pancreatic necrosis or infected fluid is present, operative debridement and drainage are indicated. Patients with sterile necrosis generally improve with nonoperative therapy including antibiotics and intensive support; however, **surgical exploration may be indicated in patients showing clinical deterioration despite appropriate nonoperative therapy.**

Patients with gallstone pancreatitis (confirmed by ultrasound) may require **endoscopic retrograde cholangiopancreatography (ERCP) if evidence of biliary obstruction persists.** The patient described in this case should undergo abdominal ultrasonography on admission and daily serum liver function test values should be measured. If the total bilirubin level does not decrease, the patient should undergo ERCP to clear the duct of stones and to prevent biliary complications. Patients with **gallstone pancreatitis usually undergo cholecystectomy prior to discharge** to prevent recurrent attacks, which occur in up to one-third of patients who do not undergo cholecystectomy.

Comprehension Questions

[32.1] A 28-year-old man is diagnosed with acute mild pancreatitis. Which of the following is the best treatment for this patient?

A. Given nothing by mouth
B. Restriction of fluids to 80cc/hour
C. Intravenous antibiotic therapy to prevent pancreatic abscess formation
D. Hypertonic glucose solution to prevent hypoglycemia

[32.2] A 42-year-old alcoholic male has chronic pancreatitis and presents with a palpable abdominal mass and a slightly elevated serum amylase level. Which of the following is the most likely diagnosis?

    A. Pancreatic cancer
    B. Pancreatic abscess
    C. Hepatic hemangioma
    D. Pancreatic pseudocyst

[32.3] A 65-year-old woman is hospitalized with gallstone pancreatitis and is noted to have significant abdominal pain, emesis, tachycardia, and tachypnea. Her amylase level is 3100 IU/L, glucose is 120 mg/dL, and calcium level is 13 mg/dL. Which of the following is most likely to correlate with poor prognosis in disease severity?

    A. The patient's age
    B. The high amylase level
    C. A glucose level below 140 mg/dL
    D. Hypercalcemia

[32.4] Patients with severe pancreatitis and infected pancreatic necrosis are best treated by which of the following?

    A. Antibiotic therapy alone
    B. Percutaneous drainage
    C. Surgical pancreatic debridement and drainage
    D. Endoscopic drainage

Answers

[32.1] **A.** Antibiotic therapy has not been shown to decrease the incidence of pancreatic complications. Nothing by mouth, parental analgesics, IV hydration, and observation for hyperglycemia are components of therapy.

[32.2] **D.** Pancreatic pseudocysts are collections of fluid and necrotic tissue around the pancreas and usually resolve over several weeks to months, but they occasionally persist, necessitating surgery.

[32.3] **A.** The level of the amylase or lipase does not correlate with disease severity. Hypoxemia, hypocalcemia, age > 55 years are some of the poor prognostic factors based on Ranson's criteria.

[32.4] **C.** Surgical debridement and drainage are indicated in the treatment of infected pancreatic necrosis.

CLINICAL PEARLS

◆ The most important element in preventing multiple-organ failure is fluid resuscitation with intensive monitoring.

◆ Serum amylase and lipase levels are useful in diagnosing acute pancreatitis, but these values correlate poorly with disease severity.

◆ Infected pancreatic necrosis and clinical deterioration in sterile necrosis are indications for operative debridement and drainage.

◆ The primary indications for surgery in chronic pancreatitis include intractable pain, bowel or biliary obstruction, and persistent pseudocysts.

REFERENCE

Mulvihill SJ. Pancreas. In: Norton JA, Bollinger RR, Change AE, et al, eds. Surgery: basic science and clinical evidence. New York: Springer, 2001: 517–552.

CASE 33

A 43-year-old woman presents with blood-tinged discharge from her right nipple. She indicates that this problem has been occurring intermittently over the past several weeks. Her past medical history is significant for hypothyroidism. She has no prior history of breast complaints. The patient is premenopausal and currently not lactating. Her medications consist of oral contraceptives and levothyroxine. On physical examination, she is found to have minimal fibrocystic changes in both breasts. There is evidence of thickening in the right retroareolar region. Small amounts of serosanguinous fluid can be expressed from the right nipple. There is no evidence of nipple discharge or a dominant mass in the left breast.

◆ **What should be your next step?**

ANSWERS TO CASE 33: Nipple Discharge (Blood-tinged)

Summary: A 43-year-old premenopausal, nonlactating woman presents with unilateral nipple discharge that is serosanguinous in nature.

◆ **Next step:** The examination should begin with bilateral mammography to evaluate for suspicious lesions and ultrasonography to evaluate the retroareolar thickening; a ductogram or biopsy should also be considered.

Analysis

Objectives

1. Become familiar with an approach to the evaluation of nipple discharge by categorizing the condition as physiologic, pathologic, or galactorrheic.
2. Appreciate the relative cancer risks of patients presenting with nipple discharge.

Considerations

This patient's history indicates that a pathologic etiology for nipple discharge should be investigated. **Characteristics of concern include** being **spontaneous** (not produced by manipulation—patients often find the discharge on their clothing), being **bloody or blood-tinged** (as opposed to milky, purulent or—as is characteristic of fibrocystic changes—yellow, brown, or green), and being **unilateral** (see Table 33–1). Although the **most common pathologic cause of bloody nipple discharge is intraductal papilloma,** prompt evaluation of this patient must be performed to exclude carcinoma. Solitary papillomas are benign and do not increase the risk of cancer; in half of all cases, they are characterized by a serous rather than a bloody discharge. **Duct ectasia (also benign) is the next most common cause of bloody nipple discharge. Carcinoma** and infection follow, with the former being one of the main reasons to pursue a diagnosis. After the history is obtained and

Table 33-1

DIFFERENTIAL DIAGNOSIS FOR NIPPLE DISCHARGE

DIAGNOSIS	HISTORY	TESTS*	TREATMENT
Pregnancy	Reproductive age and female. This diagnosis is the most common reason for nipple discharge. Milk can be secreted intermittently for as long as 2 y after breast-feeding, particularly with stimulation.	Pregnancy test.	Remember to consider this diagnosis in all women of reproductive age.
Infection and or mastitis or abscess	Purulent discharge, nipple is erythematous and tender.	Gram stain and culture of discharge. Complete blood count (CBC).	Antibiotics and or drainage for abscess.
Galactorrhea secondary to pituitary adenoma	Galactorrhea of all causes is usually characterized by bilateral milky-white discharge.	Prolactin level to rule out pituitary adenoma (if pregnancy is excluded). If pregnancy test results are negative, magnetic resonance imaging. (Tumors usually seen only for levels ~ 100 ng/mL†).	Treatment as per pituitary adenomas.
Galactorrhea secondary to medications	Patient taking phenothiazines, metoclopramide, oral contraceptives, α-methyldiphenylalanine, reserpine, or tricyclic antidepressants.		Change medications if possible and exclude other causes.

(Continues)

Table 33–1

DIFFERENTIAL DIAGNOSIS FOR NIPPLE DISCHARGE (*Continued*)

DIAGNOSIS	HISTORY	TESTS*	TREATMENT
Galactorrhea secondary to hypothyroid	May have symptoms of hypothyroidism, but may exclude with testing.	Thyroxine and thyroid-stimulating hormone levels.	If hypothyroid, treat with appropriate medications.
Fibrocystic changes	Nodularity of breasts, often varying with menstrual cycle. May have mastodynia. Discharge can be yellow, brown, or green.	Hemoccult test. Ultrasound is helpful in delineating cystic lesions and fibroglandular tissue. Mammogram may be appropriate.	If discharge is from fibrocystic changes, observe and reassure. Consider abstention from methylxanthines (caffeine) for mastodynia. If lesion is suspicious, perform a biopsy, but otherwise, there is no increased risk of breast cancer for fibrocytic changes.
Intraductal papilloma	Usually unilateral serous or bloody discharge.	Consider ductogram. Ultrasound may be helpful during workup.	Subareolar duct excision to confirm diagnosis. No increased risk of breast cancer.

Diffuse papillomatosis	Serous rather than bloody discharge, often involves multiple ducts more distant from the nipple, and can be bilateral. Discharge can recur if entire portion of ductal system is not removed.	Ductogram to identify duct system. Needle localization following ductogram may assist in excision. Ultrasound may be helpful during workup.	Excision of involved ducts. This diagnosis is associated with an increased risk of breast cancer.
Carcinoma	Bloody or serous nipple discharge (or none), newly inverted nipple, abnormal skin changes, suspicious mass on examination or mammogram.	Prior to diagnosis, consider ductogram and ultrasound in workup, or needle localization if not palpable.	Biopsy and then treatment as per breast cancer.

*Bilateral mammograms should be obtained for the evaluation of all these diagnoses except for milky discharge due to pregnancy.
†Minor elevations in prolactin without a tumor can be caused by polycystic ovary or Cushing syndrome or can be idiopathic.

a physical examination is completed, bilateral mammography should be performed to evaluate for suspicious lesions, and ultrasonography to evaluate the patient's retroareolar thickening. Ultrasonography can diagnose duct ectasia or further characterize the thickening and fibrocystic changes. Mammography is indicated in women past the age of 40 years. In this case, it can be used for both screening and diagnostic purposes. When nipple disease is suspected, such as squamous carcinoma (Bowen disease) or ductal carcinoma (Paget disease) or when a solitary mass is present, these lesions should be biopsied.

APPROACH TO BLOODY NIPPLE DISCHARGE

Definitions

Ductogram: A radiologic test with contrast injected into the duct causing the discharge.

Intraductal papilloma: A benign breast mass that is usually microscopic but may grow to 2 to 3 mm, often associated with spontaneous discharge from one nipple.

Clinical Approach

Occasionally the discharge of fibrocystic changes can be difficult to delineate from old blood. A hemoccult test can help differentiate the two. Although some advocate cytologic examination of the discharge, false-negative and -positive results are common. Awaiting results can produce further delay and cost without adding convincing data that would change the evaluation process. Therefore, it is reasonable to forgo this test and proceed to a **ductogram.** A patient must have ongoing discharge for this test to be performed. It requires a skilled radiologist, and the patient may experience discomfort during the examination. A lesion can be identified by the presence of a filling defect (a "cutoff"), an abrupt end to the duct rather than normal confluent arborization. **An abnormal ductogram generally demands a biopsy.** A ductogram can also help delineate the location of the lesion for the surgeon performing the biopsy. If the ductogram is normal, the patient can be judiciously observed with vigilance for the possibility of underlying carcinoma. A palpable dominant mass, a newly inverted nipple, skin changes, or mammographic abnormalities demand a biopsy.

Surgery is performed by either a partial or a complete duct excision, recognizing that complete excision will affect the patient's ability to breast-feed in the future. Undergoing the procedure in the operating room will help in the planning of the excision. The duct is cannulated with a fine lacrimal probe, which is used as a guide for excision. The injection of methylene blue dye into the duct with a fine angiocatheter also serves as guide in performing the excision, which is done through a circumareolar incision.

Comprehension Questions

[33.1] A 35-year-old woman with two children and no previous surgeries has noticed increased fatigue and a whitish nipple discharge. Which of the following is the next step?

    A. Determination of the thyrotropin level
    B. Imaging of the sella turcica
    C. Measurement of the human chorionic gonadotropin level
    D. Ultrasonography of the breasts

[33.2] Which of the following etiologies of nipple discharge increases the risk of breast cancer?

    A. Fibrocystic changes
    B. Diffuse papillomatosis
    C. Intraductal papilloma
    D. Pregnancy

[33.3] Which of the following findings in a workup for nipple discharge must be further evaluated?

    A. An ultrasonogram of the nipple showing duct ectasia
    B. A ductogram with no filling defects or abnormalities

C. An ultrasonogram with fibrocystic changes and a 2-mm simple cyst
D. A prolactin level of 100 ng/mL

[33.4] A 65-year-old woman who takes tricyclic antidepressants and metoclopramide has a serosanguinous discharge from her right nipple. She has no palpable masses, normal bilateral mammograms, and a right breast ultrasonogram that does not demonstrate any masses. Her ductogram shows a cutoff in an inferior lateral duct 2 cm from the right nipple. Of the following choices, which is the most appropriate approach?

A. Observation and instructions not to manipulate the nipple during self-examination
B. Change her medications
C. Check the prolactin level
D. Duct excisional biopsy

Answers

[33.1] **C.** While these can also be symptoms of hypothyroidism, the first step is to exclude pregnancy as an etiology.

[33.2] **B.** Diffuse papillomatosis increases the risk of cancer.

[33.3] **D.** A prolactin level in this range is suggestive of a pituitary adenoma, whereas the other findings are benign and can be observed.

[33.4] **D.** While the other recommendations are appropriate courses for different etiologies of nipple discharge, this patient has a demonstrated abnormality on a ductogram indicating a need for biopsy despite other possible additional sources.

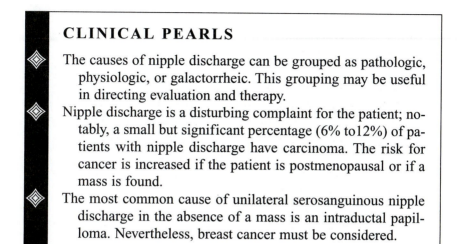

CLINICAL PEARLS

- The causes of nipple discharge can be grouped as pathologic, physiologic, or galactorrheic. This grouping may be useful in directing evaluation and therapy.
- Nipple discharge is a disturbing complaint for the patient; notably, a small but significant percentage (6% to12%) of patients with nipple discharge have carcinoma. The risk for cancer is increased if the patient is postmenopausal or if a mass is found.
- The most common cause of unilateral serosanguinous nipple discharge in the absence of a mass is an intraductal papilloma. Nevertheless, breast cancer must be considered.

REFERENCES

August DA, Sondak VK. Breast: benign breast disorders. In: Greenfield LJ. Surgery: scientific principles and practice, 2nd ed. Philadelphia: Lippincott-Raven, 1997:1370–1378.

Norton LW. Nipple discharge. In: Steigmann G, Eisman B. Surgical decision making, 4th ed. Philadelphia: WB Saunders, 2000:190–191.

CASE 34

During an office visit, a 66-year-old man tells you that several weeks ago he experienced weakness in his right hand at work that resulted in a temporary inability to write or hold a pen. These symptoms persisted for approximately 45 minutes and resolved without further recurrence. The patient's past history is significant for hypertension and coronary artery disease with stable angina. He has a history of smoking 45 packs of cigarettes per year. His medications include aspirin, nitrates, and a beta-blocker. On examination, bruits can be heard over both carotid arteries. The results from the cardiopulmonary examination and the remainder of the physical examination are unremarkable. You obtain a duplex ultrasonogram of the carotid arteries that reveals an 80% narrowing of the left carotid artery and a 95% narrowing of the right carotid artery.

◆ **What is the most likely diagnosis?**

◆ **What is the best therapy?**

ANSWERS TO CASE 34: Carotid Artery Disease

Summary: A 66-year-old man presents with signs and symptoms suggestive of a recent transient ischemic attack (TIA) involving the left cerebral hemisphere. He has evidence of severe bilateral carotid stenoses as confirmed by a duplex scan.

◆ **Most likely diagnosis:** Bilateral carotid artery stenoses with a history of a left hemispheric TIA.

◆ **Best therapy:** The patient should undergo staged bilateral carotid endarterectomies, beginning with the left carotid artery.

Analysis

Objectives

1. Understand the natural history and evaluation of asymptomatic carotid bruits.
2. Be familiar with the medical and surgical treatment of patients with asymptomatic carotid stenosis and symptomatic carotid stenosis.
3. Understand the current role of endovascular management of carotid stenosis.

Considerations

This patient provides a history that is fairly classic for TIA; however, TIA symptoms are not always easy for patients or physicians to recognize. Because the disability is frequently minor and short-lived, patients frequently attribute the symptoms to fatigue or other reasons and fail to bring them to the physician's attention. **Neurologic events arising from carotid disease are almost always unilateral, with the exception of speech impediment.** After reviewing the initial history and physical examination, it is also important to look for evidence of coronary artery disease and atherosclerotic disease involving other parts of the vascular system. This particular patient has bilateral carotid disease.

Surgical treatment should be directed toward the symptomatic side first. Once he has recovered from his left carotid endarterectomy (CEA), he should undergo an asymptomatic right CEA. As both sides meet operative stenosis criteria, the symptomatic side is addressed first as it is the higher risk lesion to leave on conservative therapy.

APPROACH TO CAROTID ARTERY DISEASE

Cerebrovascular disease involves a classic state of balancing the risks of intervention with the risks of conservative treatment. The conundrum is that the main complication of both modes of management is the same: stroke. As a general rule, the more severe the stenosis in a given situation, the higher the incidence of symptoms. **A bruit represents turbulent blood flow that resonates at an audible frequency.** Duplex ultrasonography can be very accurate in confirming the presence of significant carotid disease. However, this procedure is also operator-dependent. The accuracy of stenosis grading should be at the highest level if a surgeon plans to recommend treatment based on duplex ultrasonography alone. If there is question of stenosis grade on ultrasonography, other tests are needed to help guide the therapy. This could be a magnetic resonance angiogram, a conventional carotid angiogram, or a CT reconstruction angiogram. **An additional workup for a patient with carotid disease should include a thorough assessment of cardiopulmonary risks.**

The North American Symptomatic Carotid Endarterectomy Trial (NASCET) and the Asymptomatic Carotid Atherosclerosis Study (ACAS) have categorized the stroke-preventing potential of CEA. For high degrees of stenosis in an internal carotid artery, surgery is better at reducing the risk of stroke when compared to risk modification and antiplatelet therapy alone (Table 34–1).

The important issues in applying NASCET or ACAS data to decisions on recommending CEA are a solid knowledge of the operator's risk rate and profile. If the particular surgeon and hospital have a safety record equal to or better than the perioperative complication rates observed during the trials, recommendations based on trial stenosis grades are fair and reasonable. However, if a surgeon or hospital has a complication rate higher than 5% with symptomatic patients or higher than 2% with asymptomatic patients, CEA should not be aggressively

Table 34–1
SURGICAL VERSUS MEDICAL THERAPY
IN CAROTID DISEASE

TRIAL	STENOSIS GRADE (%)	CAROTID ENDARTERECTOMY 5-Y EVENT RATE (%)	CONSERVATIVE THERAPY 5-Y EVENT RATE (%)
NASCET, (symptomatic)	>70	7	24
ACAS (asymptomatic)	>60	5.5	11.1

recommended. Many adjuncts are available to reduce the risk of perioperative stroke. The use of an intraluminal shunt, cerebral monitoring, and a patch angioplasty closure all can make CEA safer. The majority of patients who undergo CEA are home from the hospital in less than 24 hours.

Current Status of Carotid Angioplasty/Stenting

Many surgeons can offer even lower complication rates in patients who would belong to higher risk profiles than those studied in controlled, randomized trials. However, there are a few subsets of patients who are at high risk for an open CEA and instead might be considered for carotid angioplasty/stenting (CAS). Patients who have undergone neck radiation or developed recurrent stenosis are currently two reasonable populations for possible CAS. As CAS still carries a 5% to 7% periprocedural event rate, it cannot be considered the standard of care for routine patients. However, as CAS technology evolves, this procedure may leave the realm of investigational therapy. Again, however, it is important to investigate the risk and complication profiles of the provider and hospital before offering any cerebrovascular therapy.

Comprehension Questions

[34.1] A patient has a 4-minute period of documented expressive aphasia that completely resolves. A workup reveals an 80% to 85%

left internal carotid stenosis. A 50% right internal carotid stenosis is present. Which of the following is the most appropriate care?

A. Right CEA
B. Left CEA
C. Aspirin therapy at 81 mg/d
D. Aspirin therapy at 325 mg/d

[34.2] An 84-year-old female patient with diabetes and class IV congestive heart failure presents in the office with a right neck bruit. Duplex sonography reveals a 50% to 75% stenosis in the right carotid artery. Which of the following is the most appropriate treatment?

A. Right CEA
B. Aspirin at 325 mg/d
C. Aspirin at 325 mg/d and repeated studies in 6 months
D. Confirmatory imaging with magnetic resonance angiography

[34.3] A 71-year-old male suffers a moderately dense cerebrovascular accident (CVA) affecting his right arm and leg. He initially was hemiplegic. However, over the last 3 weeks has he recovered four-fifths of the strength in his right leg and four-fifths of the strength in his right arm. It has been 8 weeks since his stroke. A workup reveals a 95% stenosis in his left internal carotid artery; his right internal carotid artery is occluded. Which of the following is the most appropriate treatment?

A. Aspirin at 325 mg/d
B. Right CEA
C. Left CEA with intraluminal shunting
D. Warfarin anticoagulation therapy

[34.4] A 66-year-old woman underwent right CEA for symptoms of cerebrovascular insufficiency (right eye visual loss and left arm weakness which resolved) confirmed by a bruit and 90%

stenosis on angiography. On postoperative day 1, the patient ex-
pired. Which of the following was the most likely cause of her
death?

A. Myocardial infarction
B. Vascular surgical failure leading to exsanguination
C. Pulmonary embolism
D. Electrolyte imbalances

Answers

[34.1] **B.** Left CEA. The patient has a high-grade stenosis in the appropriate artery distribution for his symptomatic TIA. Although
aspirin therapy is essential for both operative and nonoperative
patients with cerebrovascular disease, this patient meets the operative criteria. The definitive dose of aspirin is still debatable.

[34.2] **D.** Confirmatory magnetic resonance angiography. This is a
medically high-risk patient who has an equivocal duplex stenosis. If the stenosis actually turns out to be 75%, a careful discussion of the risks and benefits can be held with the patient.
However, it still would be prudent to continue conservative
management in this high-risk asymptomatic individual.

[34.3] **C.** Left CEA using an intraluminal shunt. This is a symptomatic
patient with significant recovery from a CVA. His highest risk
of recurrent stroke is during the first 6 months following the
first event. As such, his contralateral occlusion is not a contraindication to CEA. Based on his presentation, most surgeons
would use an intraluminal shunt for his CEA.

[34.4] **A.** Acute myocardial infarction and perioperative stroke are the
two most common severe complications following carotid CEA.

CLINICAL PEARLS

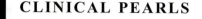

◈ The results of operative and intraluminal treatment of carotid artery disease are highly variable among providers; therefore efforts should be made to determine these results before making recommendations for treatment.

◈ Dizziness, syncope, and confusion are almost never due to carotid artery stenoses.

REFERENCES

Barnett HJ. Stroke prevention by surgery for symptomatic disease in carotid territory. Neurol Clin 1992;10(1):281–292.

Moore WS, Barnett HJ, Beebe HG, et al. Guidelines for carotid endarterectomy: a multidisciplinary consensus statement from the ad hoc committee, American Heart Association. Stroke 1995;26(1):188–201.

Mullinex PS, Anderson CA, Olsen SB, Tollefson DF. Carotid endarterectomy remains the gold standard. Am J Surg 2002;183(5):580–583.

CASE 35

A 57-year-old man has a 2-month history of a nonproductive cough. He denies weight loss or hemoptysis. His past medical history is significant for hypertension that is treated with a beta-blocker. The patient has had no known exposure to asbestos. He has a 30-pack-year history of tobacco use. On examination, the patient is afebrile and has no significant abnormalities. A chest radiograph reveals a 2-cm soft tissue mass in the perihilar region of the left lung field, which appears to be a new lesion that was not present on a chest radiograph obtained 2 years previously.

◆ **What should be your next steps?**

ANSWERS TO CASE 35: Pulmonary Nodule

Summary: A 57-year-old male smoker presents with a left lung mass that is highly suggestive of a malignancy.

◆ **Next step:** A contrast-enhanced computed tomography (CT) scan of the chest that includes the liver and adrenal gland should be obtained to better define the mass and narrow the differential diagnosis. Based on the findings, the most efficient diagnostic technique can be selected. Examples that could be offered to this patient include sputum cytology studies, bronchoscopy with or without a transbronchial biopsy, a transthoracic biopsy, or thoracotomy.

Analysis

Objectives

1. Be familiar with the strategy for the evaluation and management of a lung mass in patients with and without a known history of malignancy.
2. Be familiar with the staging and treatment of non–small cell and small cell lung cancer.
3. Understand the role of surgery in the management of pulmonary metastasis.

Considerations

This solitary pulmonary nodule most likely represents non–small cell lung cancer. The presence of a **cough, although nonspecific and common in smokers, should prompt further evaluation when it is new and persistent.** The identification of a lesion on chest radiographs not present 2 years earlier partially narrows the differential diagnosis to either an infectious or a malignant process. The absence of clinical evidence of an infection based on history or physical examination further increases the likelihood of a malignancy. A CT scan of the chest should be obtained to further delineate the mass. The presence or absence of calcifications and their radiographic pattern can assist in narrowing the differential diagnosis, and inclusion of the liver and adrenals, common sites of metastatic lung cancer involvement, can provide staging information. A tissue diagnosis will likely be required; the CT can help define the anatomic location of the mass and will assist in choosing the method of tissue procurement with the highest chance of success.

APPROACH TO LUNG MASSES

Definition

Positron emission tomography (PET) scan: Detects the increased rates of glucose metabolism (positron-emitting glucose analog) that occur commonly in malignant tumors. It can detect primary lung cancers, metastases to the lung, and mediastinal lymph nodes but may lack anatomic details.

Clinical Approach

A thorough history and physical examination allow the clinician to generate a differential diagnosis. A patient's cigarette use, known prior or concurrent neoplasms, family history of cancer, exposure to *Mycobacterium,* and symptoms of ongoing infection as well as symptoms of metastatic disease are important and may help establish the diagnosis. **Patients with a history of prior malignancies who develop a new lung mass should be assumed to have metastatic disease until proven otherwise.** Similarly, multiple primary lung cancers occur in less than 2% of patients with lung cancer; therefore the presence of multiple pulmonary tumors results in a greater likelihood of metastasis or a benign condition. **New nodules in smokers as revealed by chest radiography have a very high risk of malignancy, as high as 70% in some series, and should be approached with a high degree of suspicion.**

The initial evaluation should begin with a review of prior chest radiographs. With serial films the radiologist can determine the rate of growth, allowing a differentiation between benign and malignant

disease. **If the clinical and radiographic presentations suggest pneumonia, a 10- to 14-day course of antibiotics can be attempted with
a mandatory radiographic examination on completion. Persistence
of the mass demands further evaluation.** The next stage in evaluation

Table 35–1
DEFINITIONS OF T, N, AND M CATEGORIES
FOR CARCINOMA OF THE LUNG

CATEGORY	DESCRIPTION
T: Primary tumor	
TX	Tumor proven by the presence of malignant cells in bronchopulmonary secretions but not visualized roentgenographically or bronchoscopically, or any tumor that cannot be assessed, as in a retreatment setting.
T0	No evidence of a primary tumor.
Tis	Carcinoma in situ.
T1	A tumor that is 3.0 cm or less in greatest dimension, surrounded by lung or visceral pleura, and without evidence of invasion proximal to a lobar bronchus on bronchoscopy.[*]
T2	A tumor more than 3.0 cm in greatest dimension, or a tumor of any size that either invades the visceral pleura or has associated atelectasis or obstructive pneumonitis extending to the hilar region. On bronchoscopy, involves the lobar bronchus or at least 2.0 cm distal to the carina. Any associated atelectasis or obstructive pneumonitis must involve less than the entire lung.
T3	A tumor of any size with direct extension into the chest wall (including superior sulcus tumors), diaphragm, or mediastinal pleura or pericardium without involving the heart, great vessels, trachea, esophagus or vertebral body, or a tumor in the main bronchus within 2 cm of the carina without involving the carina, or associated atelectasis or obstructive pneumonitis of the entire lung.
T4	A tumor of any size with invasion of the mediastinum or involving the heart, great vessels, trachea, esophagus, vertebral body, or carina, or with the presence of malignant pleural or pericardial effusion,[†] or with satellite tumor nodules within the ipsilateral, primary tumor lobe of the lung.
N: Nodal involvement	
N0	No demonstrable metastasis to regional lymph nodes.
N1	Metastasis to lymph nodes in the peribronchial or the ipsilateral hilar region or both, including direct extension.

Table 35–1

DEFINITIONS OF T, N, AND M CATEGORIES
FOR CARCINOMA OF THE LUNG *(Continued)*

CATEGORY	DESCRIPTION
N2	Metastasis to ipsilateral mediastinal lymph nodes and subcarinal lymph nodes.
N3	Metastasis to contralateral mediastinal lymph nodes, contralateral hilar lymph nodes, ipsilateral or contralateral scalene or supraclavicular lymph nodes.
M: Distant metastasis	
M0	No (known) distant metastasis.
M1	Distant metastasis present.[‡] Specify site(s).

[*]An uncommon superficial tumor of any size with its invasive component limited to the bronchial wall that may extend proximal to the main bronchus is classified as T1.

[†]Most pleural effusions associated with lung cancer are due to tumor. There are, however, a few patients in whom cytopathologic examination of pleural fluid (on more than one specimen) is negative for tumor; the fluid is nonbloody and is not an exudate. In such cases where these elements and clinical judgment dictate that the effusion is not related to the tumor, the patient should be staged T1, T2, or T3 excluding effusion as a staging element.

[‡]Separate metastatic tumor nodules in the ipsilateral nonprimary tumor lobe(s) of the lung also are classified M1.

is a contrast-enhanced CT scan of the chest. The presence of specific patterns of calcifications can be pathopneumonic of a benign process, however, some calcified lesions and all noncalcified lesions require further investigation. The options, in order of increasing aggressiveness, include repeated radiographic evaluation, PET imaging, sputum cytologic studies, transthoracic fine-needle aspiration (FNA), bronchoscopic biopsy, and surgical resection.

The decision concerning which method to use is based on a wide variety of patient variables (age, smoking history, prior granulomatous disease, prior or concurrent cancers, and family history of cancers) and tumor variables (size and location). As a general rule, patients with a high risk of malignancy are evaluated with more invasive methods providing more information (ie, some form of biopsy or surgical resection), whereas those with a low risk of cancer or significant concomitant medical problems are evaluated initially with less invasive methods. PET scanning combined with CT imaging can effectively diagnose a malignancy (sensitivity, 82% to 100%; specificity, 75% to

Table 35–2
STAGE GROUPING OF TNM SUBSETS

STAGE GROUPING			
Stage 0	Carcinoma in situ		
Stage IA	T1 N0 M0		
Stage IB	T2 N0 M0		
Stage IIA	T1 N1 M0		
Stage IIB	T2 N1 M0		
	T3 N0 M0		
Stage IIIA	T3 N1 M0		
	T1 N2 M0	T2 N2 M0	T3 N2 M0
Stage IIIB	T4 N0 M0	T4 N1 M0	T4 N2 M0
	T1 N3 M0	T2 N3 M0	T3 N3 M0
	T4 N3 M0		
Stage IV	Any T	Any N	M1

100%) but is less effective with smaller lesions (<1 cm) or when concomitant infection is present. The use of sputum cytologic studies can assist in obtaining a tissue diagnosis in 10% to 15% of cases, with higher rates of detection for centrally located lesions. Transthoracic FNA and bronchoscopic biopsies are highly effective when applied to appropriately positioned lesions (peripheral and central, respectively). Finally, surgical resection can be used for patients with a high risk of malignancy and a peripherally based lesion. Although it is the most aggressive method, it does have the greatest accuracy and can simultaneously diagnose and treat an early-stage lung cancer. This advantage actually makes it relatively cost-effective in patients with a high risk of lung cancer (eg, a 65-year-old heavy smoker with hemoptysis but otherwise asymptomatic who has a new lung mass).

Once cancer is diagnosed, every effort should be made to obtain accurate clinical staging of the disease. Staging of non-small cell lung cancer utilizes the TNM system and is outlined in Tables 35–1 and 35–2. The T status is determined using CT scanning as well as any information obtained on bronchoscopy. Magnetic resonance imaging of the chest may help with lesions involving the brachial plexus and the spine. The N status is determined by physical examination, CT imaging, the results of any biopsies (FNA of palpable nodes, transbronchial FNA of mediastinal nodes, scalene node biopsy, or mediastinoscopy), and most recently PET scanning. The M status is determined by physical examination, radiographic techniques (magnetic resonance imaging of the brain, CT scanning of the chest with inclusion of the liver and adrenals) and nuclear medicine techniques (bone scanning and PET scanning). **The five most common sites of metastasis should be examined, namely, the contralateral and noninvolved ipsilateral lung, liver, adrenals, bone, and brain.** For very early-stage lesions, evaluation of the bone and brain can be reserved for patients exhibiting symptoms of metastatic involvement of these organs. However, these techniques should not preclude a thorough physical examination as lung cancer can metastasize to any location.

Small Cell Carcinoma   Staging of small cell lung cancer is much less involved because of the advanced nature of this disease at presentation. Patients have limited disease (confined entirely within the chest), extensive disease, or extrathoracic metastasis. Very rarely, small cell lung cancer is incidentally discovered at an early stage, and in these situations it can be treated using the staging system for non-small cell lung cancer.

Lung Cancer Treatment   The treatment of lung cancer is dependent on the histology (small cell versus non-small cell) and the stage of the disease. For non-small cell lung cancer, early-stage disease is primarily treated with surgery, whereas later stages are managed with chemotherapy with or without radiotherapy. However, all treatments are dependent on the physiologic reserve of the patient. Therefore, concurrent with evaluation of the tumor, a thorough examination of the pulmonary and cardiac systems should be performed. This consists of complete pulmonary function testing and in selected cases a more extensive evaluation including exercise oxygen consumption studies. Smoking cessation for at least 2 weeks is mandatory, and pulmonary function can be improved dramatically with this single intervention. Patients at risk of cardiac disease should undergo evaluation by a cardiologist, with aggressive examination and treatment of any signs or symptoms of coronary artery disease. For small cell lung cancer, limited disease is treated with combination chemotherapy and radiotherapy, whereas patients with extensive disease are offered palliative chemotherapy with radiation reserved for symptomatic relief only. An outline of the treatment of small cell and non-small cell lung cancer appears in Figure 35–1.

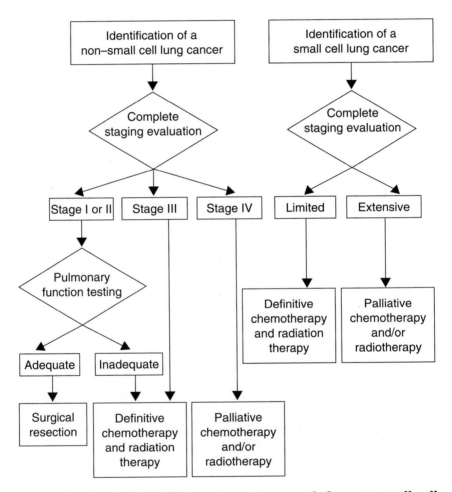

Figure 35–1. A simplified treatment approach for non–small cell and small cell lung cancer.

Management of Pulmonary Metastasis

Patients with metastatic lung disease who primarily receive chemotherapy usually have very poor outcomes. However, in very specific cases surgical extirpation can lead to a reasonable chance of cure. The minimal necessary criteria include (1) local control of the primary tumor, (2) metastatic disease confined to the lung parenchyma, (3) disease that is resectable, and (4) adequate pulmonary reserve to tolerate the planned resection. When these criteria are used, 5-year survival rates approximate 30%. Other criteria that can be considered before surgical resection is recommended include tumor doubling time, disease-free intervals, and the number of metastasis.

Comprehension Questions

[35.1] A 45-year-old nonsmoker is found to have a 2-cm soft tissue mass in the left lung. Which of the following is the most appropriate next step?

    A. Perform a CT-guided biopsy of the mass
    B. Obtain sputum samples
    C. Evaluate all previously obtained chest radiographs
    D. Obtain a repeated chest radiograph in 6 months

[35.2] Which of the following describes the main purpose of CT imaging of chest masses?

    A. Discern between a pleural effusion and transudate
    B. Differentiate between malignant and benign neoplasm
    C. Determine the anatomic location of the mass
    D. Differentiate between primary and metastatic masses

Answers

[35.1] **C.** Evaluation of all available chest radiographs is a reasonable first step in treating any patient with a newly identified lung mass.

[35.2] **C.** The primary purpose of CT imaging of chest masses is to determine the anatomic location of the lesion, and not whether it
is benign or malignant.

CLINICAL PEARLS

◈ Approximately 95% of patients with lung cancer present with
symptoms related to the disease, whereas only 5% present
with asymptomatic chest findings.

◈ Cough is the initial presenting symptoms in three-fourths of
patients with lung cancer, and this cough is produced by en-
dobronchial tumor growth causing inflammation or irritation of the airway.

◈ Approximately 10% to 20% of lung cancer patients are affected by paraneoplastic syndromes, and these syndromes
are most commonly associated with small cell and squamous carcinoma.

REFERENCE

Lau CL, Harpole DH Jr. Lung neoplasms. In: Norton JA, Bollinger RR, Chang AE,
Lowry SF, Mulvihill SJ, Pass HI, Thompson RW, eds. Surgery: basic science and
clinical evidence. New York: Springer, 2001:1189–1216.

A 58-year-old woman presents to your office complaining of generalized itching. On examination, she appears jaundiced. During your interview, you learn that she has experienced a 10-lb weight loss over the past several months and recently has noted the passage of tea-colored urine. Her past medical history is significant for type II diabetes mellitus that was diagnosed 5 months previously, and she denies any history of hepatitis. She smokes one pack of cigarettes a day but does not consume alcohol. Her temperature and the remainder of her vital signs are within normal limits. The abdomen is soft and nontender. The gallbladder is palpable but without tenderness. Her stool is hemoccult-negative. Laboratory evaluations reveals a normal complete blood count and total bilirubin 12.5 mg/dL, direct bilirubin 10.8 mg/dL, AST 120 U/L, ALT 109 U/L, alkaline phosphatase 348 mg/dL, serum amylase 85 IU/L.

◆ **What is the most likely diagnosis?**

◆ **How would you confirm the diagnosis?**

ANSWERS TO CASE 36: Periampullary Tumor

Summary: A 58-year-old woman presents with painless obstructive jaundice, weight loss, and recent-onset diabetes mellitus.

◆ **Diagnosis:** Obstructive jaundice due to a periampullary tumor.

◆ **Confirmation of diagnosis:** Begin with ultrasonography to rule out biliary stones as the source of obstruction and assess the anatomic location of the biliary obstruction. A computed tomography (CT) scan should be obtained subsequently to evaluate the periampullary region if indicated by ultrasonography findings.

Objectives

1. Be familiar with the diagnostic approach to suspected peri-ampullary tumors.
2. Be familiar with the roles and outcomes of surgical and pallia-tive therapies in the treatment of periampullary tumors.

Considerations

Mechanisms contributing to jaundice can be broadly categorized as dis-orders of bilirubin metabolism, liver disease, and biliary tract obstruc-tion. This patient's predominance of **direct bilirubinemia** suggests **bil-iary obstruction** as the cause. Her clinical presentation strongly suggests **malignant extrahepatic biliary obstruction because she has painless jaundice with a palpable, nontender gallbladder (Courvoisier sign),** weight loss, and recent-onset type II diabetes mel-litus. Ultrasonography of the right upper quadrant is an inexpensive and noninvasive imaging modality that should be used initially in this pa-tient's evaluation. The study may reveal cholelithiasis, thus suggesting choledocholithiasis as the cause of biliary obstruction. Ultrasonogra-phy may also help to identify the anatomic location of the biliary ob-struction (eg, the presence of dilated intrahepatic ducts and a nondi-lated distal common bile duct implies obstruction of the midportion of the common bile duct). If the ultrasound findings suggest obstruction not related to gallstone disease, a CT scan will be useful to further differentiate between extrinsic compression and stricture and to stage the tumor. A periampullary tumor that invades the superior mesenteric artery (SMA) is considered unresectable; similarly, the presence of distant metastasis indicates disseminated disease and precludes the possibility of a surgical cure. It has been shown **that patients with periampullary carcinoma have improved survival rates when they are treated with complete resection and adjuvant chemoradiation therapy.** It is unclear at this time whether patients receiving chemoradiation therapy prior to surgery (neoadjuvant therapy) have additional survival benefits compared to those receiving postoperative therapy.

APPROACH TO PERIAMPULLARY TUMORS

Definitions

Periampullary cancers: Commonly cancers of the pancreas, distal bile duct (cholangiocarcinoma), duodenum, and ampulla of Vater. Some less common periampullary tumors are mucinous cystic tumors of the pancreas and pancreatic lymphoma.

Pancreaticoduodenectomy (PD): A procedure involving resection of the duodenum, the head of the pancreas, the common bile duct, and sometimes the distal stomach. This operation is indicated for the treatment of patients with tumors and benign disease localized in the area surrounding the ampulla of Vater. The classic form of the operation is called a **Whipple resection.** The operative mortality of PD has improved significantly over the past decade (approaching 0% to 2%), but the complication rates are still quite high (20% to 40%).

Gemcitabine: A relatively new chemotherapy agent (a deoxycytidine analog) that has been shown to prolong the survival of patients with pancreatic carcinoma and other periampullary carcinomas. Gemcitabine is an effective radiation sensitizer; therefore it is often given in conjunction with external beam radiation therapy.

Clinical Approach

Carcinoma of the Pancreas   **Pancreatic cancer is the most common periampullary cancer,** but it carries the **worst prognosis.** Overall, carcinoma of the pancreas is an uncommon tumor, consisting of only 2% of newly diagnosed cancers in the United States. This cancer, however, is the fourth leading cause of cancer death in males and the fifth leading cause of cancer death in females; it is responsible for 5% of all cancer deaths. Tumor staging is performed according to the TNM classification (Table 36–1), which also predicts patient survival. Roughly 70% of the carcinomas are located in the head of the pancreas. Common clinical manifestations of carcinoma in the head of the pancreas include obstructive jaundice, weight loss, diabetes mellitus, abdominal pain, and gastric outlet obstruction. Patients with tumors located in the body

Table 36–1

TNM STAGING OF ADENOCARCINOMA
OF THE PANCREAS

Tumor status (T)
    TX: Primary tumor cannot be assessed
    T0:   No evidence of primary tumor
    T1:   Primary tumor limited to the pancreas and measures <2 cm in diameter
    T2:   Primary tumor limited to the pancreas and measures >2 cm in diameter
    T3:   Primary tumor involves the duodenum, bile duct, or peripancreatic tissue
    T4:   Primary tumor involves the stomach, colon, or adjacent vessels
Nodal status (N)
    NX: Regional lymph nodes cannot be assessed
    N0:   No regional lymph node involvement
    N1:   Regional lymph node involvement
Metastasis (M)
    MX: Distant metastasis cannot be assessed
    M0:   Absence of distant metastasis
    M1:   Presence of distant metastasis
Stage 1: T1–T2, N0, M0
Stage 2: T3, N0, M0
Stage 3: T1–T3, N1, M0
Stage 4A: T4, N0–N1, M0
Stage 4B: any T, any N, M1

---

and tail of the pancreas typically present only after tumor growth has caused obstruction or chronic pain from splanchnic nerve invasion. In terms of prognosis, a patient who has significant weight loss and chronic abdominal and/or back pain tends to have more advanced disease and a worse prognosis.

Patient Treatment   The initial evaluation of a patient presenting with biliary obstruction is listed in Figure 36–1. When CT imaging demonstrates a mass in the head of the pancreas without evidence of liver or intraperitoneal metastases, or a chest radiograph reveals pulmonary metastases, some groups have advocated CT-guided biopsy to confirm the diagnosis and initiate induction of chemoradiation therapy. Other investigators feel that patients with potentially resectable cancers should proceed directly to laparoscopy, followed by open exploration and resection. Proponents of neoadjuvant therapy think that chemoradiation given preoperatively is better tolerated so that patients are more likely to complete the course of therapy. It is possible that the additional benefits of neoadjuvant therapy may be in selecting out those patients whose disease rapidly progresses or undergoes clinical deterioration during therapy and therefore would not benefit from surgical resection (only one-third to one-half of patients ultimately undergo resection). Issues regarding preoperative versus postoperative systemic therapy remain unresolved at this time.

Palliative Therapy   **The majority of patients with pancreatic carcinoma have unresectable disease at the time of diagnosis,** and these patients have limited survival ranging from months to 1 to 2 years. Surgical and/or other interventions are frequently indicated to relieve biliary obstruction, gastric outlet obstruction, and pain. For patients with **locally advanced and/or metastatic disease, endoscopic placement of a biliary stent is often feasible to provide effective relief of biliary obstruction** and improves the quality of life by relieving the itching and the metabolic and cosmetic effects of the obstructive jaundice. When unfeasible, percutaneous and/or operative approaches can be used to facilitate biliary drainage. Approximately 10% to 20% of patients may develop gastric outlet obstruction and may benefit from the creation of an internal bypass (gastrojejunostomy). The development of severe, persistent abdominal and back pain is frequently seen in

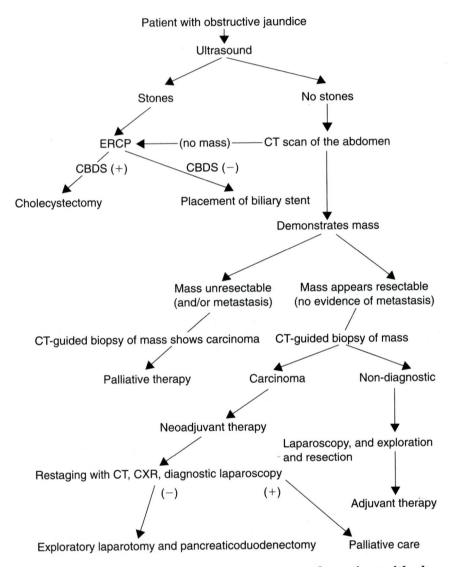

Figure 36–1. An algorithm for the treatment of a patient with obstructive jaundice. ERCP, endoscopic retrograde cholangiopancreatography; CT, computed tomography; CBDS, common bile duct stone; CXR, chest radiograph.

patients with tumor infiltration of the splanchnic nerves. This is a difficult problem to resolve. Some surgeons have reported good results with the injection of alcohol into the celiac plexus during abdominal exploration, whereas others have obtained only limited success. Alternatively, percutaneous celiac injections have been used with less effective results for nonoperative patients.

Comprehension Questions

[36.1] Which of the following is *true* regarding adenocarcinoma of the pancreas?

A. A majority of patients have unresectable tumors at presentation.
B. Anemia is a common presenting symptom.
C. Patients with isolated liver metastasis can often be cured with surgical resection.
D. It is usually associated with a predominantly elevated indirect serum bilirubin level.

[36.2] Pancreaticoduodenectomy is indicated for which one of the following patients?

A. A 55-year-old man with a history of alcoholism who presents with jaundice and an isolated mass in the head of the pancreas. Biopsy of the mass has been nondiagnostic.
B. A 60-year-old man with cirrhosis and cancer of the head of the pancreas. A CT scan indicates the presence of ascites.
C. A 40-year-old man with carcinoma of the head of the pancreas with tumor invasion of the superior mesenteric vein and artery.
D. A 50-year-old man with Gardner syndrome with an adenoma of the second portion of the duodenum.

[36.3] A 33-year-old male has been diagnosed with widely metastatic pancreatic cancer. He has severe itching and hyperbilirubinemia. Which of the following is the best therapy?

A. Administration of cholestyramine
B. Radiation therapy directed to the head of the pancreas
C. Pancreaticoduodenectomy (Whipple procedure)
D. Placement of an endoscopic stent

Answers

[36.1] **A.** Weight loss and the presence of back pain are generally indicative of disseminated and locally advanced tumors, respectively. Unlike colon cancer, pancreatic cancer is not commonly manifested by anemia, which is not a common finding until late in the course. Resection is not indicated for any metastatic disease.

[36.2] **A.** Pancreaticoduodenectomy can be performed when reasonable attempts at tissue biopsy have not revealed cancer and the clinical suspicion of cancer is high. Benign adenomas may be treated with local resection.

[36.3] **D.** A patient with widely metastatic disease will not benefit from a pancreaticoduodenectomy (Whipple procedure). The placement of an endoscopic biliary stent will bring relief with minimum morbidity and thus ameliorate the symptoms.

CLINICAL PEARLS

◈ The classic presentation of malignant extrahepatic biliary obstruction are painless jaundice and a palpable nontender gall bladder.

◈ Pancreatic cancers typically are not diagnosed until late, and are usually unresectable.

◈ In general, pancreaticoduodenectomy should be reserved for patients with localized malignancies near the ampulla of Vater.

REFERENCES

Cello JP. Pancreatic cancer. In: Feldman M, Scharischmidt BF, Sleisenger MH, eds. Sleisenger and Fordtran's gastrointestinal and liver disease, 6th ed. Philadelphia: Saunders, 1998:863–870.

Evans DB, Lee JE, Pisters PWT. Periampullary cancer. In: Cameron JL, ed. Current surgical therapy, 7th ed. St. Louis: Mosby-Year Book, 2001:558–567.

Mulvihill SJ. Pancreas. In: Norton JA, Bollinger RR, Chang AE, Lowery SF,

Mulvihill SJ, Pass HI, Thompson RW, eds. Surgery: basic science and clinical evidence. New York: Springer, 2001:517–552.

A 52-year-old woman underwent a comprehensive health evaluation as part of an application for a life insurance policy. She was noted to have a history of hypertension that was controlled with dietary modification. She was otherwise healthy, and no problems were identified. The results of her physical examination were unremarkable. Routine screening blood work was obtained, and she was noted to have a serum calcium level of 11.8 mg/dL (8.4 to 10.4 mg/dL), phosphate level of 1.9 mg/dL (2.5 to 4.8 mg/dL), and chloride level of 104 mmol/L (95 to 109 mmol/L). The other electrolyte levels determined, a complete blood count, a urinalysis, a chest radiograph, and a 12-lead electrocardiogram were all normal.

◆ **What is the most likely cause of this patient's hypercalcemia?**

◆ **How would you confirm the diagnosis?**

◆ **What is the most appropriate therapy?**

ANSWERS TO CASE 37: Hyperparathyroidism

Summary: A 52-year-old woman is found to have incidental hypercalcemia and hypophosphatemia.

◆ **Cause of hypercalcemia:** Primary hyperparathyroidism.

◆ **Confirmation of diagnosis:** An elevated serum parathyroid hormone (PTH) level and the absence of a familial pattern of hypercalcemia.

◆ **Treatment:** The treatment for primary hyperparathyroidism is surgery.

Analysis

Objectives

1. Formulate a differential diagnosis for hypercalcemia.
2. Describe the diagnosis and treatment of primary hyperparathyroidism.
3. Appreciate the natural history and long-term consequences of untreated primary hyperparathyroidism.

Considerations

The differential diagnosis of hypercalcemia is extensive. Primary hyperparathyroidism and malignancy account for 90% of all cases. In the **ambulatory setting, primary hyperparathyroidism is by far the most common cause of hypercalcemia.** In this patient, the chloride/phosphate ratio is greater than 33:1, suggesting hyperparathyroidism. The diagnosis can be confirmed by a serum PTH assay and a low level of calcium excreted in the urine.

APPROACH TO HYPERCALCEMIA AND HYPERPARATHYROIDISM

The differential diagnosis for hypercalcemia is extensive (Table 37–1). **Primary hyperparathyroidism and malignancies** account for 90% of all causes of hypercalcemia. **In the ambulatory setting, primary hyperparathyroidism is the most common cause of hypercalcemia, accounting for 50% to 60% of all cases.** Hypercalcemia is the hallmark of primary hyperparathyroidism. Patients may also have a low or low-normal serum phosphorus level, a high or high-normal serum chloride level, and mild metabolic acidosis. This is a result of the inhibitory effects of PTH on the reabsorption of phosphorus and bicarbonate in the renal tubule. Because of the increased amount of bicarbonate excreted, more chloride is reabsorbed with sodium in order to maintain electroneutrality. **A chloride/phosphorus ratio of greater than 33:1 is consistent with a diagnosis of primary hyperparathyroidism.** A definitive diagnosis of hyperparathyroidism is made by documenting an elevated serum intact PTH level by an immunoradiometric or chemiluminescence assay. **With the exception of familial hypocalciuric hypercalcemia, which may be associated with a mild increase in serum PTH levels, all other causes of hypercalcemia are associated with suppressed PTH levels.**

Since the introduction of automated laboratory methods in the early 1970s, in most patients primary hyperparathyroidism is diagnosed after incidental hypercalcemia is detected on routine blood testing. The clinical manifestations of primary hyperparathyroidism are protean (Table 37–2). Most patients admit to nonspecific symptoms such as weakness, fatigue, or constipation. **Kidney stones are the most common metabolic complication,** occurring in 15% to 20% of patients with primary hyperparathyroidism. The potential development of skeletal manifestations such as generalized demineralization, osteoporosis, and pathologic fractures are of particular concern for postmenopausal women. Gastrointestinal manifestations include peptic ulcer disease and pancreatitis. Patients may experience joint manifestations related to gout or pseudogout, as well as a wide variety of psychiatric symptoms. **Hyperparathyroidism is also associated with certain well-described cardiovascular effects including an**

Table 37–1
DIFFERENTIAL DIAGNOSIS FOR HYPERCALCEMIA

Hyperparathyroidism
   Primary
   Tertiary (occurs as a result of autonomous parathyroid function that develops in
   patients with long-standing secondary hyperparathyroidism, usually from chronic
   renal failure; also refers to hyperparathyroidism that develops after renal
   transplantation)
Malignancy
   Tumor metastases to bone
   Pseudohyperparathyroidism (secretion of parathyroid hormone–related peptide by
   renal cell carcinoma, squamous cell carcinoma of the lung, carcinoma of the
   urinary bladder)
   Hematologic malignancies (multiple myeloma, lymphoma, leukemia)
Other endocrine disorders
   Hyperthyroidism
   Hypothyroidism
   Adrenal insufficiency
   Pheochromocytoma
   VIPoma
   Acromegaly
Granulomatous diseases
   Tuberculosis
   Sarcoidosis
   Fungal infection
   Leprosy
Exogenous agents
   Calcium
   Vitamin D
   Vitamin A
   Thiazide diuretics
   Lithium
   Milk alkali
Immobilization
Paget disease
Familial hypocalciuric hypercalcemia (an autosomal dominant disorder characterized
by hypercalcemia, hypocalciuria, none of the complications of hypercalcemia, and a
urinary calcium clearance of <0.010 mmol/24 h)

Source: Reproduced, with permission, from McHenry CR. The parathyroid glands and hyperparathyroidism II. Hospital Physician, General Surgery Board Review Manual 7(1):1–11, 2001.

Table 37–2
CLINICAL MANIFESTATIONS OF PRIMARY HYPERPARATHYROIDISM

SYMPTOMS	METABOLIC CONDITIONS
Skeletal	
Bone pain	Osteitis fibrosa cystica
Pathologic fractures	Osteopenia
Joint pain	Osteoporosis
Joint swelling	Gout
	Pseudogout
	Hyperuricemia
Renal	
Colic	Nephrolithiasis
Hematuria	Nephrocalcinosis
Polyuria	Hypercalciuria
Polydipsia	Reduced creatinine clearance
Nocturia	
Gastrointestinal	
Constipation	Peptic ulcer disease
Abdominal pain	Pancreatitis
Nausea	
Vomiting	
Psychiatric	
Lethargy	Depression
Memory loss	Psychosis
Confusion	Coma
Hallucinations	
Delusions	
Neuromuscular	
Fatigue	
Muscle weakness	
Malaise	
Cardiovascular	Hypertension
	Left ventricular hypertrophy
	Heart block
	Cardiac calcifications
Dermatologic	
Brittle nails	
Pruritus	

Source: Reproduced, with permission, from McHenry CR. The parathyroid glands and hyperparathyroidism II. Hospital Physician, General Surgery Board Review Manual 7(1):1–11, 2001.

increased prevalence of hypertension, left ventricular hypertrophy, and calcification of the myocardium and the mitral and aortic valves.

A hypercalcemic crisis may occur in 1.6% to 3.2% of patients with primary hyperparathyroidism. It is manifested by **marked hypercalcemia,** with serum calcium levels usually **greater than 15 mg/dL,** and an **altered mental status.** Patients may present with nausea, vomiting, dehydration, lethargy, and confusion or frank coma.

Long-Term Effects

Untreated hyperparathyroidism has been reported to reduce patient survival by approximately 10% when compared to age- and gender-matched control subjects without hyperparathyroidism. **This increased risk for premature death is primarily due to cardiovascular disease** and less commonly to malignancy or renal failure, and it can be reversed with parathyroidectomy.

Indications and Preparation for Parathyroidectomy

Currently, the **only definitive treatment for primary hyperparathyroidism is parathyroidectomy.** There is consensus in the literature that parathyroidectomy is indicated for all **symptomatic patients** and for **asymptomatic patients younger than 50 years of age** with one or more of the following: a serum **calcium level greater than 11.5 mg/dL, a 24-hour urine calcium excretion greater than 400 mg, a creatinine clearance reduced more than 30% for the age group in the absence of another cause, or a bone mineral density greater than two standard deviations below normal** for age-, gender-, and race-matched controls. Because parathyroidectomy may improve the vague nonspecific symptoms and render survival benefits in patients with primary hyperparathyroidism, many experts advise that in the absence of prohibitive operative risk, all patients with primary hyperparathyroidism be treated with parathyroidectomy.

Comprehension Questions

[37.1] A 60-year-old postmenopausal woman with osteoporosis has a serum calcium level of 11.4 mg/dL, a serum phosphorus level of 2.0 mg/dL, and a 24-hour urine calcium excretion of 425 mg. What serum test is most likely to establish the cause of her hypercalcemia?

    A. Chloride/phosphorus ratio
    B. PTH-related polypeptide
    C. Urine calcium clearance
    D. Intact PTH level

[37.2] You are asked to evaluate a patient in the hospital with hypercalcemia. A diagnosis of hyperparathyroidism has been excluded. What is the most likely cause?

    A. Familial hypocalciuric hypercalcemia
    B. Sarcoidosis
    C. Induced by medication
    D. Malignancy

[37.3] Which of the following is the most common metabolic complication of primary hyperparathyroidism?

    A. Kidney stones
    B. Osteoporosis
    C. Pancreatitis
    D. Gout

[37.4] Which of the following abnormalities is most likely to be caused by hyperparathyroidism?

    A. Hypocalcinuria
    B. Hyperphosphatemia
    C. Hyperchloremia
    D. Elevated serum bicarbonate

Answers

[37.1] **D.** An intact PTH level, to assess for hyperparathyroidism.

[37.2] **D.** Malignancy is the most common cause of hypercalcemia encountered in patients in the hospital setting, particularly when hyperparathyroidism is ruled out.

[37.3] **A.** Kidney stones are the most common metabolic complications associated with hyperparathyroidism, occurring in 15% to 20% of patients with the disease.

[37.4] **C.** Hyperparathyroidism is associated with high secretion of calcium in urine (hypercalcinuria), low serum phosphate, high serum chloride, and low serum bicarbonate levels.

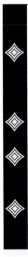

CLINICAL PEARLS

❖ Support for parathyroidectomy in an asymptomatic patient is based on the increase in cardiovascular complications and 10% survival reduction associated with patients with untreated primary parathyroidism

❖ The two most common causes of hypercalcemia are hyperparathyroidism and malignancy.

❖ Hypercalcemia with hypophosphatemia is suggestive of hyperparathyroidism. The diagnosis is confirmed by an elevated PTH level.

❖ The best treatment for primary hyperparathyroidism is surgery.

REFERENCES

McHenry CR. The parathyroid glands and hyperparathyroidism II. Hospital Physician, General Surgery Board Review Manual 2001;7(1):1–11.

Udelsman R. Primary hyperparathyroidism. In: Cameron JL, ed. Current surgical therapy, 7th ed. St. Louis: Mosby-Year Book, 2001:662–667.

A 66-year-old woman is seen in the outpatient clinic for an evaluation of weight loss. The patient says that 6 months ago her weight was 155 lb but over the past several months has steadily declined to 105 lb. The patient attributes her weight loss to an inability to eat. She indicates that whenever she tries to eat a meal, she develops intense abdominal pain that is severe and diffuse throughout the entire abdomen. To avoid this pain, the patient has limited herself to small meals and soups. She denies any fever, malaise, nausea, vomiting, or constipation. Her past medical history is significant for hypertension for which she takes an angiotensin-converting enzyme inhibitor. She smokes approximately one pack of cigarettes per day and consumes two glasses of wine per day. The physical examination reveals a thin woman in no distress. Her skin and sclera are nonicteric, and bilateral carotid bruits are present. The results of her cardiopulmonary examination are unremarkable. The abdomen is flat, nontender, and without masses. Her stool is hemoccult-negative. Her femoral pulses are diminished, with audible bruits bilaterally. The pulses are diminished in both lower extremities. Laboratory evaluations are obtained revealing a normal complete blood count and normal electrolyte levels. The serum urea nitrogen, creatine, and glucose values are within the normal range, as are the results from a urinalysis. The 12-lead electrocardiogram reveals a normal sinus rhythm.

◆ **What is the most likely diagnosis?**

◆ **What is the most likely mechanism causing the problem?**

◆ **What is the best treatment?**

ANSWERS TO CASE 38: Mesenteric Ischemia

Summary: A 66-year-old woman with carotid and femoral artery bruits presents with signs and symptoms consistent with mesenteric angina leading to "food fear" and massive weight loss.

◆ **Diagnosis:** Postprandial abdominal pain, massive weight loss, and signs of advanced atherosclerotic changes suggest possible chronic mesenteric ischemia.

◆ **Mechanism causing the problem:** Occlusion of the mesenteric arteries due to atherosclerotic changes.

◆ **Best treatment:** Aortomesenteric bypass grafting.

Analysis

Objectives

1. Know the causes, presentations, diagnosis, and treatment of mesenteric ischemia.
2. Become familiar with the diagnosis and treatment of patients with mesenteric angina due to mesenteric occlusion.

Considerations

The patient presents with the classic symptom complex of **food fear with postprandial pain and significant weight loss,** which are the hallmarks of **chronic mesenteric ischemia.** However, a thorough workup for other conditions causing abdominal pain is important because mesenteric revascularization is a procedure associated with some morbidity. When more common causes of upper and lower intestinal sources of abdominal pain are ruled out (either by strong clinical impression, endoscopy, or imaging studies), the mesenteric arteries can be studied. At centers with high-quality vascular laboratories, duplex ultrasonography is an excellent screening test. In this setting, **a normal study performed both before and after a food challenge can accurately rule out proximal mesenteric artery vascular disease.** Magnetic resonance angiography can give an accurate assessment of the superior mesenteric and celiac artery origins. Selective arteriography with lateral aortic projections remains the gold standard for definitive diagnosis and therapy planning. **The best treatment for chronic mesenteric ischemia is operative revascularization.**

APPROACH TO MESENTERIC ISCHEMIA

Chronic Mesenteric Ischemia

The most common cause of chronic mesenteric ischemia is atherosclerotic occlusive disease of the mesenteric arteries. Typically, a patient has occlusion of two of the three vessels (Table 38–1), with significant disease in the remaining mesenteric vessel. In atherosclerotic mesenteric ischemia, arteriography can be useful in guiding the therapy. Rarely, younger patients develop celiac artery compression causing an ischemic syndrome.

In selected high-risk patients, angioplasty can be a useful treatment. However, definitive revascularization with antegrade aortomesenteric bypass or perivisceral aortic endarterectomy are the best options. In the face of higher operative risks or complicating aortic atherosclerosis, a retrograde bypass from an alternative arterial source (such as the iliac artery) have a role. Advanced age and the presence of typical cardiovascular comorbidities increase the morbidity and mortality associated with mesenteric reconstructions.

Table 38–1
VISCERAL BLOOD SUPPLY

Celiac artery	Hepatic, splenic, left gastric artery
Superior mesenteric artery	Small bowel, ascending and transverse colon
Inferior mesenteric artery	Distal colon

Acute Mesenteric Ischemia

Acute mesenteric ischemia is a surgical emergency. It can be caused by an acute embolus in the superior mesenteric artery (SMA) or the celiac arteries (Figure 38–1). There is usually no history of chronic symptoms. **Arteriography can aid in the diagnosis but may lead to treatment delay;** thus, clinical judgment should be exercised in deciding whether imaging should be performed prior to emergent laparotomy. On laparotomy, the bowel can range in appearance from frankly necrotic (a late presentation) to dusky and nonmotile. With an embolus,

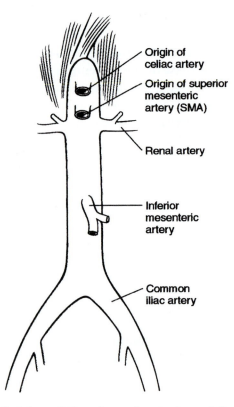

Figure 38–1. Origins of the visceral arteries arising from the abdominal aorta.

the proximal jejunum is spared because of small proximal collaterals. The embolus tends to lodge in the more distal main SMA trunk. Embolectomy may be all that is required. However, a **second-look laparotomy** should be strongly considered if the resultant bowel does not appear perfectly viable.

Less Common Causes of Mesenteric Ischemia

Nonocclusive mesenteric ischemia, associated with low-flow states, can develop in a setting of critical illness or as a result of vasospastic medications. Mesenteric venous thrombosis is uncommon and can occur as the result of advanced infectious processes due to gastrointestinal tract pathology, such as appendicitis and diverticulitis. Also, mesenteric venous thrombosis has been seen as a manifestation of a hypercoagulable state.

Comprehension Questions

[38.1] A 66-year-old man is admitted to the coronary care unit because of new-onset atrial fibrillation. After 24 hours, he develops the acute onset of abdominal pain and distension, and on examination is found to have diffuse peritonitis. The patient undergoes exploratory laparotomy with resection of necrotic bowel. Which of the following is the most important postoperative treatment for this patient?

A. Intraarterial thrombolytic therapy with streptokinase
B. Cardioversion
C. Systemic heparinization
D. Early oral feeding to stimulate intestinal lengthening

[38.2] Which of the following clinical presentations is the most typical of mesenteric angina?

A. Diarrhea that occurs following fatty meals, steatorrhea, and chronic epigastric and back pain

    B. Daily postprandial abdominal pain, associated with a 40-lb weight loss

    C. Recurrent, intermittent epigastric abdominal pain that occurs approximately 1 hour after meals

    D. Chronic, persistent abdominal and back pain of 1-month duration and a 10-lb weight loss

Answers

[38.1] **C.** This patient likely has a mural thrombus of the left atrium, which has embolized to the SMA, leading to bowel necrosis. Initiation of intravenous heparin is important to stabilize and prevent further extension of the clot. Other important steps include antibiotic therapy to prevent sepsis, echocardiography to assess for an intracardiac thrombus, and possibly a second look laparotomy to evaluate the viability of the remaining bowel. Thrombolytic therapy is not indicated in this case.

[38.2] **B.** Mesenteric angina produces symptoms after increase in GI tract workload such as meals, and weight loss because the patient learns to avoid this challenge. Answer A is more consistent with chronic pancreatitis with pancreatic exocrine insufficiency. Answer C is more typical of biliary tract disease, and answer D correlates with pancreatic malignancy.

CLINICAL PEARLS

❖ A patient with chronic mesenteric ischemia almost always has significant unexplained weight loss. If there is no weight loss, the diagnosis should be questioned.

❖ An abdominal bruit is a very nonspecific finding. It does not pay to be dogmatic about its presence or absence.

❖ Acute mesenteric ischemia is a surgical emergency.

Exposure of the SMA for embolectomy is accomplished via the root of the small bowel mesentery.

REFERENCES

Kazmers A. Chronic mesenteric ischemia. In: Cameron JL, ed. Current surgical therapy, 7th ed. St. Louis: Mosby-Year Book, 2001:970–977.

Park WM, Cherry KJ Jr, Chua HK, et al. Current results of open revascularization for chronic mesenteric ischemia: a standard for comparison. J Vasc Surg 2002;35(5):853–859.

A 68-year-old man undergoes evaluation for the treatment of an 8-cm abdominal aortic aneurysm. His past medical history is significant for unstable angina that was treated by coronary artery angioplasty and stenting 8 months ago. Since that time, he has been doing well without angina. His other medical problems include hypertension and gout. His medications are metoprolol, allopurinol, and aspirin. Recently, he has been active and walks 1 mile daily. He had a 60-pack-year smoking history but quit 8 months ago, and he consumes alcohol socially. He denies any nocturnal dyspnea or pulmonary symptoms. On physical examination, he appears well nourished. His blood pressure is 138/82, and his heart rate is 66/min. There is no jugular venous distension or carotid bruits. The lungs are clear bilaterally, and the heart sounds are normal. A nontender, pulsatile mass is present in the abdomen. No cyanosis or edema is noted in the extremities. Laboratory evaluations reveal a normal complete blood count and normal electrolyte levels. The serum urea nitrogen and serum creatinine levels are 40/1.2 mg/dL. The urinalysis reveals trace proteinuria. The electrocardiogram (ECG) reveals a normal sinus rhythm and left ventricular hypertrophy.

◆ **What are the risks associated with surgical treatment of this patient's problem?**

◆ **What can be done to optimize the patient's condition?**

ANSWERS TO CASE 39: Preoperative Risk Assessment and Optimization

Summary: A 68-year-old man with a large abdominal aortic aneurysm, hypertension, coronary artery disease, gout, and mild chronic renal insufficiency requires risk assessment and optimization prior to elective abdominal aortic aneurysm repair.

◆ **Surgical risk factors:** The risks include the usual procedural risks, postoperative pulmonary, renal, and cardiac complications.

◆ **Optimizing the status of the patient:** A complete cardiac risk assessment should be made to define the current cardiac status and identify and quantify any end-organ dysfunction caused by hypertensive and cardiac disease. Optimization of patient status can include pharmacologic therapy, coronary revascularization, and perioperative hemodynamic monitoring.

Analysis

Objective

1. Become familiar with a general approach to preoperative cardiac risk assessment.
2. Understand the principles of optimization of the medical problems of surgical patients.

Considerations

The goals of preoperative patient evaluation are to prevent perioperative complications, avoid unnecessary delays in surgical therapy, and avoid unnecessary risks to patients from testing procedures. **Elective repair of abdominal aortic aneurysms** is associated with a **postoperative mortality rate of 2% to 6%, with cardiac and renal complications being the most common causes of death.** This patient has a history of coronary artery disease and hypertension and subtle evidence of chronic renal insufficiency (proteinuria). It is vital to thoroughly assess his cardiac and renal status prior to surgery. A favorable factor in the history is that his cardiac symptoms have resolved since the coronary artery stent placement. The **risk of perioperative cardiac death or myocardial infarction is extremely low** when a patient has **completed surgical coronary revascularization within 5 years or has undergone coronary angioplasty from 6 months to 5 years prior, and** if the clinical status of the patient has remained stable **without recurrent symptoms of ischemia.** Further formal cardiac evaluation may not be required in this setting.

For this patient, the cardiac evaluation begins with a complete history, a physical examination, and direct communication with the patient's cardiologist or primary physician. Other important issues are the adequacy of the hypertensive control and the quantification of the renal insufficiency. If not obtained previously, a 24-hour urine collection to determine creatinine clearance may be helpful because the serum creatinine level in an elderly patient may not accurately reflect renal clearance functions because of the smaller muscle mass. This information may prove useful in the perioperative period for dose adjustment of medications. **Control of systolic hypertension has been shown to reduce perioperative cardiac complications,** and this should be accomplished prior to any elective surgery. Patients with **moderate cardiac risks have less frequent cardiac complications when adequate beta-blockade** is established during the perioperative period; therefore, if this patient had not been taking a beta-blocker (metoprolol), one would have been prescribed preoperatively. Further preparations during the perioperative period include preoperative hydration to prevent hypotension during anesthesia induction, monitoring of blood pressure by an arterial line, monitoring of intravascular volume status by central venous pressure measurement, and monitoring of cardiac status by a pulmonary artery catheter or transesophageal echocardiography.

PREOPERATIVE ASSESSMENT OF HIGH-RISK PATIENTS

Definitions

Metabolic demand (MET): An arbitrary measure of the aerobic demands of specific activities. The perioperative cardiac and long-term risks are increased for patients unable to meet a 4 MET demand during most of their daily living. (Example: Activities of daily living such as dressing and cooking require from 1 to 4 MET; climbing a flight of stairs, walking at 6 mi/h, and scrubbing the floor require from 4 to 10 MET).

Resting left ventricular function: Generally assessed by echocardiography. A patient with a left ventricular ejection fraction (LVEF) of less than 35% has a significantly increased risk of perioperative cardiac complications; however, a LVEF greater than 35% does not reliably rule out the development of cardiac complications.

Dobutamine stress echocardiography: Provocative testing under a controlled setting involving the administration of high-dose intravenous dobutamine to evaluate the cardiac status of patients who are unable to undergo an exercise stress test. Test results are positive when the patient develops symptoms and/or wall motion abnormalities as revealed by echocardiography. Vascular surgery patients with positive test results have a 7% to 23% risk for a perioperative myocardial infarction (MI) (high false-positive rate/low specificity). A dobutamine stress test with negative results is associated with a 0% to 7 % risk of perioperative MI (low false-negative rate/high sensitivity).

Clinical Approach

When preparing a patient with significant medical conditions for elective surgery, it is essential that the **patient's comorbidity problems be clearly defined and addressed during the perioperative period.** An assessment of comorbidity has been found to be **particularly important** for patients undergoing **vascular surgery procedures.** Advanced vascular disease is frequently associated with long-standing diabetes, atherosclerosis, and hypertension, and these factors may cause multiple end-organ damage and reduce the patient's physiologic reserve. The assessment of cardiac risk consists of the eight steps listed in Table 39–1. Several major, intermediate, and minor clinical predictors can be used to determine patient risks (Table 39–2). Clinical history, the **patient's current symptoms, and the level of physical activity** are important in determining the patient's risk. Notably, in vascular surgery patients, **coronary artery disease may be clinically silent because of limited**

Table 39–1
CONSIDERATIONS IN PREOPERATIVE
CARDIAC RISK ASSESSMENT

Step 1	What is the urgency of the surgical procedure? (If emergent, short-term medical optimization and perioperative monitoring may be indicated.)
Step 2	Has the patient undergone coronary revascularization during the past 5 y, and if so, have the symptoms resolved? (If yes, low risk.)
Step 3	Has the patient undergone an adequate cardiac evaluation during the past 2 y? (If yes and the results are favorable, then repeated studies are unnecessary.)
Step 4	Does the patient have an unstable coronary syndrome or a major clinical predictor of risk? (If yes, the elective procedure should be postponed until these issues can be addressed.)
Step 5	Does the patient have an intermediate predictor of risk? (If yes, consideration of functional capacity and procedural risk are important in identifying patients who may benefit from further noninvasive testing.)
Step 6	(a) Intermediate-risk patients with moderate or excellent functional capacity generally undergo intermediate-risk procedures with low cardiac morbidity. (b) Further noninvasive testing may benefit patients with poor to moderate functional capacity undergoing high-risk procedures.
Step 7	Patients with neither major nor intermediate clinical predictors and who have moderate to excellent functional capacity ($\geq$4 MET) can generally tolerate noncardiac surgery; additional noninvasive testing is performed on an individual basis.
Step 8	(a) The results of noninvasive testing often identify the need for preoperative coronary intervention or cardiac surgery. (b) In general, cardiac intervention is undertaken if the morbidity associated with these interventions is less than that of the planned surgery. (c) If the morbidity of cardiac preoperative intervention exceeds the morbidity of the planned surgical procedures, coronary intervention is indicated only if it also significantly improves the patient's long-term prognosis.

Table 39–2

CLINICAL PREDICTORS OF CARDIAC RISK[*]

MAJOR CLINICAL PREDICTORS	INTERMEDIATE CLINICAL PREDICTORS	MINOR CLINICAL PREDICTORS
Unstable coronary syndrome Decompensated CHF Significant arrhythmias Severe valvular disease	Mild angina pectoris Prior myocardial infarction Compensated CHF or prior CHF Diabetes mellitus	Advanced age Abnormal electrocardiogram Rhythm other than sinus Low functional capacity History of stroke Uncontrolled systemic hypertension

[*]CHF, congestive heart failure.

activity and/or coexisting diabetes mellitus. The other major component in risk assessment is stratification of the cardiac risk associated
with the proposed operative procedure. The combination of patient risk
and procedural risk is used to determine if additional testing, coronary
intervention, or perioperative monitoring is indicated.

Additional cardiac evaluation ranges from noninvasive tests such as
24-hour Holter monitoring, echocardiography, exercise stress testing,
pharmacologic stress testing, and invasive examinations such as cardiac
catheterization. Generally, patients with **moderate clinical risks** who
are to undergo moderate- to high-risk procedures may benefit from
noninvasive stress testing. High-risk patients who are to undergo high-
risk procedures may benefit from coronary angiography and possibly
coronary revascularization when their condition does not improve with
medication adjustments and when it is determined that revascularization provides long-term survival benefits.

Comprehension Questions

[39.1] A 63-year-old man desires elective repair of an asymptomatic
inguinal hernia because it interferes with his golf game. He has
a history of hypertension controlled with an angiotensin-

converting enzyme inhibitor and suffered an MI 4 years ago. He underwent coronary artery bypass 4 years ago and has been asymptomatic since that time. Which of the following is the most appropriate preoperative plan?

A. Review of the history, physical examination, ECG, and routine laboratory tests prior to surgery
B. Review of the history, physical examination, ECG, laboratory tests, and a stress test prior to surgery
C. Review of the history, physical examination, ECG, laboratory tests, and coronary angiography to document the patency of bypass grafts
D. Review of the history, physical examination, ECG, laboratory tests, and V/Q scan prior to surgery

[39.2] A 55-year-old patient with a history of unstable angina presents with acute abdominal pain. He is found to have diffuse peritonitis, tachycardia, and chest pain. The ECG shows ischemic changes in the anterior leads. An upright chest radiograph reveals a pneumoperitoneum. Based on these findings, a perforated peptic ulcer is suspected. Which of the following is the most appropriate treatment?

A. Antibiotics therapy and immediate cardiac catheterization
B. Antibiotics therapy and nonoperative care
C. Antibiotics therapy, invasive monitoring, maximal treatment for his cardiac disease, and surgery when he is stabilized in 48 hours
D. Antibiotics therapy, invasive monitoring, and early surgical intervention

[39.3] Which of the following is true of dobutamine echocardiography?

A. It is highly specific in identifying patients who will develop perioperative cardiac complications.
B. It is highly sensitive in identifying patients who will develop perioperative complications.

C. When positive, it reliably predicts the occurrence of perioperative complications.
D. It is of limited use in patients with moderate clinical risk
   who have poor functional capacity and are undergoing high-
   risk procedures

Answers

[39.1] **A.** History, physical examination, laboratory tests, and an ECG
are sufficient evaluation for this patient who underwent surgical revascularization of the coronary vessels 4 years ago and has
had no recurrence of symptoms.

[39.2] **D.** A perforated ulcer is a surgical emergency. Early supportive
care, invasive monitoring, and operative therapy are indicated
for this patient with intra-abdominal sepsis and evolving cardiac
ischemia because the underlying septic process is presumably
contributing to the cardiac complication.

[39.3] **B.** Dobutamine echocardiography has a sensitivity of 93% to
100% in identifying patients with coronary artery disease, but
perioperative MI is seen in only 7% to 23% of patients with positive stress test results (low specificity).

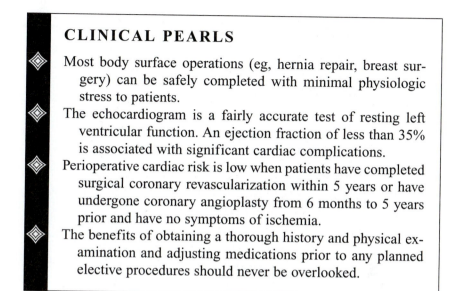

CLINICAL PEARLS

◈ Most body surface operations (eg, hernia repair, breast surgery) can be safely completed with minimal physiologic stress to patients.

◈ The echocardiogram is a fairly accurate test of resting left ventricular function. An ejection fraction of less than 35% is associated with significant cardiac complications.

◈ Perioperative cardiac risk is low when patients have completed surgical coronary revascularization within 5 years or have undergone coronary angioplasty from 6 months to 5 years prior and have no symptoms of ischemia.

◈ The benefits of obtaining a thorough history and physical examination and adjusting medications prior to any planned elective procedures should never be overlooked.

REFERENCE

Eagle KA, Brundage BH, Chatman BR, et al: Guidelines for perioperative cardiovascular evaluation for noncardiac surgery: reports of the American College of Cardiology/American Heart Association Task Force on Practice Guidelines. Circulation 1996;93:1278–1347.

A 45-year-old man presents with a 2-month history of epigastric abdominal pain. He describes the pain as burning and says that it occurs at night or early in the morning. The patient has found that eating food generally improves these symptoms. The patient admits to having had similar symptoms intermittently during the past several years, and over-the-counter H2 antagonists have always resolved his symptoms. He denies any weight loss, vomiting, or melena. He has no family history of significant medical problems. The patient's physical examination reveals a normal head and neck, and cardiopulmonary examinations show no abnormalities. The abdomen is nondistended, minimally tender in the epigastrium, and without masses. A rectal examination reveals hemoccult-negative stool. Laboratory studies reveal normal values for the white blood cell (WBC) count, hemoglobin and hematocrit levels, platelet count, electrolyte levels, serum amylase level, and liver function tests.

◆ **What is your next step?**

◆ **What is the most likely diagnosis?**

◆ **What are the treatment options?**

ANSWERS TO CASE 40: Peptic Ulcer Disease

Summary: A 45-year-old man has signs and symptoms consistent with peptic ulcer disease (PUD). The patient has self-medicated with H_2-receptor antagonists in the past with success, but the symptoms are currently unrelieved with medication.

◆ **Next step:** Perform diagnostic esophagogastroduodenoscopy (EGD).

◆ **Most likely diagnosis:** Peptic ulcer disease.

◆ **Treatment options:** Testing for *Helicobacter pylori* should be performed, and if positive results are obtained, treatment should be administered. If the *H. pylori* status is negative, conventional treatment for PUD should be administered (see below).

Analysis

Objective

1. Be familiar with the five types of gastric ulcers and their implications in pathogenesis and treatment.
2. Be able to discuss the relationship between *H. pylori* and PUD.
3. Become familiar with the mechanisms of action and the efficacy of medications used for the treatment of PUD.
4. Become familiar with the indications for surgery in the treatment of ulcer disease.

Considerations

The case presented is fairly convincing for PUD that is refractory to medical management. However, whenever such a patient is encountered, the initial step should be to evaluate for other disease processes (ie, pancreatitis, gastric malignancy, biliary colic). In this case, upper gastrointestinal (GI) endoscopy is indicated to assess the ulcer disease, as well as the esophagus, stomach, and duodenum. When indicated, ultrasonography and computed tomography (CT) imaging of the abdomen may be useful. When it is confirmed that the patient is indeed suffering from PUD, it is important to question the patient to see if he has been compliant with the medical therapy. Failure of optimal medical therapy may be influenced by the presence of *H. pylori,* high gastrin levels, or noxious stimuli such as nonsteroidal anti-inflammatory drugs (NSAIDs).

APPROACH TO ULCER DISEASE

Despite advances in medical therapy for the inhibition of acid secretion and the eradication of *H. pylori,* surgery remains important in treating patients suffering from PUD. Moreover, the introduction of more effective antiulcer medications has not decreased the mortality from PUD, as it has remained stable or risen slightly. Furthermore, with the high recurrence rate of ulcers following the discontinuation of medical therapy, there has been a renewed interest in operative therapy. There has been a change in the type of surgery performed on patients with PUD in the *H. pylori* era. Specifically, gastric resections are less frequently used, and **vagotomy procedures with or without drainage seem to be most effective.**

Pathophysiology of Peptic Ulcer Disease

Benign Gastric Ulcer   The number of hospitalizations and operations for patients with benign gastric ulcers may be increasing slightly because of the greater use and abuse of NSAIDs, particularly in women. As shown in Table 40–1, there are five types of gastric ulcers. **The most common, accounting for 60% to 70% of these ulcers, are type 1 ulcers located on the greater curvature at or proximal to the incisura.** Hypersecretion of acid is generally not a causative factor, but acid likely plays a permissive role in ulcer development and accentuates their progression once they occur. Evidence also suggests that *H. pylori* has a role in ulcer pathogenesis, although the etiologic role is not as strong as in the case of duodenal ulcers. In general, hemorrhage is infrequent in this setting although penetration with or without perforation

Table 40–1
TYPES OF GASTRIC ULCERS

TYPE	LOCATION	ACID SECRETION
I	Gastric body, usually lesser curvature	Low
II	Gastric body, in association with a duodenal ulcer	High
III	Prepyloric region	High
IV	High on lesser curvature	Low
V	Anywhere in the stomach	Nonsteroidal anti-inflammatory drugs

is not uncommon. **Type 2 ulcers** account for about 20% and are in the **same location as type 1 lesions** but **are also associated with duodenal ulcer disease and excessive acid secretion.** Hemorrhage, obstruction, and perforation are frequently seen with this type of gastric ulcer. **Type 3 gastric ulcers are** located **within 2 cm of the pylorus (ie, prepyloric) and are also associated with excess acid secretion.** Again, hemorrhage and perforation are frequent with this type of gastric ulcer. **Type 4 gastric ulcers are rarely encountered** but are situated **within 2 cm of the gastroesophageal junction,** are associated with **hypochlorhydria,** and carry a **significant operative mortality risk.** Hemorrhage is uncommon in this type of ulcer, although penetration is frequent. The **fifth type of gastric ulcer can occur anywhere in the stomach and is a direct result of chronic ingestion of aspirin or NSAIDs.**

Duodenal Ulcers   The number of hospitalizations and elective operations for duodenal ulcer disease has decreased dramatically over the past three decades. However, the number of urgent operations appears to be increasing; also, because patients tend to be older than previously, there is increased perioperative morbidity and mortality. Duodenal ulcer disease has multiple etiologies. The only relatively absolute requirements are secretion of acid and pepsin in conjunction with an *H. pylori* infection or the ingestion of NSAIDs. Gastric acid secretory rates are usually increased in patients with duodenal ulcer disease.

There is strong evidence for an association between gastric antral infestation with *H. pylori* and duodenal ulcer disease, particularly in ulcers that are resistant to or recur after standard antisecretory therapy. Moreover, in patients infected with *H. pylori,* complete eradication of the organism results in extraordinarily high healing rates and low recurrence rates of about 2%.

Treatment of Uncomplicated Peptic Ulcer Disease

Following a review of the patient's history, a physical examination, and routine laboratory studies, endoscopy is generally performed (Figure 40–1). In addition, testing for *H. pylori* should be performed as *H. pylori* is present in most gastric ulcer patients (60% to 90%) and those who are not infected tend to be NSAID users. *H. pylori* is found in more than 90% of patients with duodenal ulcer disease. Nearly all of the currently available tests for detecting *H. pylori* have good sensitivity and specificity. Noninvasive testing includes a serologic study and a urea breath test. Useful invasive tests include the rapid urease assay or a histologic study and cultures in conjunction with endoscopy. For an initial diagnosis without endoscopy, a serologic study is the test of choice. With endoscopy, the rapid urease assay and a histologic examination are both excellent options, although the rapid urease test is less expensive. If patients test positive for *H. pylori,* treatment should be instituted. **Failure to eradicate *H. pylori* leads to an annual relapse of roughly 58%, as opposed to roughly 2% when *H. pylori* has been eradicated.** In general, triple therapy regimens are more successful than dual therapy or monotherapy for eradicating *H. pylori.* Three promising triple regimens are currently available: OAC, OMC, and OAM (*O,* omeprazole or a protein pump inhibitor [PPI]; *A,* amoxicillin; *C,* clarithromycin; and *M,* metronidazole). These medications are used for 1 to 2 weeks, do not contain bismuth, and are taken twice daily. For patients who are *H. pylori*–negative, conventional treatment should be administered.

The agents available for the medical treatment of gastric ulcers are shown in Table 40–2 along with their mechanism of action. In general, drugs can heal ulcers by neutralizing acid secretion or by restoring mucosal defenses. While both histamine-2-receptor antagonists and PPIs inhibit acid secretion, PPIs block all types of acid secretion because of

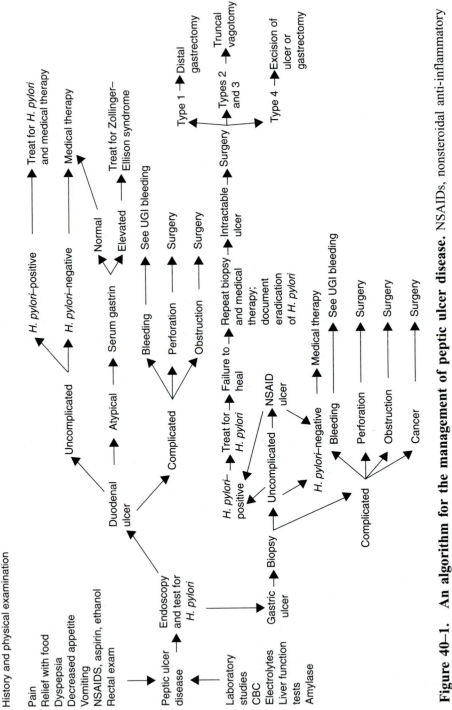

Figure 40–1. An algorithm for the management of peptic ulcer disease. NSAIDs, nonsteroidal anti-inflammatory drugs; UGI, upper gastrointestinal; CBC, complete blood count.

Table 40–2

MEDICAL THERAPY FOR PEPTIC ULCER DISEASE

AGENT	MECHANISM OF ACTION
Antacids	Neutralize gastric acidity and decrease activity of pepsin
Histamine-2 antagonist	Block parietal cell histamine-2 receptor
Proton pump inhibitors	Inhibits H^+-K^+-adenosine-triphosphatase pump
Sucralfate	Complexes with pepsin and bile salts and binds to proteins in mucosa
Prostaglandins	Inhibit, acid secretion, increase endogenous mucosal defense

their direct inhibition of the proton pump. As a result, they also produce more prolonged inhibition of acid secretion than histamine-2 blockers.

A gastric ulcer should be treated for 8 to 12 weeks and then evaluated for healing. If it has not healed, a biopsy should be repeated to rule out malignancy. If it has healed, maintenance therapy should be considered provided the patient is not taking NSAIDs and does not have *H. pylori* infection.

In the setting of NSAID use, it is best to discontinue these drugs if possible while the ulcer is being treated. Ulcer therapy is still initiated with an antiacid secretory agent, preferably a PPI. *Helicobacter pylori* infection should also be treated if present. For NSAID-dependent patients, cotherapy with misoprostol, a prostaglandin analog, should be considered, or switching to a safer NSAID that selectively inhibits the inducible isoform of cyclooxygenase (ie, COX-2).

Surgical Therapy

In both gastric and duodenal ulcer disease, surgery is indicated for the complications of PUD. Gastrointestinal hemorrhage, perforation, intractable pain, and obstruction are indications for surgical intervention. Ulcers are considered **intractable if they persist for more than 3 months despite active drug therapy, the ulcer recurs within 1 year after initial healing despite maintenance therapy,** or if the ulcer disease is characterized by **cycles of prolonged activity with brief**

remissions. Gastric ulcers should undergo biopsy early in the evaluation process because of **the risk for carcinoma.** Thus, for intractable gastric ulcers, excision of the ulcer should be performed in conjunction with proximal gastric vagotomy or some type of gastrectomy. For a type 1 gastric ulcer in the setting of intractability, elective distal gastrectomy with gastroduodenal (Billroth I) anastomosis is usually performed. The ulcer should be included in the antrectomy specimen. For type 2 gastric ulcers, antrectomy that includes the gastric ulcer is generally performed in conjunction with a truncal vagotomy to further reduce acid secretion and remove the gastric mucosa at risk for ulcer as well as the ulcer itself. The type of reconstruction, gastroduodenostomy (Billroth I) or gastrojejunostomy (Billroth II) depends on how badly the duodenum is inflamed. An alternative is truncal vagotomy and gastrojejunostomy. A third option is vagotomy and pyloroplasty. For type 3 gastric ulcers, a vagotomy and antrectomy that includes the ulcer is usually performed. As previously mentioned, type 4 gastric ulcers are difficult to treat, and the choice of operation depends on a number of factors. These include the size of the ulcer and the degree of surrounding inflammation, as well as the distance of the ulcer from the gastroesophageal junction. **Type 5 gastric ulcers rarely require surgery,** and if this type of ulcer does not heal rapidly with the standard medical therapy mentioned above, malignant disease must be excluded.

For treatment of perforated duodenal ulcers, when there is no prior history of ulcer disease or if they are *H. pylori*–positive, an omental patch closure may be performed and treatment for *H. pylori* administered. If the patient has an underlying history of ulcer disease or is known to be *H. pylori*–negative, and is hemodynamically stable at the time of the procedure, a highly selective vagotomy is another option in addition to closure of the perforation. For the treatment of perforated gastric ulcers, the possibility of malignancy still must be addressed as well as the possibility of *H. pylori* infection. Thus, depending on the type of gastric ulcer, the area requires biopsy with closure of the perforation. Alternatively, the ulcer can also be excised and/or resected with primary repair or a Billroth I or II reconstruction. For an obstruction, the patient can be treated with antrectomy and gastroduodenostomy, although if scarring is so severe as to preclude a safe anastomosis, gastrojejunostomy in conjunction with a truncal vagotomy should be performed.

Comprehension Questions

[40.1] Which of the following best describes a characteristic of gastric ulcers?

    A. Type 1 gastric ulcers are usually not associated with excess acid secretion
    B. Type 1 gastric ulcers are usually located in the prepyloric region of the stomach
    C. Type 2 gastric ulcers are usually associated with esophageal disease
    D. Type 5 is a gastric ulcer associated with chronic steroid use

[40.2] Which of the following best describes characteristics of duodenal ulcer disease?

    A. It is rarely associated with hypersecretion of acid
    B. It is a disease of multiple etiologies
    C. Complete erradication of *H. pylori* is difficult and associated with frequent recurrences
    D. *H. pylori* infestation usually occurs in the gastric cardia

[40.3] Which of the following is correct regarding medical therapy of peptic ulcer disease?

    A. Proton pump inhibitors and histamine antagonists have approximately equal efficacy in controlling ulcer disease.
    B. Prostaglandin compounds such as misoprostol promote resolution of gastric ulcers by decreasing acid production.
    C. NSAID induced ulcers are sometimes associated with *H. pylori* and require antibiotic therapy.
    D. Histamine 1 receptors are associated with gastric acid secretion.

[40.4] A 35-year-old male is diagnosed with a duodenal ulcer. He asks about the indications for surgical therapy versus medical treatment. Which one of the following conditions would necessitate surgical therapy?

A. Development of diabetes mellitus
B. Persistent *H. pylori* infection
C. Gastric outlet obstruction
D. Need for taking NSAIDs

Answers

[40.1] **A.** Type 1 gastric ulcers are usually not associated with excess acid secretion and usually are located on the lesser curvature of the stomach. Type 5 gastric ulcers are associated with chronic NSAID or aspirin use.

[40.2] **B.** Duodenal ulcer disease has multiple etiologies, and is commonly associated with acid hypersecretion. Antacid therapy results in a high rate of ulcer resolution but the eradication of *H. pylori* helps to maintain long-term ulcer cure.

[40.3] **C.** Patients with NSAID induced ulcers not uncommonly also have *H. pylori* involvement, and when *H. pylori* is documented, those affected require antibiotic therapy to promote complete healing. In general, proton pump inhibitors have superior efficacy over H2 blockers.

[40.4] **C.** Gastric outlet obstruction due to chronic duodenal ulcer is an indication for surgical therapy, as is inability to exclude malignancy, intractable symptoms, and perforation.

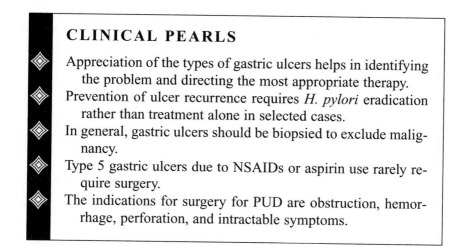

CLINICAL PEARLS

- Appreciation of the types of gastric ulcers helps in identifying the problem and directing the most appropriate therapy.
- Prevention of ulcer recurrence requires *H. pylori* eradication rather than treatment alone in selected cases.
- In general, gastric ulcers should be biopsied to exclude malignancy.
- Type 5 gastric ulcers due to NSAIDs or aspirin use rarely require surgery.
- The indications for surgery for PUD are obstruction, hemorrhage, perforation, and intractable symptoms.

REFERENCES

Armstrong CP, Blower AL. Non-steroidal anti-inflammatory drugs and life threatening complications of peptic ulceration. Gut 1987;28:527–532.

Dempsey D, Ashley S, Mercer D, Sillin L. Peptic ulcer surgery in the *H. pylori* era: indications for operation. Contemp Surg 2001;57:433–441.

Griffin MR, Ray WA, Schaffner W. Nonsteroidal anti-inflammatory drug use and death from peptic ulcer in elderly persons. Ann Intern Med 1988;109:359–363.

Ng EK, Lam YH, Sung JJ, et al. Eradication of *Helicobacter pylori* prevents recurrence of ulcer after simple closure of duodenal ulcer perforation: randomized controlled trial. Ann Surg 2000;231:153–158.

Soll AH. Pathogenesis of peptic ulcer and implications for treatment. New Engl J Med 1990;322:909–916.

Taylor TV. Deaths from peptic ulceration. BMJ 1985;291:653–654.

Tygat GNJ: Treatments that impact favorably upon the eradication of *Helicobacter pylori* and ulcer recurrence. Aliment Pharmacol Ther 1994;8:359–368.

CASE 41

A 23-year-old man was the restrained driver of an automobile involved in a high-speed head-on collision with an 18-wheeler that drifted across the highway divider. According to the paramedics, the front-seat occupant in the patient's automobile was found dead at the scene. Extrication of the patient required approximately 30 minutes. His vital signs at the scene were pulse rate 110/min, blood pressure 90/60, respiratory rate 14/min, and Glasgow Coma Score (GCS) 6. The paramedics performed endotracheal intubation, placed a peripheral intravenous line and initiated ventilation, and administered intravenous fluids during transportation to your trauma center. His vital signs on arrival at the emergency center are temperature 36.2C° (97.2°F), pulse 112/min, blood pressure 88/70, assisted respiratory rate 20/min, and GCS 6 (4 + 1 + 1). A forehead hematoma, multiple facial lacerations and abrasions, and a bony deformity of the left cheek are present. The breath sounds are diminished on the left, with soft tissue crepitance in the left anterior chest wall. The abdomen is distended, with diminished bowel sounds. The bony pelvis is stable to palpation. Examination of the extremities reveals a markedly swollen, tender left thigh with a 10-cm laceration over the left knee. The peripheral pulses are present in all the extremities. No spontaneous movements in the lower extremities are identified.

◆ **What should be the next steps in the treatment?**

◆ **What are the most likely mechanisms causing the patient's current clinical picture?**

ANSWERS TO CASE 41: Blunt Trauma (Multiple)

Summary: A 23-year-old restrained driver is involved in a high-speed motor vehicle collision (MVC). He presents with tachycardia, hypotension, and a GCS of 6. The patient's initial assessment suggests the following injuries: closed head injury, left pneumothorax, possible intra-abdominal injury, and left femur fracture. The exact cause of the hypotension is undetermined at this time.

◆ **Next steps:** Placement of a left chest tube (tube thoracostomy) should be performed to treat the suspected left pneumothorax, which should improve his breathing and address a potential cause of the hemodynamic instability.

◆ **Responsible mechanisms:** The possible causes of the tachycardia, hypotension, and unresponsiveness in this patient include hemorrhagic shock and left tension pneumothorax; less likely causes are spinal shock, primary cardiac dysfunction, and severe closed head injury.

Analysis

Objectives

1. Understand the priorities and principles in treating patients with multiple injuries, including blunt chest injury, blunt abdominal injury, closed head injury, orthopedic injury, and spinal cord injury.
2. Recognize the causes of hemodynamic instability in a trauma patient and learn the methods of diagnosis for these problems.

Considerations

A young man is injured in a high-speed MVC and presents with tachycardia, hypotension, a GCS of 6, a clinically suspicious left pneumothorax, and a left femur fracture. It is vital to approach any patient with multiple injuries or the potential for multiple injuries in a systematic fashion to ensure that serious injuries are identified and treated in the timeliest manner. **The evaluation begins by learning the details of the collision from the patient, eyewitnesses, or paramedics to gain insight into the injury mechanism and severity.** With an initial **GCS of 6, a severe closed head injury should be strongly suspected, and therefore early airway control is essential for oxygenation, ventilation, and minimizing the possibility of secondary brain injury.**

On arrival of the patient at the emergency department, the primary survey should begin with reassessment of the airway to make certain that the endotracheal tube has been secured in the correct position. The presence of **left chest wall crepitance, diminished breath sounds, and hypotension are highly suggestive of pneumothorax** or possibly tension pneumothorax; therefore, a **left chest tube should be placed even prior to confirmation** by chest radiography. If the patient remains hemodynamically unstable following chest tube insertion, the cause of the hypotension is most likely hemorrhage. Treatment should then be directed toward restoring intravascular volume, and simultaneous attempts should be made to identify the source of blood loss. It is important to recognize that other causes of hypotension in the acute traumatic setting are possible but less likely, and these include cardiac dysfunction, cardiac tamponade, and neurogenic shock. Because these other causes of shock are far less common than hemorrhagic shock, **hypotension in a polytrauma patient should be presumed to be the result of hemorrhage until bleeding from all possible sources can be ruled out. The potential locations of major blood loss to be considered include external, pleural space, intraperitoneal, retroperitoneal, pelvic, and soft tissue.** A survey of the patient's body for open wounds and clothing for blood is usually helpful in identifying external blood loss. A chest radiograph or bilateral chest tubes are useful in locating pleural space blood loss. A pelvic radiograph can identify bony fractures and/or dislocations, which are the primary cause of extraperitoneal pelvic blood loss.

Intraperitoneal bleeding can be readily identified by diagnostic peritoneal lavage (DPL) or focused abdominal sonography for trauma (FAST) performed during the secondary survey of unstable patients. Major long bone fractures are the result of large kinetic energy transfers and are associated with destruction and bleeding from the surrounding soft tissue; this type of bleeding is generally identified by physical examination and radiography. Retroperitoneal blood loss without pelvic fracture occurs rarely and can be identified by FAST. **Injuries to the cervical or upper thoracic spinal cord can disrupt sympathetic functions** and lead to **neurogenic shock.** The majority of spinal cord injuries occur in the presence of bony fractures and/or dislocations; therefore, plain radiographs of the spine can be utilized to screen for these injuries. Rarely, cardiac dysfunction can result from blunt injury, which is generally recognized by echocardiography or elevated right heart filling pressures measured through central venous catheters or pulmonary artery catheters. **In a hemodynamically unstable patient, it is important to identify life-threatening problems in a timely fashion without having to transport the patient to the radiology suite. Therefore, the use of a computed tomography (CT) scan is not indicated in the evaluation of unstable trauma patients.**

APPROACH TO MULTIPLE TRAUMA

Definitions

Focused abdominal sonography for trauma: A quick ultrasound examination performed during the secondary survey. The four views examined are subxiphoid, right and left upper quadrant, and pelvic. The FAST procedure is sensitive in identifying intraperitoneal fluid and pericardial fluid, and it is most useful for the rapid assessment of unstable patients.

Diagnostic peritoneal lavage: A bedside invasive diagnostic procedure performed during the secondary survey in unstable patients. This study is highly sensitive in identifying intraperitoneal blood. Positive results are defined as 10 ml of gross blood or enteric content aspirate or a red blood cell (RBC) count of more than 100,000/mL or a white blood cell (WBC) count of more than 500/mL. The primary limitation of DPL is its lack of specificity. In hemodynamically stable patients, laparotomies performed on the basis of microscopically positive DPL result in nontherapeutic laparotomies in up to 30% of patients.

Abdominal computed tomography scans: A sensitive, specific diagnostic modality for solid organ injuries, retroperitoneal injuries, and peritoneal fluid in the blunt trauma setting. Because of the time required for completion and the need to transport patients to an uncontrolled environment, CT imaging is contraindicated for unstable patients.

Clinical Treatment

The **initial treatment** begins with a primary survey consisting of **airway (A), breathing (B), and circulation (C)** assessment and optimization. The primary survey focuses on immediate life-threatening problems, which should be promptly treated. Once the ABC's have been addressed satisfactorily, a **secondary survey** is conducted via a **thorough head-to-toe examination and an inventory of all possible injuries.** Plain nasogastric tubes and urinary catheters are placed as needed. After completion of the primary and secondary surveys, the next step in treating the patient can generally be determined. If the patient is stable, additional radiographic studies can be completed in the radiology suite as indicated. It is important to remember that **whenever a patient develops any significant change in clinical condition, a thorough reevaluation beginning with the ABC's should be immediately performed.** For patients with identifiable bleeding, neurosurgical injuries, and orthopedic injuries, the problem of ongoing bleeding should be addressed first if it causes hemodynamic instability. Damage control operations are abbreviated surgeries to control bleeding and may be useful to allow timely management of severe neurosurgical injuries. Generally, the treatment of major orthopedic injuries not associated with significant bleeding can be delayed until after an initial period of stabilization ($>$24 to 48 hours). **Most hemodynamically stable patients with hemoperitoneum, liver, spleen, or kidney injuries can be treated nonoperatively with close observation.**

Comprehension Questions

[41.1] A 73-year-old man is seen after falling down a flight of stairs. He arrives on a backboard with a C-collar in place. His initial pulse rate is 70/min, blood pressure 160/80, respiratory rate 10/min, and GCS 6. He has a large scalp hematoma, a dilated, nonreactive left pupil, and a large bruise over his left flank. Which of the following is the *most appropriate* treatment?

A. Provide an O_2 face mask and intravenous (IV) fluids, obtain a head and abdomen CT scan, and request a neurosurgical consultation.
B. Perform endotracheal intubation, provide IV fluids, obtain an abdomen CT scan, and request a neurosurgical consultation.
C. Perform endotracheal intubation, provide IV fluids, perform a FAST examination, request a neurosurgical consultation, and prepare to perform bedside decompressive craniectomy.
D. Perform endotracheal intubation, provide IV fluids, perform a FAST examination, obtain a head CT scan, and request a neurosurgical consultation.

[41.2] An abdominal CT scan for blunt trauma patient evaluations is

A. Costly and time-consuming, thus should not be used when DPL is available.
B. Highly sensitive and specific for solid organ injuries but lacks sensitivity for retroperitoneal and hollow viscus injuries.
C. Highly sensitive and specific for solid organ injuries but lacks sensitivity for hollow viscus injuries.
D. Highly sensitive and specific for solid organ injuries and intraperitoneal blood and useful for both stable and hypotensive patients.

Answers

[41.1] **D.** In a hemodynamically stable patient with signs of severe closed head injury with a left hemispheric mass effect as demonstrated by the nonreactive and dilated left pupil, airway management with controlled ventilation can minimize secondary brain injury. A CT scan of the head is vital to help the neurosurgeon define the problem so that the appropriate surgical intervention can be performed. A blindly performed craniectomy is never indicated.

[41.2] **C.** A CT scan of the abdomen is very accurate in identifying solid organ and retroperitoneal injuries, but it lacks sensitivity for hollow viscus injuries. Fortunately, hollow viscus injuries are unusual following blunt trauma and occur in only 1% to 5% of cases.

CLINICAL PEARLS

◈ Airway, breathing, and circulation should be reassessed whenever clinical deterioration develops in a trauma patient.

◈ Obtaining a detailed description of the traumatic event helps to identify the injury mechanisms and direct the evaluation process.

◈ A closed head injury is rarely the cause of hemodynamic instability in a trauma patient; therefore the evaluation should be directed toward identification of the bleeding source.

◈ A low GCS score in a patient with profound shock may result from cerebrospinal fluid hypoperfusion, and the usual sequence of approach should not be altered.

REFERENCES

Hoyt DB, Coimbra R, Winchell RJ. Management of acute trauma. In: Townsend CM, Beauchamp RD, Evers BM, Mattox KL, eds. Textbook of surgery: the biological basis of modern surgical practice, 16th ed. Philadelphia: Saunders, 2001:311–344.

Spector SA, Rabinovici R. Initial evaluation and resuscitation of the trauma patient. In: Cameron JL, ed. Current surgical therapy, 7th ed. St. Louis: Mosby-Yearbook, 2001:1050–1062.

A 44-year-old women is found to have an incidental anterior mediastinal mass as revealed by a preemployment chest radiograph. The patient has no known medical problems, and she denies respiratory and gastrointestinal symptoms. On examination, she is found to have mild bilateral ptosis and no neck masses. The results of the cardiopulmonary examination are unremarkable, and there is no generalized lymphadenopathy. The neurologic examination reveals normal sensation and diminished muscle strength in all the extremities with repetitive motion against resistance. A computed tomography (CT) scan of the chest reveals the presence of a 4.5-cm, well-circumscribed solid mass in the anterior mediastinum.

◆ **What is the diagnosis?**

◆ **What is the best therapy?**

ANSWERS TO CASE 42: Thymoma and Myasthenia Gravis

Summary: A 44-year-old woman has an 4.5-cm anterior mediastinal mass and symptoms suggestive of myasthenia gravis.

◆ **Most likely diagnosis:** An incidentally identified thymoma in a patient with class IIA myasthenia gravis (MG).

◆ **Best therapy:** The best treatment for thymoma is complete resection.

Analysis

Objectives

1. Know the pathogenesis and the medical management of MG.
2. Learn the role of thymectomy in the treatment of MG, with and without the presence of a thymoma.
3. Learn the strategies for diagnosing anterior mediastinal masses.

Considerations

Myasthenia gravis is a disorder of the neuromuscular junction resulting from autoimmune damage to the nicotinic cholinergic receptor. Symptoms **include weakness that worsens after exercise and improves after rest.** Other symptoms include ptosis, diplopia, dysarthria, dysphagia, and respiratory complications. Myasthenia gravis is evidenced by history and physical examination **and can be confirmed by provocative testing (the Edrophonium-Tensilon test).** The Osserman classification is a commonly used system for characterizing the severity of MG (Table 42–1). Medical management of MG varies depending on the response of the patient, including the response to anticholinesterase drugs, glucocorticoids (prednisone), and immunosuppressive drugs (azathioprine, cyclophosphamide). Acute exacerbations or myasthenic crises are treated medically and with plasmapheresis. **Thymectomy should be avoided during an acute crisis.**

Table 42–1

OSSERMAN CLASSIFICATION FOR SEVERITY
OF MYASTHENIA GRAVIS

CLASS	SYMPTOMS
I	Occular involvement only (diplopia, ptosis)
IIA	Generalized muscle weakness without respiratory impairment
IIB	More bulbar manifestation than in class IIA
III	Rapid onset and progression of bulbar and generalized weakness including respiratory muscle weakness
IV	Severe generalized weakness, progressive myasthenic symptoms
V	Muscle atrophy requiring mechanical ventilation

Myasthenia gravis occurs in 30% to 50% of patients with thymoma; 15% of myasthenic patients have thymoma. Pathologic staging of thymoma relies on both the surgical assessment at the time of resection and the microscopic evaluation (Table 42–2).

Diagnostic sampling of anterior mediastinal masses suspected to be thymoma is usually unnecessary. Biopsy of anterior mediastinal masses may prove useful for patients with very extensive anterior mediastinal masses causing invasion of adjacent vital structures and for patients in whom lymphoma is suspected. **The primary treatment of thymoma remains surgical resection via a median sternotomy.** Complete thymectomy includes removal of the entire thymus gland, pericardial fat, and thymoma *en bloc.* If macroscopic invasion of the thymoma is encountered, adjacent structures may be sacrificed (eg, pericardium, lung, a single phrenic nerve [but never both], great vessels), understanding that the best prognosis relies on a complete resection. Adjuvant therapies can be utilized accordingly.

Surgical Outcome   At 5 years postresection, 25% to 30% of patients show complete remission of MG; 35% to 60% have an improvement in symptoms with a decrease in their medication requirement; 20% show no change in status; and 10% to 15% have a worsening of their symptoms.

Table 42–2

STAGING AND PROGNOSIS OF THYMOMA

STAGE	DESCRIPTION	TREATMENT*	5-Y PROGNOSIS (%)
I	Completely encapsulated, no invasion	Surgical resection	90
II	Macroscopic invasion to fat or pleura or microscopic invasion through capsule	Radical surgical resection	70–80
III	Macroscopic invasion to adjacent structure: pericardium, great vessels, lung or intrathoracic metastasis	Radical surgical resection and/or XRT	50–60
IV	Extrathoracic metastasis	Chemotherapy, XRT	20–30

*XRT, radiotherapy.

Evaluation and Treatment of an Anterior Mediastinal Mass

The mediastinum is divided into three compartments: anterior (superior), middle, and posterior. Neurogenic tumors (20%), usually located in the posterior mediastinum, are the most common mediastinal tumor, followed by thymomas (15% to 20%), which are located in the anterior mediastinum. Twenty-five percent to 40% of mediastinal masses are malignant.

Evaluation of an anterior mediastinal mass always begins with a review of the history, a physical examination, and a screening chest radiograph demonstrating a mediastinal mass. Particular attention should be given to identifying symptoms and findings that indicate thyroid pathology and to detecting the presence of diffuse adenopathy suggesting the possibility of lymphoma. A CT scan of the chest is often helpful in identifying the exact location, the invasion of adjacent structures, associated lymphadenopathy, and intra- or extrathoracic metastasis. When germ cell tumors (seminomatous and nonseminomatous) are suspected, serum marker, α-fetoprotein, and human chorionic gonadotropin measurements should be obtained (see Table 42–3 for a summary of treatment recommendations).

Indications for Biopsy   Patients with mediastinal masses are often referred for tissue diagnosis, but fine-needle aspiration (FNA) is seldom helpful. Open resection can be performed directly for most anterior mediastinal masses. If lymphoma or stage III or IV thymoma is suspected, open biopsy via an anterior mediastinotomy or video-assisted thoracoscopy is indicated.

Table 42–3
EVALUATION AND TREATMENT OF ANTERIOR
MEDIASTINAL MASSES*

TUMOR	DIAGNOSIS	TREATMENT
Thymoma	Surgical resection	Surgical resection, possible XRT, chemotherapy
Lymphoma	Open mediastinotomy, video-assisted thoracoscopy if fine-needle aspiration biopsy is equivocal	Chemotherapy or XRT, depending on cell type

Germ cell tumor
  Teratoma
  Seminoma
  Nonseminoma
	Surgical resection
	PE
	PE, positive β-human chorionic gonadotropin and α-fetoprotein tests
		Surgical resection
		XRT
		Chemotherapy

Parathyroid adenoma	Hyperparathyroidism, CT scan, Sestimibi scan	Surgical resection
Aberrant thyroid	CT scan	Surgical resection if symptomatic
Lipoma, hemangioma, thymic cyst	CT scan, magnetic resonance imaging	Surgical resection if symptomatic or to rule out malignancy

*XRT, radiotherapy; PE, physical examination; CT, computed tomography.

Comprehension Questions

[42.1-3] Match the following locations within the mediastinum (A-C) to the disorders.

    A. Anterior
    B. Middle
    C. Posterior

[42.1] Neurogenic tumors

[42.2] Thymomas

[42.3] Teratomas

[42.4] Staging of thymoma is determined primarily by which of the following?

    A. Surgical evaluation
    B. Pathologic immunohistochemistry
    C. Magnetic resonance imaging evaluation
    D. CT scan evaluation

Answers

[42.1] **C.** Neurogenic tumors are usually located in the posterior mediastinum.

[42.2] **A.** Thymomas are usually found in the anterior mediastinum.

[42.3] **A.** Germ cell tumors (such as teratomas) are also usually found in the anterior mediastinum.

[42.4] **A.** Thymoma staging is based on the pathologic and histologic characteristics of the tumor.

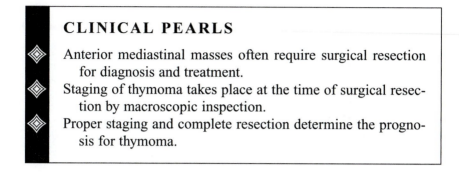

CLINICAL PEARLS

◈ Anterior mediastinal masses often require surgical resection for diagnosis and treatment.

◈ Staging of thymoma takes place at the time of surgical resection by macroscopic inspection.

◈ Proper staging and complete resection determine the prognosis for thymoma.

REFERENCES

Benfield JR. Chest. Surg Clin North Am 1992;2:12–23.

Wilkins EW Jr, Grillo HC, Scannell JG, et al. Role of staging in prognosis and management of thymoma. Ann Thorac Surg 1991;51:888–892.

A 20-year-old male reports that he has had a nontender, heavy sensation in his scrotal area for 2 months. He jogs several miles every day but denies lifting heavy objects. He does not recall trauma to the area and has no urinary complaints. He is healthy and does not smoke. On examination, his blood pressure is 110/70 and his heart rate is 80/min; he is afebrile. The results from his heart and lung examinations are normal. There is no back tenderness. His abdomen is nontender and without masses. The external genitalia reveal a 2-cm nontender mass in the right testis. Transillumination shows no light penetration. The findings from a rectal examination are unremarkable.

 What is the most likely diagnosis?

 What is the best therapy for this patient?

ANSWERS TO CASE 43: Testicular Cancer

Summary: A 20-year-old male is noted to have had a nontender heavy sensation in the scrotal area for 2 months. He jogs several miles every day but denies lifting heavy objects. He denies trauma to the area and has no urinary complaints. A 2-cm, nontransilluminating, nontender mass in the right testis is noted. The results from a rectal examination are unremarkable.

◆ **Most likely diagnosis:** Testicular cancer.

◆ **Best therapy for this patient:** Surgery (radical orchiectomy) with possible chemotherapy.

Analysis

Objectives

1. Know that a nontender, nontransilluminating testicular mass in a young male should be considered testicular cancer unless proven otherwise.
2. Understand that knowledge of the correct pathologic diagnosis or cell type(s) is crucial in directing therapy.
3. Know that a testicular carcinoma can be cured; however, patient compliance with treatment and surveillance protocols is important.

Considerations

Testicular carcinoma affects young men, usually between the ages of 15 and 40 years, with an incidence of 3 to 5 per 100,000 males. It is more common in Caucasian males than in black males. Thus, this patient matches the most common profile. While a **painless scrotal mass is the most common presentation,** references are often made to a trivial traumatic event that may have brought the scrotal mass to the patient's attention. Further, an incorrect clinical diagnosis such as varicocele, spermatocele, hydrocele, epididymitis, or testicular torsion may further delay appropriate evaluation and treatment. Regular scrotal self-examination is advocated but rarely performed; rather, an element of **embarrassment often delays presentation.**

The next step for this individual is a complete examination at the time of presentation to search for evidence of metastatic disease. There are tumor markers for many of cell types, most prominently β-human chorionic gonadotropin (β-hCG) and α-fetoprotein (AFP). A radical orchiectomy would be the best therapy. **Tumor cell types** are generally divided to **seminoma and nonseminomatous germ cell tumors.** Treatment protocols rely on an accurate diagnosis of the cell type(s) within the tumor. A skilled pathologist often reviews many slides from the surgical specimen, using special stainings when necessary to obtain a diagnosis.

APPROACH TO TESTICULAR MASSES

Definitions

Radical orchiectomy: A surgical procedure in which an inguinal incision is made over the cord leading to the testicle to be removed. The surgical specimen includes testis, epididymis, and spermatic cord taken at the internal iliac ring. Care is taken not to incise the scrotum itself during the surgical procedure.

Retroperitoneal lymphadenectomy: A surgical procedure performed to remove the lymph nodes draining the testicle. **Testicular cancer often progresses in an orderly fashion up the lymphatic drainage of the testis.** Testicular lymphatics flow from the testis through the spermatic cord following the testicular artery into the retroperitoneum where they drain into nodes around the vena cava and aorta.

Germ cell tumor: **Ninety percent of cancers of the testis are derived from the germinal epithelium** (sperm-forming elements) of the testis. Subtypes include **choriocarcinoma, embryonal carcinoma, seminoma, teratoma, and yolk sac tumor.** The other 10% of testicular tumors are made up of what is known as gonadal stromal tumors, secondary tumors of the testis such as lymphoma, and metastatic tumors to the testis.

Clinical Approach

When a male presents with a chief complaint of a testicular mass, a detailed examination of the genitalia should be performed, delineating the **character of the mass, painful versus painless, hard versus soft, and transilluminating versus nontransilluminating.** Palpation of the **lymph nodes,** examination of the male breasts, and a general survey of the signs and symptoms related not only to the genitourinary system but also to the **endocrine and neurologic systems** are important.

Radical (inguinal) orchiectomy should be performed when it is confirmed that the lesion within the scrotum is a **solid mass.** An **ultrasound of the scrotum is helpful** in making this determination. Preoperative testing should also include tumor markers such as **β-hCG** and **AFP.** Lactic acid dehydrogenase and placental alkaline phosphatase are also useful tumor markers. A **chest radiograph** should be obtained preoperatively to rule out metastatic disease that may influence the anesthetic method.

Once the diagnosis of testicular cancer is confirmed, further metastatic evaluation such as a CT scan of the abdomen and chest is warranted. Therapeutic decisions depend first on an accurate pathologic diagnosis of the cell type(s) within the tumor. **Often there is more than one cell type, hence the term "mixed germ cell tumor."** Other important factors determining therapeutic decisions include the extent of disease (tumor stage), risk factors (known characteristics of the tumor type or extent that are often associated with an aggressive prognosis), and compliance of the patient.

Although testicular cancer has played a part in one of the modern medical success stories, where the terms "cure" and "cancer" can be used honestly in the same sentence, it does strike men at a time when they are otherwise healthy and are not used to medical intervention. **Compliance with the aggressive regimens of chemotherapy, radiation therapy, and/or surgery is key to avoiding tumor relapse and to detecting disease progression as early as possible.**

Pure seminoma is treated differently than other nonseminomatous germ cell tumors primarily because of its **exquisite sensitivity to radiation therapy and its response to chemotherapy** when the disease is bulky and advanced. Residual testicular tumor following chemotherapy is treated with surgery, most often retroperitoneal lymphadenectomy.

After successful treatment of a testicular tumor, patients will need life-long surveillance of their remaining testicle as the incidence of carcinoma becomes greater by a manyfold factor.

Comprehension Questions

[43.1] Which one of the following is most likely to be associated with testicular cancer?

A. XY gonadal dysgenesis
B. Androgen insensitivity
C. Turner syndrome
D. Noonan syndrome

[43.2] Physical examination of a young man with testicular cancer during a routine surveillance visit reveals a hard mass just above the left clavicle. Which of the following is the most likely diagnosis?

A. Chemotherapy sclerosis of the subclavian vein
B. Metastatic testicular cancer
C. Second primary cancer of head and neck origin
D. Pathologic fracture of the clavicle

[43.3] Which of the following best describes the fertility of a patient before treatment for testicular cancer?

A. Below normal on average
B. Same as that of his peers
C. Above average
D. Far worse than average

Answers

[43.1] **A.** Although both androgen insensitivity and XY gonadal dysgenesis have propensity to become malignant, the nonfunctional dysgenetic gonad has the greater risk.

[43.2] **B.** The Virchow node is palpated in this clinical question. This physical finding indicates a metastatic tumor within the lymph node. This supraclavicular lymph node is a harbinger of more extensive disease and may be the only clinical finding of more extensive retroperitoneal metastases. Palpation of this region is an essential part of the initial and follow-up examinations of men with testicular cancer because of the lymphatic predilections of the disease.

[43.3] **A.** For reasons not yet clear, the fertility of men at the time of diagnosis of testicular cancer is abnormal as assessed by a semen analysis. Certainly, surgery, radiation, and chemotherapy greatly further reduce the fertility of men with testicular cancer. The likelihood of reduced fertility and the side effects of treatments on fertility must be discussed with men who receive a diagnosis of testicular cancer.

CLINICAL PEARLS

◈ Nearly all testicular cancers are of germ cell origin, and approximately half are caused by seminomas. Many cancers have multiple cell types, the delineation of which is crucial for the therapy.

◈ Cryptorchidism (undescended testicle) significantly increases the risk of a germ cell tumor even if the maldescended testicle is surgically corrected.

◈ An inguinal incision is made for a radical orchiectomy to avoid disruption of the lymphatic drainage of the testicle, which normally does not involve the scrotum itself.

◈ A testicular mass that is solid (does not transilluminate) in a young man should be assumed to be testicular cancer until proven otherwise.

REFERENCES

Walsh PC, Wein AJ, Vaughan EDJ, Retik AB (eds). Campbell's urology, 8th ed. Philadelphia: Saunders, 2002.

Tanagho EA, McAninch JW. Smith's general urology, 15th ed. New York: Lange Medical Books/McGraw-Hill, 2000.

A 35-year-old man presents with a 3-week history of perianal pain. The patient describes intermittent pain produced by defecation, and these episodes of pain generally last for 15 to 20 minutes. Because of his pain, the patient has been unable to defecate over the past 3 days. He denies any fever, difficulty with urination, or previous episodes of pain. His past medical history is unremarkable. He does not take any medications. On physical examination, his temperature is 37.7°C (99.9°F), pulse rate 100/min, and blood pressure 140/90. Examination of the perirectal region reveals an anal skin tag located in the posterior 12 o'clock position. There are no masses, erythema, or tenderness in the perianal or buttock region. During an attempted digital rectal examination, the patient had exquisite tenderness, resulting in an inadequate evaluation. The laboratory findings revealed a normal white blood cell (WBC) count, normal hemoglobin and hematocrit values, and a platelet count within the normal range.

◆ **What is the most likely diagnosis?**

◆ **What is the most likely mechanism for this condition?**

◆ **What are your next steps?**

ANSWERS TO CASE 44: Anorectal Disease

Summary: A 35-year-old man presents with severe anorectal pain associated with defecation. He has no fever. The examination is incomplete because of patient discomfort and reveals a perianal skin tag but no erythema, mass, or swelling.

◆ **Diagnosis:** Anal fissure.

◆ **Mechanisms:** Causes include trauma to the anal canal from the passage of large, firm stool and regional ischemia of the mucosa due to a hypertonic internal sphincter.

◆ **Next steps:** At this juncture, a complete rectoanal examination should be performed. Severe pain frequently prevents this examination from being completed, and most patients require sedation or a topical, local, or general anesthetic.

Analysis

Objectives

1. Learn the differential diagnosis for anorectal pain.
2. Become familiar with the approach to diagnosis and treatment of common anorectal diseases.

Considerations

The case presented is classic for an anal fissure. Hemorrhoids, fistula-in-ano, and perirectal abscess are the more commonly encountered anorectal complaints seen in clinical practice, but these diagnoses are unlikely in the absence of bleeding, erythema, or tenderness in the perianal and buttock region. In order to treat this patient, a thorough physical examination must be performed either under regional anesthesia or with sedation. Anal fissures are commonly found in the posterior midline position and associated with a skin tag. The symptom most typical of anal fissure is intense pain accompanying defecation. Many patients with fissures have constipation, which can contribute to the problem but may develop as the patient refuses to defecate in an effort to avoid the pain. An anal fissure may present as an acute or chronic problem and is a tear in the lining of the anal canal from the dentate line to the anal verge (anoderm). It is produced by trauma due to the passage of hard stool and the presence of elevated resting internal sphincter pressures. Nonoperative treatment should be attempted for this patient with an acute anal fissure, including sitz baths, bulking agents, a stool softener, and topical nitroglycerine ointment. When patients with chronic and recurrent fissures are encountered, local injection of botulinum toxin or operative therapy to reduce the resting sphincter tone (internal sphincterotomy) may be indicated.

APPROACH TO ANORECTAL COMPLAINTS

Definitions

Hemorrhoids: Abnormal enlargement of the hemorrhoidal venous plexus caused by constipation or diarrhea, obesity, and increased intra-abdominal pressure. Internal hemorrhoids are located above the dentate line; external hemorrhoids are located below the dentate line. Internal hemorrhoids can be classified as follows.

Grade I—prominent hemorrhoids on inspection or on anoscopy

Grade II—hemorrhoids that prolapse but reduce spontaneously

Grade III—hemorrhoids that require manual reduction

Grade IV—nonreducible hemorrhoids

Fistula-in-ano: Abnormal communication between the anal canal and the perineum. Fistulas represent the end result of perianal abscesses. Most fistulas arise from infections in the anal canal glands at the dentate line and track into different spaces and planes. They may appear as an abscess or as a draining sinus. Their location based on whether they are between the internal or the external sphincter above or below the levator ani muscle, gives them their respective names, that is, intersphincteric, transsphincteric, and so on.

Goodsall rule: Used to find the internal opening of a fistula. Most fistulas located anteriorly to a transverse anal imaginary line, that is, an anterior hemicircumference of the anus, track **straight directly** to the dentate line. Fistulas in the posterior portion or hemicircumference track in a **curved line** toward the posterior midline or commissure of the anal canal.

Clinical Approach

Most patients with perianal, anal, or rectal disease self-medicate with over-the-counter products, and they consult a physician only when the symptoms worsen or become complicated. It is therefore imperative to obtain a thorough, detailed history regarding symptom duration and prior treatments. An anorectal examination is performed with the patient in the left lateral decubitus with knees flexed to provide the most privacy and comfort. The examination consists of a careful inspection of the anus followed by a digital examination and anoscopy with or without sedation. When indicated, rigid proctosigmoidoscopy or flexible sigmoidoscopy may provide additional information but generally requires additional preparations and a separate visit to the office or outpatient endoscopy suite. During inspection, one should look for lesions, rashes, discharge, or other defects. Digital palpation is performed to identify any masses, gauge sphincter tone, and establish the presence of bleeding (Table 44–1). **A malignancy and inflammatory bowel disease should always be considered in the differential diagnosis when patients present with chronic and/or recurrent anal and/or rectal complaints, and biopsies should be strongly considered during the evaluation.** Anoscopy is performed to visualize an anal tear and to inspect and evaluate palpable lesions and hemorrhoids. During anoscopy, visualization of the dentate line marks the division between the rectal and the anal mucosae. The lack of somatic innervation above the dentate line makes lesions above this area less painful.

Symptoms

Anal fissure: Severe anal pain with defection, bleeding, itching, and minimal drainage.

Table 44–1
EXAMINATION FINDINGS AND TREATMENT

SOURCE	APPEARANCE	PALPATION	ANOSCOPY
Anal fissure	Superficial tear in anoderm, sentinel tag	Tear increased sphincter tone, hypertrophic anal papilla.	Tear, bleeding, hypertrophic anal papilla
Hemorrhoids	Blue or purple mass at anus	Enlarged soft mass	Prominent veins above or below dentate line
Fistula-in-ano	Purulent drainage, erythema, ulcer, fluctuant mass	Fluctuant mass, induration	Small, rough areas in anus

Hemorrhoids:
  Grade I—painless bleeding
  Grade II—mild pain, bleeding, and pruritus
  Grade III—pain and bleeding
  Grade IV—painful, nonreducible hemorrhoids
Perianal abscess: Painful, fluctuant perianal mass or ulcer associated with fever and/or purulent drainage.
Fistula-in-ano: Patients may complain of pain, but the more common complaint is mucous or minimal stool soilage on their undergarments.

Treatment

  Anal fissure: Sitz baths, stool softeners, suppositories, bulking agents, and nitroglycerin ointment. Chronic fissures can be treated with botulinum toxin injection or internal sphincterotomy (see Table 44-2).
  Hemorrhoids:
    Grade I—diet changes (increase bulk and fluid intake)
    Grade II—diet changes, rubber band ligation, infrared coagulation

Table 44–2

ANORECTAL DISEASES AND TREATMENT

	SYMPTOMS	FINDINGS	TREATMENT
Fissure-in-ano	Anal pain with defecation, bleeding, itching, drainage	Tear in anoderm. Spastic sphincter tone sentinel tag, hypertrophic anal papilla	Sitz baths, stool softeners, suppositories, nitroglycerin; partial internal sphincterotomy
Hemorrhoids Grade I	Painless bleeding	Engorged hemorrhoids	Diet changes
Grade II	Bleeding, pruritus, mild pain	Hemorrhoid prolapses	Diet, band ligation, infrared coagulation
Grade III	Pain, bleeding	Prolapsing hemorrhoids, manual reduction	Rubber band ligation hemorrhoidectomy
Grade IV	Nonreducible hemorrhoids, severe pain	Bleeding, strangulation	Hemorrhoidectomy
Fistula-in-ano	Ulcer, painful fluctuant mass, purulent	Scarred tract from dentate line to external opening	Draining and/or fistulotomy

Grade III—rubber band ligation or hemorrhoidectomy
Grade IV—hemorrhoidectomy
Fistula-in-ano: Abscess drainage and/or fistulotomy.

Comprehension Questions

[44.1] Which of the following findings suggest the diagnosis of an anal fissure?

A. Fever, a fluctuant mass, obesity, and diarrhea
B. Painless rectal bleeding, a purple anal mass, and an ulcer

C. Presence of a purulent sinus, erythema, and a fluctuant mass
D. Severe anal pain, a tear in the posterior anoderm, bleeding, and increased sphincter tone

[44.2] The differential diagnosis for an anal fissure should include which one of the following?

A. Rectocele
B. Condyloma
C. Rectal polyp
D. Crohn's disease, ulcerated hemorrhoid, malignancy

[44.3] Which of the following is the most appropriate next step after establishing a diagnosis for a patient suspected of having an anal fissure?

A. Obtain a barium enema, followed by a colonoscopy
B. Rectoanal examination under sedation, anoscopy, and proctoscopy
C. Anal biopsy, anoscopy in the office, and a barium enema
D. Rectoanal examination in the office without sedation, anal biopsy, and fissurectomy.

[44.4] Which of the following is considered the most appropriate treatment for acute anal fissure?

A. Infrared coagulation, sitz baths, and oral antibiotics
B. Rubber band ligation, suppositories, and topical antibiotics
C. Increased dietary bulk, sitz baths, suppositories, stool softeners, and nitroglycerin ointment
D. Infrared coagulation and fissurectomy.

Answers

[44.1] **D.** Severe anal pain, a tear in the posterior anoderm, bleeding, and increased sphincter tone are findings compatible with anal fissure.

[44.2] **D.** Crohn's disease, ulcerated hemorrhoid, and malignancy should be included in the differential diagnosis when evaluating an anal fissure.

[44.3] **B.** Examination under anesthesia, anoscopy, and proctoscopy are appropriate steps in evaluating a patient clinically suspected of having an anal fissure.

[44.4] **C.** Conservative management of an anal fissure consists of increasing dietary bulk and using sitz baths, stool softeners, and nitroglycerin ointment.

CLINICAL PEARLS

◈ Patients may be reluctant to volunteer information regarding bowel habits, duration of symptoms, and sexual behavior; therefore it is important to be specific in questioning the patient during the interview.

◈ Anorectal carcinoma may manifest as severe perianal pain and tenderness and must be considered part of the differential diagnosis.

◈ Patients with anal fissure characteristically have severe anal pain, a tear in the posterior anoderm, bleeding, and increased sphincter tone.

◈ A nonhealing anal fissure or a fissure located anywhere other than in the posterior area of the anus should alert the clinician to the possibility of Crohn's disease or a malignancy.

◈ A thrombosed external hemorrhoid not responding to medical therapy should be treated by excisional thrombectomy instead of incision and drainage.

REFERENCES

Kaufman HS. Anal fissure. In Cameron JL, ed. Current surgical therapy, 6th ed. St. Louis: Mosby-Year Book, 1998:272–274.

Welton ML, Varma MG, Amerhauser A. Colon, rectum, and anus. In Norton JA, Bollinger RR, Chang AE, Lowery SF, Mulvihill SJ, Thompson RW, ed. Surgery: basic science and clinical evidence. New York: Springer, 2001:667–762

A healthy 53-year-old woman was involved in a low-speed automobile collision and was brought to the emergency department 4 weeks ago. Her physical examination revealed mild, diffuse abdominal tenderness. She underwent a computed tomography (CT) scan of her abdomen, which revealed an incidental 3.5-cm solid mass in the left adrenal gland. The patient was discharged from the emergency department with instructions to follow up for an outpatient evaluation of the left adrenal mass. During her office visit, she indicates that she is feeling well, and she is asymptomatic. Her heart rate is 70/min and her blood pressure 128/72. Her physical examination reveals no abnormal findings.

◆ **What is the differential diagnosis for an incidental adrenal mass?**

◆ **What are the important elements of the history and physical examination *in* a patient with an adrenal mass?**

◆ **Most likely diagnosis?**

ANSWERS TO CASE 45: Adrenal Incidentaloma

Summary: A 53-year-old woman is found to have an incidental 3.5-cm solid adrenal mass.

◆ **Differential diagnosis:** May include a variety of primary malignant tumors, metastatic tumors, and benign functioning and nonfunctioning tumors.

◆ **History and physical examination:** The history should describe symptoms of hypertension, previous malignancies, prior endocrinopathies, and previous imaging studies, as well as family medical history. The physical examination should include an abdominal examination and a blood pressure reading and the patient's general appearance should be noted.

◆ **Most likely diagnosis:** Nonfunctioning adenoma.

Analysis

Objectives

1. Appreciate the prevalence of clinically inapparent adrenal masses otherwise referred to as adrenal incidentalomas.
2. To become familiar with nonfunctioning and functioning adrenal tumors as well as the other clinical entities that may manifest as an incidentaloma.
3. Know the diagnostic evaluation and management of an adrenal incidentaloma.

APPROACH TO ADRENAL INCIDENTALOMAS

The term "adrenal incidentaloma" refers to a clinically inapparent adrenal mass that is discovered inadvertently in the course of diagnostic testing for other conditions. Incidental adrenal masses are found in

0.7% to 4.3% of patients undergoing abdominal CT scans and in 1.4% to 8.7% of patients at autopsy. **Most adrenal incidentalomas are non-functioning adenomas, accounting for 55% to 94% of all cases.** Functioning tumors, which include pheochromocytoma, aldosterone-producing adenoma, and cortisol-producing adenoma, are less common. Other adrenal tumors that can appear as incidentaloma are ganglioneuroma, adrenocortical carcinoma, and metastases. The differential diagnosis also includes myelolipoma, cysts, and hemorrhage, which are entities that can be diagnosed on the basis of CT criteria alone. An adrenal hematoma is not an infrequent finding in a patient whose sustains abdominal trauma, and the diagnosis is confirmed with resolution of the mass on follow-up CT scanning.

The evaluation of a patient with an adrenal incidentaloma consists of obtaining a history, performing a physical examination, and making a functional and anatomic assessment of the adrenal mass. Specific signs and symptoms of excess catecholamines, aldosterone, cortisol, and androgens should be actively sought in the history and on physical examination. At minimum, patients should be asked about a history of hypertension and whether or not they have been experiencing headaches, palpitations, profuse sweating, abdominal pain, or anxiety. All patients should be questions about a prior history of malignancy. When present, adrenal masses are metastases in up to 75% of patients. In addition to obtaining a resting heart rate and a blood pressure reading, patients should be examined for features suggestive of Cushing syndrome such as truncal obesity, moon facies, thin extremities, prominent fat deposition in the supraclavicular areas and the nape of the neck, hirsutism, bruising, abdominal striae, and facial plethora.

The functional assessment consists of the following: measurement of plasma-free metanephrine levels; a 24-hour urine collection for detection of vanillylmandelic acid, metanephrine, and normetanephrine to evaluate for pheochromocytoma; a serum potassium test; measurement of aldosterone and plasma renin activity to evaluate for an aldosterone-producing adenoma; and a overnight 1-mg dexamethasone suppression test to evaluate for hypercortisolism.

Once it has been determined whether an adrenal mass is functioning or nonfunctioning, the next step is an anatomic assessment, preferably with unenhanced CT or magnetic resonance imaging. Positron emission tomography (PET) scanning is used for the evaluation of an adrenal mass in a patient with a known extra-adrenal cancer because it is of value in separating benign lesions from metastases. It is also important in excluding the presence of other metastases. Myelolipomas, cysts, and hemorrhage of the adrenal gland can be identified on the basis of CT criteria alone. CT imaging has been less useful in differentiating benign from malignant lesions. However, there are certain imaging characteristics that are suggestive of adrenocortical carcinoma, including irregular margins, inhomogeneous density, scattered areas of decreased attenuation, and local invasion. Other CT criteria that increase the probability of malignancy include large tumor size and tumor enlargement over time. **Primary adrenocortical carcinomas are rare, and the majority of them are larger than 6 cm.**

For nonfunctioning tumors of the adrenal gland, selecting a tumor size for which surgery will be recommended requires a determination of the risks and benefits. The larger the size threshold for surgery, the lower the number of unnecessary operations on patients with benign disease; however, rare patients with small adrenocortical carcinomas will be missed. The smaller the tumor threshold, the greater the likelihood that all carcinomas will be resected but at the expense of performing unnecessary operations on a large majority of patients with benign disease. No consensus exists for a recommended size cutoff for surgery. In patients with adrenal incidentaloma, **surgery is recommended for all functioning tumors, nonfunctioning tumors 4 cm or larger, tumors** that are less than 4 cm that are **enlarging,** tumors of any size with imaging characteristics **suggestive of carcinoma,** and a **solitary adrenal metastasis.**

Treatment in Patients With Other Malignancies

The adrenal gland is well recognized as a site of metastasis. **The most common tumor metastasizing to the adrenal gland is lung carcinoma.** Other tumors include carcinoma of the breast, kidney, colon, and stomach, and melanoma. The patient with adrenal incidentaloma and a prior history of malignancy should undergo a biochemical assessment to exclude a functioning tumor. Whole-body PET scanning is performed in patients with a nonfunctioning tumor to exclude the presence of other metastases. Surgery is recommended for a solitary lesion 4 cm **or larger. Fine-needle aspiration biopsy is reserved for a soli-**

tary nonfunctioning lesion <4 cm because the result will alter treatment. Patients with negative results from a fine-needle aspiration biopsy are treated nonoperatively. Finally, nonsurgical treatment is recommended for patients with diffuse metastases.

Follow-up

A patient with a nonfunctioning adrenal incidentaloma less than 4 cm in size usually undergoes follow-up CT scans at 3 and 15 months. If there is no change in the size of the mass, the patient is followed annually by reviewing the history and performing a physical examination. Repeated biochemical testing is reserved for abnormal findings from the history or the physical examination.

Comprehension Questions

[45.1] Which of the following is a *true* statement regarding adrenal incidentalomas?

A. They are uncommon.
B. They are most often nonfunctioning adrenal adenomas.
C. They are routinely evaluated with fine-needle aspiration biopsy.
D. They are surgically removed whether benign or malignant.

[45.2] A 3.5-cm right adrenal mass was incidentally discovered on an abdominal CT scan obtained for a 62-year-old man who was a victim of motor vehicular trauma. His medical history was notable for a right upper lobe lung resection 3 years previously for a stage I carcinoma. He is asymptomatic. Which of the following is the next most appropriate step in the evaluation?

A. Fine-needle aspiration biopsy of the adrenal mass
B. Repeated CT scanning in 3 months
C. A functional assessment of the adrenal mass
D. Magnetic resonance imaging of the adrenal gland

[45.3] Which of the following entities can be diagnosed on the basis of CT criteria alone?

A. Ganglioneuroma
B. A solitary metastasis
C. Myelolipoma
D. Pheochromocytoma

Answers

[45.1] **B.** 55% to 94% of adrenal incidentalomas are nonfunctioning adenomas. Surgical excision is indicated when there is a concern for malignancy or if the lesion is functional.

[45.2] **C.** The initial step in evaluating an adrenal mass is performing functional studies.

[45.3] **C.** Myelolipoma can be recognized by CT criteria alone.

CLINICAL PEARLS

◈ Assessment of functional studies is the first step in the evaluation of any patient with an adrenal mass.

◈ Biopsy of an adrenal mass is indicated only when the mass is suspected of being a metastatic lesion.

◈ The most common tumor metastasizing to the adrenal gland is lung carcinoma. Other tumors include carcinoma of the breast, kidney, colon, and stomach, and melanoma.

◈ The functional assessment consists of evaluation for pheochromocytoma, aldosterone-producing adenoma, and a cortisol-producing tumor.

REFERENCES

Graham DJ, McHenry CR. Diagnosis of tumors of the adrenal gland. Hospital Physician. General Surgery Board Review Manual 2001;7(2):1–12.

Graham DJ, McHenry CR. Management of tumors of the adrenal gland. Hospital Physician. General Surgery Board Review Manual 2001;7(3):1–12.

Graham DJ, McHenry CR. The adrenal incidentaloma: guidelines for evaluation and recommendations for management. Surg Oncol Clin North Am 1988;7(4): 749–764.

A 36-year-old man presents with a 1-day history of right groin pain. The patient indicates that the pain developed during a tennis match the previous evening and that on returning home he noticed swelling in the area. His past medical history is unremarkable. The patient denies any history of medical problems or similar complaints. He has not undergone any previous operations. The physical examination reveals a well-nourished man. The results from the cardiopulmonary examination are unremarkable, and the abdominal examination reveals a nondistended, nontender abdomen. Auscultation of the abdomen reveals normal bowel sounds. Examination of the right inguinal region reveals no inguinal mass. There is a 2 × 2 cm nonerythematous swelling on the medial thigh just below the right inguinal ligament. Palpation reveals localized tenderness. The lower extremities are otherwise unremarkable. Laboratory findings reveal a white blood cell count of 6500/mm^3 and normal hemoglobin and hematocrit levels. Electrolyte concentrations are within the normal range, as the results from a urinalysis. Radiographs of the abdomen demonstrate no abnormalities.

◆ **What is the most likely diagnosis?**

◆ **What are the complications associated with this disease process?**

◆ **What is the best therapy?**

ANSWERS TO CASE 46: Hernias

Summary: A 36-year-old man complains of a new-onset, painful mass in the groin region present since he played tennis the previous day.

◆ **Diagnosis:** Incarcerated femoral hernia.

◆ **Complications:** Strangulation of the hernia sac contents with resulting sepsis.

◆ **Best therapy:** Operative exploration of the right groin to evaluate, reduce the hernia sac contents, and repair the femoral hernia.

Analysis

Objectives

1. Know the presentations of inguinal, femoral, and umbilical hernias.
2. Recognize the anatomic landmarks of the different types of hernias.
3. Understand the pros and cons of the different approaches to hernia repair.

Considerations

The differential diagnosis of groin pain and/or mass includes inguinal hernia, femoral hernia, muscle strain, and adenopathy. Although many patients believe that the sudden development of pain or a mass in the groin is the classic and usual presentation for a groin hernia, this particular clinical picture is in fact more suggestive of muscle injury. Patients with inguinal hernias generally describe a long history of intermittent groin pain or "heaviness" that is more prominent when standing and during physical activity. **The sudden development of a painful**

groin mass, such as in a patient with a known hernia, suggests hernia incarceration. In particular, this patient's presentation is compatible with that for an incarcerated femoral hernia. Because a femoral hernia usually is a small, well-defined anatomic defect, there may be few or no long-term symptoms and acute incarceration may be the initial presenting symptom. The diagnosis in this case can be established on the basis of the history and the results from a physical examination. In the event of clinical uncertainty, ultrasonography or computed tomography (CT) imaging may be helpful in differentiating an incarcerated hernia from lymph nodes, hematomas, or abscesses. Once the diagnosis is made, **a patient with an incarcerated hernia should undergo urgent surgical repair to relieve the symptoms and to prevent strangulation of hernia sac contents.**

APPROACH TO HERNIAS

Definitions

Indirect hernia: An inguinal hernia in which the abdominal contents protrude through the indirect inguinal ring through a patent processus vaginalis into the inguinal canal. In men, they follow the spermatic cord and may appear as scrotal swelling, whereas in females they may manifest as labial swelling.

Direct hernia: An inguinal hernia that protrudes through the Hesselbach triangle medial to the inferior epigastric vessels.

Femoral hernia: A hernia that protrudes through the femoral canal, bounded by the inguinal ligament superiorly, the femoral vein laterally, and the pyriformis and pubic ramus medially. Unlike inguinal hernias, these hernias protrude below, rather than above, the inguinal ligament.

Umbilical hernia: A hernia resulting from improper healing of the umbilical scar. Eighty percent of pediatric umbilical hernias close by age 2 years. In adults, defects are often exacerbated by conditions that increase intra-abdominal pressure, such as ascites.

Littre hernia: A groin hernia that contains a Meckel diverticulum or the appendix.

Richter hernia: Herniation of part of the bowel wall through a defect in the anterior abdominal wall. Bowel obstruction does not occur, although the constricted bowel wall may become ischemic and subsequently necrotic.

Spigelian hernia: A hernia just lateral to the rectus sheath at the semilunar line, the lower limit of the posterior rectus sheath.

Obturator hernia: Herniation through the obturator canal alongside the obturator vessels and nerves. This hernia occurs mostly in women, particularly elderly women with a history of recent weight loss. A mass may be palpable in the **medial thigh,** particularly with the hip flexed, externally rotated, and abducted (Howship–Romberg sign).

Sliding hernia: A hernia in which one wall of the hernia is made up of an intra-abdominal organ, most commonly the sigmoid colon, ascending colon, or bladder.

Clinical Approach

Abdominal wall hernias are protrusions of abdominal contents through a defect in the abdominal wall. **Incarceration** occurs if the abdominal contents become trapped. **Strangulation** occurs when the blood supply to the trapped contents becomes compromised, leading to ischemia, necrosis, and ultimately perforation. **Intestinal obstruction can occur in an incarcerated or strangulated hernia.** Abdominal wall defects that develop following surgical procedures not related to a hernia are referred to as incisional hernias and are addressed elsewhere.

Anatomy

Knowledge of the regional anatomy is essential for the diagnosis and repair of hernias. In the groin, the inguinal ligament divides inguinal hernias from femoral hernias. Inguinal hernias are further divided into indirect and direct hernias based on their relationship to the inferior epigastric vessels. The **Hesselbach triangle, defined by the edge of the rectus medially, the inguinal ligament inferolaterally, and the inferior epigastric vessels superolaterally, is the site of direct hernias (Figure 46–1).** In this triangle, the peritoneum and transversalis

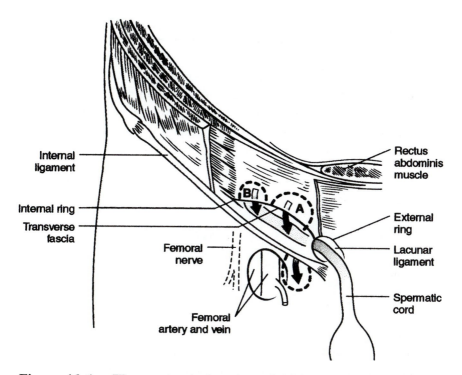

Figure 46–1.   The anatomic location of groin hernias. (A) Direct hernia, (B) indirect hernia, (C) femoral hernia (right groin from an anterior view).

fascia are the only components of the anterior abdominal wall. **Indirect hernias are lateral to the inferior epigastric vessels.** The Cooper ligament, or the pectineal ligament, extends from the pubic tubercle laterally and passes posteriorly to the femoral vessels.

Approach to an Incarcerated Hernia

Reduction should be attempted in a patient with an incarcerated hernia. This procedure is best accomplished by elongating the neck of the hernia sac while judiciously applying pressure to reduce the hernia. **If reduction is unsuccessful, the patient should be prepared for urgent operation.** In a patient with a bowel obstruction, volume depletion and abnormalities in electrolyte levels are common. These conditions should be corrected before operative intervention. Urgent repair requires an incision over the incarcerated hernia, close inspection of any contents, and **tension-free reapproximation.** For inguinal hernias, the transversus abdominus is sutured to either the Cooper ligament or the shelving edge of the inguinal ligament. For femoral hernias, a Cooper

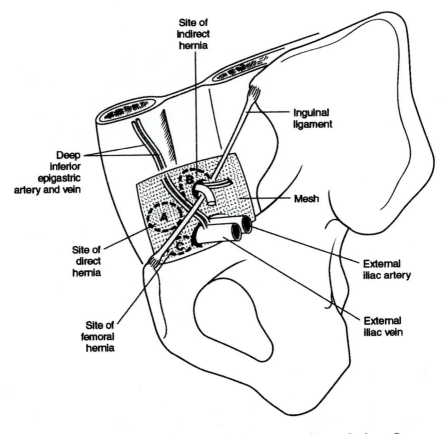

Figure 46–2.   Right groin anatomy by pre-peritoneal view. Operative repair of (A) a direct hernia, (B) an indirect hernia, and (C) a femoral hernia using a prosthetic mesh in a posterior (preperitoneal) approach.

ligament repair must be used. **With a compromised bowel, a prosthetic mesh should be avoided because of the infection risk.**

Indications for Repair

The majority of hernias should be repaired when discovered, as the mortality increases 9- to 10-fold with emergent compared to elective repair. Elective repair via an open approach can be performed under local, spinal, or general anesthesia. It can also be done laparoscopically, which requires a general anesthetic. In addition to the elective or urgent/emergent nature of the repair, anesthetic choice, patient preference, and the primary or recurrent nature of the hernia factor into the decision regarding the operative approach. A laparoscopic approach or an open preperitoneal approach is best for recurrent or bilateral hernias (Figure 46–2). For unilateral primary groin hernias, the approaches have similar recurrence rates, similar disability times, and similar costs. Patients who undergo laparoscopy seem to have less pain and may be able to return to work sooner.

Comprehension Questions

[46.1] A 20-year-old man complains of a bulge in his right groin that has become increasingly bothersome over the last 3 months. On examination, you feel a bulge in his groin that is exacerbated by coughing. His left groin is without any abnormalities. What type of hernia is most likely in this patient?

    A. Femoral
    B. Indirect inguinal
    C. Direct inguinal
    D. Obturator

[46.2] Which is the most appropriate treatment for the above patient?

    A. Admit him for urgent repair of his hernia.
    B. Schedule him for elective repair of his hernia.

C. Provide a truss for him to wear.

D. Inform him that most hernias close on their own.

[46.3] An 80-year-old woman who resides at a nursing home has lost several pounds over the last 3 months. For the last 3 days she has not been able to eat anything, has been vomiting, and was found in bed this morning confused and quite ill. The results from her abdominal examination are fairly unremarkable, revealing no previous scars, and she has a mass in her medial thigh. Her radiographs show a dilated small bowel. Which of the following is the most likely diagnosis?

A. Inguinal hernia

B. Adhesive bowel obstruction

C. Cancer

D. Obturator hernia

E. Femoral hernia

[46.4] What is the appropriate treatment for the above patient?

A. Schedule her for an elective operation.

B. Request a barium enema.

C. Take her straight to the operating room.

D. Hospitalize her for volume and electrolyte replacement and urgent operation.

Answers

[46.1] **B.** Indirect inguinal hernia is by far the most common hernia.

[46.2] **B.** Elective repair is the most appropriate management for a young, healthy individual with an inguinal hernia.

[46.3] **D.** Obturator hernia. These hernias are extremely unusual, but when occur, they most commonly occur in thin, elderly females.

[46.4] **D.** Resuscitation and urgent repair are indicated for patients with a bowel obstruction due to a hernia.

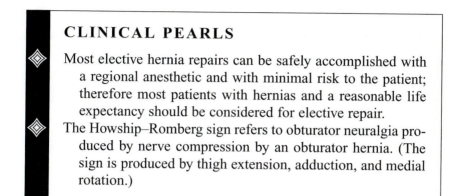

CLINICAL PEARLS

◈ Most elective hernia repairs can be safely accomplished with a regional anesthetic and with minimal risk to the patient; therefore most patients with hernias and a reasonable life expectancy should be considered for elective repair.

◈ The Howship–Romberg sign refers to obturator neuralgia produced by nerve compression by an obturator hernia. (The sign is produced by thigh extension, adduction, and medial rotation.)

REFERENCES

Beets GL, Dirksen CD, Go PMNYH, Geisler FEA, Baeten CGMI, Kootstra G. Open or laparoscopic preperitoneal mesh repair for recurrent inguinal hernia? A randomized controlled trial. Surg Endosc 1999;13:323–327.

Brooks DC. A prospective comparison of laparoscopic and tension-free open herniorrhaphy. Arch Surg 1994;129:361-366.

Maddern GJ, Rudkin G, Bessell JR, Devitt P, Ponte L. A comparison of laparoscopic and open hernia repair as a day surgical procedure. Surg Endosc 1994;8: 1404–1408.

Paganini AM, Lezoche E, Carle F, et al: A randomized, controlled clinical study of laparoscopic vs open tension-free inguinal hernia repair. Surg Endosc 1998;12: 979–986.

Payne JH, Grininger LM, Izawa MT, Podoll EF, Lindahl PJ, et al. Laparoscopic or open herniorrhaphy? A randomized prospective trial. Arch Surg 1994;129: 973–981.

Stoker DL, Spiegelhalter DJ, Singh R, Wellwood JM. Laparoscopic versus open inguinal hernia repair: randomized prospective trial. Lancet 1994;343:1243–1245.

Wellwood J, Sculpher MJ, Stoker D, et al. Randomised controlled trial of laparoscopic versus open mesh repair for inguinal hernia: outcome and cost. BMJ 1998;317:103–110.

A 48-year-old man with a history of alcoholism and cirrhosis undergoes evaluation for severe left leg pain and fever. The patient says his symptoms began after he scraped the lateral aspect of his knee at home 3 days ago. During the past 2 days he has had subjective fevers and noticed decreased urinary frequency. The patient has been self-medicating with aspirin for these symptoms. He consumes approximately 16 oz of whiskey per day and smokes one pack of cigarettes per day. On physical examination, his temperature is 39.2°C (102.6°F), pulse rate 110/min, blood pressure 115/78, and respiratory rate 28/min. His skin is mildly icteric. The findings from his cardiopulmonary examination are unremarkable. The abdomen is soft and without hepatosplenomegaly or ascites. The left leg is edematous from the ankle to the upper thigh. The skin is tense and exquisitely tender; however, it is without erythema, fluctuance, necrosis, or vesicular changes. Examination of the other leg reveals normal findings. Laboratory studies demonstrate a white blood cell count of 26,000/mm^3 and normal hemoglobin and hematocrit values. Other laboratory studies revealed sodium 128 mEq/L, glucose 180 mg/dL, total bilirubin 3.8, and direct bilirubin 1.5 mg/dL. Radio-graphs of the left leg reveal no bony injuries and no evidence of soft tissue air.

◆ **What is the most likely diagnosis?**

◆ **What is the best therapy for this condition?**

ANSWERS TO CASE 47: Necrotizing Soft Tissue Infections

Summary: A 48-year-old man with alcoholic cirrhosis presents with necrotizing soft tissue infection (NSTI) following a trivial injury to the left leg.

- ◆ **Most likely diagnosis:** Necrotizing soft tissue infection.

- ◆ **Best therapy:** Early initiation of appropriate antibiotics and radical surgical debridement of necrotic tissue. The treatment outcome is adversely affected by delays in therapy.

Objectives

1. Learn to recognize the clinical presentation and diagnostic strategies for NSTI.
2. Understand that rapid, aggressive surgical debridement is crucial in the treatment of NSTI.
3. Become familiar with the bacteriology of NSTI and appropriate antimicrobial choices for these conditions.

Considerations

A patient with alcohol-induced cirrhosis, in an immunocompromised state, presents with a high fever, soft tissue edema, and leg pain out of proportion to the physical findings, all of which strongly suggest the possibility of severe soft tissue infection. These findings are not specific for NSTI and may be compatible with a deep-seated abscess. The patient reports receiving minor trauma to his leg prior to the onset of leg pain, which favors the diagnosis of NSTI over that of an abscess. The development of NSTI following trivial soft tissue trauma is typical of infections caused by gram-positive skin flora, including group A β-hemolytic *Streptococcus*. Because NSTI frequently involves mixed bacterial organisms, the initial antibiotic regimen for this patient should include broad-spectrum antibiotics directed against gram-positive, gram-negative, and anaerobic bacteria. Following initial resuscitation, the patient should undergo examination of the leg with exploration of the subcutaneous tissue for infection and tissue viability. Once the bacteriologic findings from the operative drainage/debridement become available, the antibiotic regimen can be modified to cover the specific pathogens identified.

Distant end-organ dysfunction such as acute respiratory insufficiency, acute renal insufficiency, and acute liver insufficiency may occur with NSTI; therefore, most patients should be treated in the intensive care unit with careful monitoring and maximal supportive care. The systemic consequences of NSTI can develop because of overwhelming sepsis and from circulating toxins (associated with *Staphylococcus* and group A *Streptococcus* toxic shock syndrome [TSS]).

Surgical debridement for this patient should begin with an incision over the involved soft tissue and an inspection of the subcutaneous tissue for gross evidence of necrosis and adherence to the underlying fascia. **Easy separation of the subcutaneous tissue from the underlying fascia indicates microvascular thrombosis and necrosis** and should be treated by tissue debridement.

Because of the rich blood supply to the skin, patients with NSTI generally do not develop skin necrosis and bullous changes until late in the disease process. **It should be recognized that the absence of skin abnormalities is one of the leading factors contributing to delays in the recognition of NSTI.** When identified, all necrotic tissue should be excised. The fascia commonly serves as a natural barrier to the infectious processes; involvement below the fascia occurs infrequently except during infections by *Clostridium* species. Patients whose conditions do not respond appropriately to supportive care, antibiotics therapy, and surgical debridement should be reassessed; the **lack of improvement may be due to inadequate debridement and/or inappropriate antibiotic selection (source control).**

APPROACH TO SOFT TISSUE INFECTION

Definitions

Cellulitis: A milder form of soft tissue infection without the association of microvascular thrombosis and necrosis. Clinically, patients do not have evidence of systemic toxicity and can be adequately treated with antibiotic therapy.

Necrotizing soft tissue infection: Soft tissue infection that affects primarily the dermis and subcutaneous tissue. **Early manifestations include the extension of edema beyond the spread of erythema and severe pain.** Late clinical manifestations may include crepitance, the formation of skin vesicles, cutaneous anesthesia, and focal necrosis. Computed tomography (CT) scans and magnetic resonance imaging (MRI) are helpful in differentiating NSTI from cellulitis. The diagnosis of NSTI in most cases can be established on the basis of clinical evaluation (see Table 47–1). Adjunctive imaging studies should not be obtained if they would lead to additional delays in surgical therapy. A definitive diagnosis can be achieved on the basis of needle aspiration of the involved tissue, Gram stain evaluation, or exploration and visualization of the subcutaneous tissue under anesthesia. **The infection**

Table 47–1

CLINICAL MANIFESTATIONS OF NECROTIZING
SOFT TISSUE INFECTION

CLINICAL SETTING	ORGANISMS	CLINICAL MANIFESTATIONS	ANTIBIOTICS
Acquired after contact with fish or seawater	*Vibrio* species	Rapid progression of soft tissue infection, fever, rigors, and hypotension	Ceftazidime plus quinolone or tetracycline
Mixed synergistic infection; progression of perirectal infection or complications of gastrointestinal surgery	Mixed gram-negative aerobes and anaerobes	Clinical progression over several days; may involve perineum and abdominal wall	Multiple regimens developed to cover gram-negative and anaerobes
Gas gangrene may complicate trauma or ischemia	Clostridrial species	Swollen, tense skin, crepitus, and skin vesicles; frequently present with systemic toxic therapy	Penicillin (questionable benefit with hyperbaric therapy)

is associated with spreading thrombosis of the blood vessels in the subcutaneous fat and dermis, leading to tissue necrosis and poor antibiotic penetration into the affected tissue. NSTI can involve a variety of bacterial organisms. Optimal treatment consists of systemic antibiotic administration, surgical debridement, and supportive care.

Group A β-hemolytic *Streptococcus* soft tissue infection: Referred to in the lay press as the "flesh-eating infection," this form of NSTI frequently occurs in patients with a compromised immune status (alcoholics, diabetic patients, and the malnourished); however, it can also occur in healthy individuals following trivial soft tissue trauma. About 75% of cases are community-acquired. Bacteremia and/or TSS develops in approximately 50% of patients. The local process generally spreads rapidly over the course of hours to days. The combination of clindamycin and penicillin has been touted to produce superior results compared to the use of the penicillins alone. There is limited evidence suggesting that therapy with intravenous immunoglobulins (Ig) neutralizes the bacteria-produced superantigens and may improve patient outcome.

Toxic shock syndrome: A clinical syndrome caused by pyrogenic toxin superantigens produced by staphylococcal organisms or group A β-hemolytic *Streptococcus*. The binding of superantigens to major histocompatibility complex class III molecules leads to T-cell clonal expansion and a massive release of proinflammatory cytokines by macrophages and T cells. Patients with TSS frequently develop mental obtundation, hyperdynamic shock, and multiple-organ dysfunction syndrome. The systemic findings in TSS frequently do not correlate with the local extent of the soft tissue (vaginal) infection and thus can cause a delay in diagnosis and treatment.

Fournier gangrene: A specific form of scrotal gangrene first described by Fournier in 1883. Anaerobic streptococci are the predominant causative organisms, with secondary infection caused by gram-negative organisms. Strictly speaking, the term "Fournier gangrene" refers to the anaerobic *Streptococcus*-related scrotal infection but is frequently inappropriately applied to gram-negative synergistic soft tissue infections of the perineum and groin.

Comprehension Questions

[47.1] A 55-year-old diabetic man presents with a swollen, painful right hand that developed 1 day after he sustained a puncture wound to the hand while fishing in the Gulf of Mexico. His temperature is 39.5°C (103.1°F), pulse rate 120/min, and blood pressure 95/60. His right hand and forearm are swollen, and a puncture wound with surrounding ecchymosis is present on the hand. There is drainage of brown fluid from the wound. Which of the following therapies is most appropriate?

A. Supportive care, penicillin G, and hyperbaric treatment
B. Supportive care, penicillin G/tetracycline/ceftazidime, and surgical debridement
C. Supportive care, penicillin G /tetracycline/ceftazidime, surgical debridement, and hyperbaric treatment
D. Supportive care, penicillin G + clindamycin, and intravenous Ig

[47.2] A 62-year-old diabetic man returns to the emergency center 3 days after undergoing incision and drainage of a perirectal abscess. The patient is complaining of fever and malaise. Evaluation of the perirectal area reveals an open, draining wound with a 20-cm area of surrounding induration, erythema, localized areas of blister formation, and skin necrosis. The infection has extended to involve the perineum, scrotum, and anterior abdomen. The process in this patient most likely represents.

A. Fournier gangrene
B. Clostridial gas gangrene
C. NSTI due to group A β-hemolytic *Streptococcus*
D. Polymicrobial synergistic NSTI

Answers

[47.1] **B.** Supportive care, penicillin G/tetracycline/ceftazidime, and debridement are appropriate initial treatment for a patient who develops severe NSTI in an injury with the potential for *Vibrio* infection (acquired while fishing).

[47.2] **D.** Polymicrobial synergistic infection is the most likely diagnosis based on the duration of events and the distribution of soft tissue infection.

CLINICAL PEARLS

◈ The most common findings in a patient with NSTI are local edema and pain in the presence of systemic signs such as high fever (in some patients hypothermia), tachycardia, and frequently mental confusion.

◈ When NSTI is strongly suspected, exploration of the wound through a limited skin incision may help establish the diagnosis in a rapid fashion.

◈ Rapid, aggressive surgical debridement is the most important treatment for NSTI.

◈ Lack of improvement after treatment of NSTI may be due to inadequate debridement and/or inappropriate antibiotic selection (source control).

REFERENCES

Lewis RT. Soft tissue infection. In: Wilmore DW, Cheung LY, Harken AH, Holcroft JW, Meakin JL, Soper NJ, eds. ACS surgery: principles and practice. New York: WebMD, 2001;313–333.

Majeski J. Necrotizing infections of the skin and soft tissue. In: Cameron JL, ed. Current surgical therapy, 7th ed. St. Louis: Mosby-Year Book, 2001:1246–1250.

Ten days following exploratory laparotomy and small bowel resection for a strangulating bowel obstruction, a 45-year-old man is noted to have tachycardia, tachypnea, abdominal distention, and a total urine output of 130 mL over the past 8 hours. He appears confused and complains of shortness of breath and abdominal discomfort. His temperature is 39.0°C (102.2°F), pulse rate 125/min, blood pressure 100/70, and respiratory rate 34/min. The pulmonary examination reveals labored respirations with diminished breath sounds in the lung bases. The abdomen is distended and mildly tender. The skin incision is erythematous, with moderate amount of enteric contents leaking between the skin staples near the midportion of the wound. Laboratory studies reveal a white blood cell (WBC) count of 23,000/mm^3 and a hemoglobin level of 12 g/dL. The pulse oximeter registers 88% oxygen saturation with a 100% nonrebreathing mask. You decide to perform endotracheal intubation, which is successfully accomplished using rapid sequence induction including Etomidate, lidocaine, and succinylcholine. Immediately following intubation, the patient's blood pressure is noted to be 70/40, with a pulse rate of 110/min.

◆ **What is the most likely cause of the acute hypotension?**

◆ **What are the most appropriate next steps in treatment?**

◆ **What are the potential complications associated with this process?**

ANSWERS TO CASE 48: Septic Shock

Summary: A postoperative patient presents with an enterocutaneous fistula, fever, confusion, and hypotension consistent with septic shock.

◆ **Cause of hypotension:** The hypotension is most likely due to the combination of volume redistribution associated with sepsis and the abrupt removal of sympathetic response associated with the medications given for intubation.

◆ **Next steps:** Restore the intravascular volume with fluids and determine the cause of sepsis.

◆ **Complications:** Septic shock may cause decreased tissue perfusion leading to immediate or delayed organ dysfunction.

Analysis

Objectives

1. Understand the basic principles of resuscitation, infection source control, and metabolic support in the treatment of patients with sepsis.
2. Understand the concept and determinants of tissue oxygen delivery.

Treatment of a critically ill septic patient consists of three major components: (1) source control, (2) restoration of oxygen delivery, and (3) metabolic support. As with advanced cardiac life support, considerations of airway, adequate ventilation, and adequate oxygen transport take priority in the initial treatment of this patient.

Hypotension immediately following intubation is not uncommon after the urgent intubation of septic patients. This condition is related to the loss of sympathetic tone. **Sepsis results in increased vasodilation in the vascular beds and can acutely cause an impairment in cardiac contractility.** These effects are exacerbated after intubation because of a decrease in the sympathetic stimulus in a patient who is no longer struggling to breathe. This effect is further enhanced by the medications used to facilitate intubation. Nearly all sedative agents contribute to some degree of hypotension in the postintubation setting. The treatment of hypotension in this situation should consist of **intravascular volume repletion with fluids** administered rapidly via a large-bore intravenous line. There is currently no proven benefit of colloid as compared to crystalloid resuscitation with respect to outcome.

Despite the restoration of oxygen delivery, **inattention to source control invariably leads to the death of the patient** (see Table 48–1 for common infectious sources). This patient should undergo a computed tomography (CT) scan to evaluate the enterocutaneous fistula for adequacy of drainage, followed by surgery or another procedure to obtain control of small intestinal drainage. An important adjunctive measure is broad-spectrum antibiotic therapy directed toward common organisms. Once the patient is resuscitated and the infectious source controlled, attention should be turned toward metabolic support to avoid and prevent the effects of catabolism on the recovery process.

APPROACH TO SEPTIC SHOCK AND RESUSCITATION

Resuscitation

The primary goal of resuscitation is restoration of oxygen delivery to vital tissues. Oxygen is needed by cells to convert glucose to adenosine

Table 48–1
SOURCES OF INFECTION IN SURGICAL PATIENTS

Catheter-related sepsis (indwelling intravenous lines)
Surgical site infection (superficial, deep)
Clostridium difficile enterocolitis
Urinary tract infection
Sinusitis (with long-term nasogastric or endotracheal tube)
Acalculous cholecystitis
Perforated peptic ulcer
Diverticulitis

---

triphosphate (ATP) aerobically, yielding 36 molecules of ATP per molecule of glucose rather than only 2 molecules of ATP via anaerobic glycolysis. Oxygen delivery to the tissues is dependent on three major factors: (1) adequate oxygen in the blood, (2) a sufficient number of carrier molecules (hemoglobin) to carry oxygen to the tissues, and (3) sufficient blood flow (cardiac output) to deliver oxygen and hemoglobin to the tissues (see Table 48–2 for description of volume therapies). Oxygen delivery is difficult to measure with current technology short of invasive monitoring with pulmonary artery catheterization. Invasive monitoring using pulmonary artery catheterization should be considered for patients who do not respond appropriately to the initial therapy with stabilization of organ function and vital signs.

Table 48–2
COMMON INTRAVENOUS FLUID THERAPY FOR RESUSCITATION

TYPE OF FLUID	INDICATION	CLASS*	COST	INFECTIOUS RISK
Isotonic crystalloid (eg, normal saline, Ringer's lactate)	Volume expansion	Crystalloid	Very low	Nil
Hetastarch	Volume expansion	Colloid	Moderate	Nil
Human albumin	Volume expansion	Colloid	Moderate to high	Very low
Packed red blood cells	Improve oxygen-carrying capacity	Colloid	High	Moderate
Fresh frozen plasma	Coagulopathy	Colloid	High	Moderate
Platelets	Thrombocytopenia	Colloid	High	Moderate to high

*Crystalloid: significant volume of distribution outside the intravascular space, typically 1 part intravascular to 3 parts extravascular at equilibrium. Colloid: remains (more or less) in intravascular space at equilibrium.

Source Control

A key concept in the management of most postsurgical patients is that often operative intervention in addition to antibiotics is required to obtain adequate source control and treatment of the infection. An aggressive search for the site of infection should be carried out in cases where the source is not immediately apparent.

Metabolic Support

The final important aspect of caring for critically ill patients is the need for metabolic support. Nutritional support is indicated in all patients with an illness significant enough to require intubation and ventilatory support and an anticipated hospital stay of longer than 3 days. When available, the enteral route through a surgically placed jejunostomy or the nasojejunal route is preferred. Nutrition should be provided only after successful initial source control and restoration of oxygen delivery have been accomplished. Peripheral parenteral nutrition has no role in metabolic support of patients and should not be used. If the parenteral route is chosen, nutrition should be delivered via catheter (either a central line or a peripherally inserted central catheter) into a central vein.

Comprehension Questions

[48.1] A 56-year-old male with peritonitis from a perforated diverticulum undergoes emergency surgery for source control. He is given ventilatory assistance and returned to your intensive care unit (ICU). He is noted to have a blood pressure of 85/55 and a heart rate of 110/min. His urine output was 15 mL over the last hour, and his hemoglobin level is 12 g/dL. Which of the following is most likely to be *inappropriate for* this patient's treatment at this time?

A. Placement of a nasojejunal feeding tube and initiation of tube feedings
B. Placement of a pulmonary artery catheter

    C. Administration of intravenous fluid boluses
    D. Initiation of broad-spectrum antibiotic therapy

[48.2] A 51-year-old woman has undergone an open elective cholecystectomy five days previously. She has fever of one-day duration
and complains of shortness of breath and cough. Her pulse rate
is 120/min, temperature 39.5°C (103.1°F), respiratory rate of
46/min, blood pressure of 110/70 mmHg, and O_2 saturation
level 89% on 60% O_2 by face mask. She has crackles in the left
lung base and her leukocyte count is 17,000 cells/mm3. Her
chest radiograph shows left lower lobe subsegmental infiltrate.
Which of the following is correct regarding this patient's care?

    A. A higher FiO_2 should be avoided so that oxygen toxicity is
       avoided.
    B. Intravenous streptokinase for pulmonary embolus should be
       initiated.
    C. Mechanical ventilation and transfer to the ICU is likely
       indicated.
    D. A perinephric abscess is the most likely diagnosis.

[48.3] Which of the following statements regarding fluid resuscitation
is *true?*

    A. Packed red blood cells should be transfused when hemoglo-
       bin values are less than 12 g/dL.
    B. Colloid resuscitation is preferable to crystalloid resuscita-
       tion in patients with a need for acute volume expansion.
    C. At equilibrium, approximately one-fourth of administered
       crystalloid remains in the intravascular space.
    D. Hetastarch distributes to the extracellular space at equilib-
       rium.

Answers

[48.1] **A.** Nutritional support should be initiated only after appropriate
resuscitation and source control. This individual is still hypotensive.

[48.2] **C.** This patient has significant hypoxemia and tachypnea despite high levels of oxygen; this portends the possible need for mechanical ventilation. The differential diagnosis includes subphrenic abscess, postoperative pneumonia, and pulmonary embolism. Intravenous heparin (and not intravenous streptokinase) would be the treatment in pulmonary embolism.

[48.3] **C.** At equilibrium, only one-fourth of isotonic crystalloid remains in the intravascular space; thus, 3 mL of crystalloids is usually infused for every 1 mL of blood lost. Hetastarch is a colloid solution and tends to remain in the intravascular space at equilibrium.

CLINICAL PEARLS

◈ The initial treatment of all clinically unstable patients includes appropriate airway management.

◈ The **initial therapy** for hypotension in most patients in whom sepsis is suspected should be aggressive fluid resuscitation—**not vasopressors!**

◈ Source control in patients with a surgical illness frequently requires appropriate procedures to adequately control infection (eg, drainage, debridement, bowel resection). For these types of patients antibiotics alone **are not** usually adequate for source control.

◈ Invasive monitoring using pulmonary artery catheterization should be considered for patients who do not respond appropriately to initial therapy with stabilization of organ function and vital signs.

REFERENCES

Marino P. The ICU book, 2nd ed. Philadelphia: Lippincott Williams & Wilkins, 1997.

Irwin RS, Cerra FB, Rippe JM, eds. Intensive care medicine, 4th ed. Philadelphia: Lippincott-Raven, 1998.

A 4-year-old boy informed his mother that he had just passed some blood in his urine. Hematuria was confirmed by the mother, who brought the boy in for evaluation. The child denied any significant recent trauma, and he had been in good health. His past medical history is unremarkable. He is in the 56th percentile in height and in the 43rd percentile in weight. On physical examination, the patient appears healthy and has normal vital signs. Findings from the cardiopulmonary examinations are within normal limits. A 10-cm mass is identified in the left upper quadrant of the abdomen. This mass is firm and nontender. No abnormalities are noted in the extremities. Laboratory studies reveal a normal complete blood count (CBC) and electrolyte levels with the normal range. The urinalysis reveals 50 to100 red blood cells per high-power field.

◆ **What is the most likely diagnosis?**

◆ **What is the best therapy?**

ANSWERS TO CASE 49: Wilms Tumor
(Pediatric Abdominal Mass)

Summary: A 4-year-old boy presents with hematuria and an abdominal mass

◆ **Diagnosis:** Wilms tumor involving the left kidney.

◆ **Best therapy:** The management of a Wilms tumor depends on the findings from the imaging studies. If the tumor is massive or bilateral and an intracaval extension of tumor extends proximally to the hepatic veins, preoperative multiagent chemotherapy is utilized initially. These findings are uncommon, and the majority of Wilms tumors, even if large at the initial presentation, can be completely resected prior to chemotherapy. Almost all patients receive chemotherapy following nephrectomy. Radiation therapy is given if there has been tumor spillage, either from a preoperative capsular rupture or from an intraoperative tumor spill.

Analysis

Objectives

1. Become familiar with the common presentation, differential diagnosis, and initial evaluation of an abdominal mass in newborns and pediatric patients.
2. Understand the management and outcome of a Wilms tumor and neuroblastoma.

Considerations

Wilms tumors are renal embryonal neoplasms that occur with a peak incidence in children between 1 and 5 years of age; thus, at age 4 years this patient is within this group. These tumors usually manifest as asymptomatic abdominal or flank masses, although hematuria is often seen. Before surgery, imaging evaluation is important to determine the extent of the tumor, and in this patient it should include abdominal ultrasonography and a computed tomography (CT) scan of the abdomen and chest. If the tumor is unilateral and appears that it can be safely removed, surgical exploration and resection should be attempted.

APPROACH TO AN ABDOMINAL MASS IN THE PEDIATRIC PATIENT

The etiology of an abdominal mass in a pediatric patient depends to a large extent on the age of the patient at presentation. Knowing the age of the patient, the details of a directed history obtained from the child and the parents, and the results from a routine physical examination allow one to develop a focused differential diagnosis. Based on this list of possible etiologies, imaging studies and selected laboratory findings will then allow a more definitive diagnosis to be made. The most likely etiologies of an abdominal mass are listed in Table 49–1 for neonates (<1 month of age) and in Table 49–2 for older infants and children.

Clinical Approach

With the information in Tables 49–1 and 49–2, the etiology of the majority of abdominal masses can usually be determined with a high degree of certainty. A careful history should be obtained from the patient and the family that includes the length of time the mass has been present (or noticed), associated pain or other symptoms, changes in eating habits, changes in bowel or bladder function, associated fatigue or night sweats, associated bleeding or bruising, and other related conditions. An important consideration for neonates is the maternal prenatal history, especially data from prenatal ultrasound and information about the presence or absence of polyhydramnios. **Maternal polyhydramnios may be the first sign of a neonatal bowel obstruction, which then may appear as an abdominal mass.** The physical examination should document the location, size, consistency, and mobility of the mass, as well as associated lymphadenopathy or tenderness.

Table 49–1
ABDOMINAL MASSES IN NEONATES
(BIRTH TO 1 MONTH)[*]

Renal
    Hydronephrosis, eg, from obstruction (ureteropelvic junction, obstruction, posterior urethral valves, other)
    Multicystic dysplastic kidney
    Polycystic kidney disease
    Mesoblastic nephroma
    Wilms tumor
Genital
    Hydrometrocolpos
    Ovarian mass, simple cyst, teratoma, torsion
Gastrointestinal
    Duplication cyst
    Complicated meconium ileus
    Mesenteric or omental cyst
Retroperitoneal
    Adrenal hemorrhage
    Neuroblastoma
    Teratoma
    Rhabdomyosarcoma
    Lymphangioma
    Hemangioma
Hepatobiliary
    Hemangioendothelioma
    Hepatic mesenchymal hamartoma
    Choledochal cyst
    Hepatoblastoma

[*]The most common etiologies of an abdominal mass in a neonate can be categorized as shown here (from most common to least common).

Radiographic Evaluations

Initially, plain abdominal radiographs are obtained to rule out gastrointestinal obstruction, to assess bowel gas patterns, and to determine the presence or absence of calcifications. Intra-abdominal calcifications in a neonate with an abdominal mass are often associated with complicated cystic meconium ileus. Calcifications in a different distribution can lead to the diagnosis of neuroblastoma, especially in an older in-

Table 49–2
ABDOMINAL MASSES IN INFANTS AND CHILDREN
(1 MONTH TO 18 YEARS)[*]

Renal
  Wilms tumor
  Hydronephrosis, eg, from obstruction (ureteropelvic junction, obstruction, posterior urethral valves, other)
  Rhabdoid tumor
  Clear cell sarcoma
  Polycystic kidney disease
Retroperitoneal
  Neuroblastoma
  Rhabdomyosarcoma
  Teratoma
  Lymphoma
  Lymphangioma
  Hemangioma
Gastrointestinal
  Appendiceal abscess
  Intussusception
  Duplication cyst
  Functional constipation
  Hirschsprung disease
  Mesenteric or omental cyst
  Lymphoma
Hepatobiliary
  Hepatoblastoma
  Hepatocellular carcinoma
  Benign liver tumors
  Choledochal cyst
Genital
  Ovarian mass, eg, simple cyst, teratoma, torsion
  Hydrometrocolpos
  Undescended testicle, neoplasm, or torsion

[*]Note that although many of the specific etiologies of an abdominal mass are the same as listed for neonates, the most likely causes change with older children.

fant. If the findings from plain abdominal radiography are nonspecific, which is often the case, abdominal ultrasound is the next imaging modality of choice. Ultrasonography can usually identify the organ of origin, the mass can be classified as cystic or solid, and vascular flow characteristics can be determined using Doppler ultrasound techniques.

Sonographic interpretation is very operator-dependent and may be inaccurate in children.

CT scans are typically obtained if the ultrasonogram is either nondiagnostic or shows a solid tumor. CT imaging can provide additional anatomic detail and can be diagnostic. As many of these conditions ultimately require operative intervention, a CT scan can provide an accurate preoperative assessment of the etiology of the mass and the involvement of adjacent structures; it can also detect the distant spread in case of neoplasms. The disadvantages of obtaining CT scans for children include the need for sedation in many cases and the unknown long-term effects of this level of ionizing radiation.

After the history is recorded, a physical examination performed, and selective imaging studies obtained, a short differential diagnosis is compiled. Very selective laboratory analyses can then be used to verify the diagnosis. For example, if the most likely diagnosis based on imaging is neuroblastoma, then a CBC and a urine test for catecholamines should be obtained. If, however, the most likely diagnosis is hepatoblastoma, the level of α-fetoprotein should be evaluated prior to resection of the liver tumor.

Comprehension Questions

[49.1] A previously healthy 9-month-old male is brought to the emergency room with severe, intermittent abdominal pain. During the attacks, which are episodic and occur every 10 to 15 minutes, the child draws his legs up to his abdomen. The child is vomiting and has heme-positive stools. On physical examination a tender, mobile, sausage-shaped mass is found in the midabdomen. Which of the following is the most likely diagnosis?

    A. Intussusception
    B. Jejunal atresia
    C. Neuroblastoma
    D. Intestinal duplication cyst

[49.2] A 5-year-old female presents with a 7-cm, vague, left-sided abdominal mass. The patient has also experienced recent weight loss and failure to thrive. The mass is hard and fixed. A plain radiograph reveals fine calcifications in the region of the mass, and a CT scan shows an irregular, solid mass arising from the left adrenal gland. Which of the following conditions is the most likely?

A. Adrenal hemorrhage
B. Adrenal adenoma
C. Neuroblastoma
D. Wilms tumor

[49.3] A 15-year-old male presents to the emergency room with a fever of 102°F, a firm, fixed mass in the right lower quadrant of the abdomen, and a chief complaint of abdominal pain. The patient has been ill for the past 2 weeks but has not sought medical care until now. Which of the following findings is a CT scan of the abdomen most likely to demonstrate?

A. Neoplasm arising in an undescended testicle
B. Right hydronephrosis
C. Lymphoma
D. Abscess from a perforated appendix

[49.4] A 12-year-old female presents with left lower quadrant pain, pelvic pain, and a vague fullness on physical examination. She is otherwise healthy and has no associated symptoms. The most likely imaging modality that would identify the etiology of the mass is which of the following?

A. Plain abdominal radiograph
B. Upper gastrointestinal tract contrast study
C. Magnetic resonance imaging of the abdomen and pelvis
D. Ultrasound of the abdomen and pelvis

Answers

[49.1] **A.** This is a classic and severe presentation of intussusception (when the bowel telescopes on itself). This infant should be treated with intravenous hydration followed by a barium or air

contrast enema to both diagnose the condition and attempt to reduce the intussusception. If it cannot be reduced with the enema, an emergent operation is indicated.

[49.2] **C.** Children with neuroblastoma are often symptomatic at presentation and suffer from failure to thrive. This is in contrast to
children with Wilms tumor who usually appear to be healthy.
Patients with neuroblastoma usually require tumor biopsy followed by neoadjuvant chemotherapy prior to tumor resection,
again in contrast to the situation with Wilms tumor. The outcome with neuroblastoma depends on the biology of the tumor
and the stage of disease, but overall is much worse than for
Wilms tumor.

[49.3] **D.** An abdominal mass in a previously healthy adolescent with
a fever and signs of systemic illness is most commonly an abscess from a perforated appendix, especially if it is located in
the right lower quadrant. CT imaging or ultrasound can readily
identify this as the likely diagnosis, and image-guided abscess
drainage can be employed with plans for a delayed-interval appendectomy. This management option is preferable to urgent
appendectomy and abscess drainage in this inflammatory
condition.

[49.4] **D.** This patient probably has an ovarian tumor, most likely benign. The most common of these tumors is an ovarian teratoma,
which can easily be identified with pelvic ultrasound to fully ex-
amine the adnexa. None of the other imaging modalities would
be the procedure of choice for this patient.

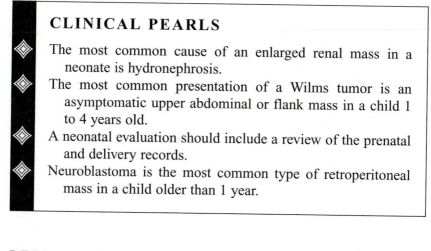

CLINICAL PEARLS

- The most common cause of an enlarged renal mass in a neonate is hydronephrosis.
- The most common presentation of a Wilms tumor is an asymptomatic upper abdominal or flank mass in a child 1 to 4 years old.
- A neonatal evaluation should include a review of the prenatal and delivery records.
- Neuroblastoma is the most common type of retroperitoneal mass in a child older than 1 year.

REFERENCES

Ashcraft KW, Holder TM, ed. Pediatric surgery, 2nd ed. Philadephia: Saunders, 1993.

O'Neill JA, Rowe MI, Grosfeld JL, et al, eds. Pediatric surgery, 5th ed. St. Louis: Mosby-Year Book, 1998.

A 38-year-old morbidly obese woman presents to the clinic for evaluation and management of venous insufficiency in the lower extremities. During your conversation with the patient, she tells you that she has been extremely overweight ever since childhood. She has tried many different dietary modifications, hypnosis, and medications but has not been able to achieve sustained weight loss. She is concerned about her health status because of a recent diagnosis of type II diabetes mellitus and a history of coronary artery disease in several immediate family members. The patient is married and without children. She works as a computer programmer. She does not consume tobacco or alcohol. Her current medications are an oral hypoglycemic agent and NPH insulin. On examination, she is found to be 5 ft 3 in and weighs 280 lb. Her body mass index (BMI) is 47 kg/m^2. Her pulse rate is 95/min and her blood pressure is 158/86. The findings from her cardiopulmonary examination and abdominal examination are unremarkable. Examination of the lower extremities reveals mild edema, diffuse varicosity, and venous stasis dermatitis bilaterally. The patient indicates that she is not interested in surgical therapy for her venous disease but would like your opinion regarding operative intervention for management of her obesity.

◆ **Is surgical therapy a reasonable treatment option in this patient?**

◆ **What are the complications associated with morbid obesity?**

ANSWERS TO CASE 50: Obesity (Morbid)

Summary: A 38-year-old morbidly obese woman (BMI 47 kg/m^2) with obesity-associated complications (diabetes and venous stasis) is inquiring about the surgical treatment of obesity.

✦ **Surgical therapy:** Surgical therapy is a reasonable option in this patient.

✦ **Complications associated with morbid obesity:** Diabetes mellitus, hypertension, hyperlipidemia, atherosclerosis, cardiomyopathy, sleep apnea syndrome, gallstones, arthritis, and infertility are disease processes associated with morbid obesity.

Analysis

Objectives

1. Become familiar with the complications associated with morbid obesity and the effectiveness of bariatric operations on these complications.
2. Become familiar with the short- and long-term outcomes in weight reduction achieved with operative treatment.

Considerations

This patient falls within the National Institutes of Health (NIH) class III (see Table 50-1) category of clinically severe obesity and on the basis of weight/height ratio alone is a candidate for surgical therapy. Her co-morbidities, diabetes and venous stasis, add further evidence of the advanced nature of her disease. Her blood glucose level should be carefully monitored during the postoperative period, and the venous disease in her lower extremities treated prophylactically during surgery with mini-heparin and sequential compression stockings.

Table 50–1
NIH CLASSIFICATION OF OBESITY (REVISED)

DESCRIPTION	BMI (kg/m^2)	OBESITY CLASS	DISEASE RISK
Normal	18.5–24.9		
Overweight	25.0–29.9		Increased

Obesity
  Mild
  Moderate
  Severe
	
	30.0–34.9
	35.0–39.9
	>40
		
		I
		II
		III
			
			High
			Very high
			Extremely high

Superobese	>50		Extremely high

Source: Adapted from NIH Conference on Gastrointestinal Surgery for Severe Obesity: Consensus Development Conference Panel. Ann Intern Med 1991;115:956–961.

APPROACH TO SURGICAL TREATMENT OF MORBID OBESITY

Definitions

Body mass index: The ratio of weight in kilograms (kg) to height in meters squared (m^2). It is calculated by dividing the weight (in kg) by the height (in m^2) or by multiplying the weight in pounds (lb) by 704 and dividing by the height in inches squared (in^2).

Clinically severe obesity: BMI greater than 40 kg/m^2.

Obesity-related comorbidities: Various diseases are considered to be caused by obesity: hypertension, diabetes, coronary and hypertrophic heart disease, gallstones, gastroesophageal reflux disease (GERD), sleep apnea, asthma, reactive pulmonary disease, osteoarthritis, lumbosacral disk disease, urinary incontinence, infertility, polycystic ovarian syndrome, and cancer. This list attests to the serious nature of this problem.

Gastric restrictive procedures: Operations that involve the creation of a small pouch at the upper end of the stomach that communicates directly with the intestine or the stomach.

Malabsorptive procedures: Surgeries that decrease the contact of food with the digestive juices and the absorptive surface of the small intestine.

Clinical Approach

Obesity is increasing in epidemic proportions and qualifies as one of the leading medical problems among Americans. The adverse health effects associated with obesity may reduce patient quality of life and longevity. Because of concerns about the prevalence of obesity and its associated health problems, two NIH consensus conferences have taken

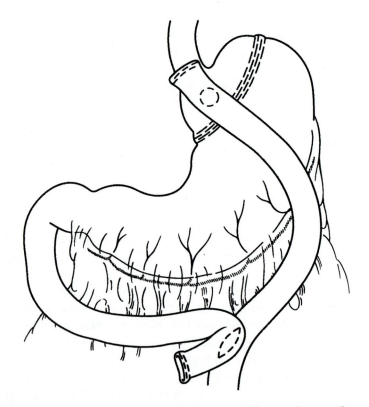

Figure 50–1.   Gastric bypass showing a small gastric pouch anastomosis with a Roux-en-Y limb.

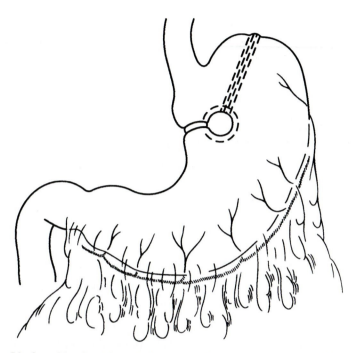

Figure 50–2. Vertical banded gastroplasty creates a small gastric pouch with a narrow outlet.

place to address the surgical treatment of morbid obesity. At the 1991 conference, Roux-en-Y gastric bypass (RYGB) (Figure 50–1) and vertical banded gastroplasty (VBG) (Figure 50–2) were recommended for appropriately selected patients. Based on more recent results, an updated statement indicates a **preference for RYGB** compared to VBG becauseVBG does not result in adequate sustained weight loss and is associated with complications. The treatment goals of any patient with morbid obesity should be focused on weight loss as well as on the reduction of comorbidities (Tables 50–2 to 50–4). It is important for the patient and the physician to have realistic expectations about surgical treatment outcome; **most successfully treated patients achieve a reduction in weight that is frequently sustainable; however, patients**

Table 50–2

OPERATIONS USED TO TREAT CLINICALLY
SEVERE OBESITY

OPERATION	DESCRIPTION
Roux-en-Y small-pouch gastric bypass	Proximal pouch to Roux limb of jejunum
Vertical banded gastroplasty	Proximal lesser curve pouch to main stomach with circumferential band at communication
Adjustable lap band	Band around upper stomach with circumferential balloon accessible by subcutaneous port
Duodenal switch	Stomach reduction with division of duodenum at the pylorus. The distal small bowel is attached to the gastric tube, and the proximal small bowel is attached to the lower ileum.

rarely achieve the ideal body weight proscribed in standard height-weight tables. Most patients experience an improvement in obesity-related complications following successful surgery, however, increased longevity has not been demonstrated. The success and the patient satisfaction associated with surgical therapy are further augmented when

Table 50–3

TREATMENT RESULTS AND COMPLICATIONS

METHOD	RESULTS	COMPLICATIONS
Vertical banded gastroplasty	Sustained weight loss is difficult, especially with "sweets eaters"	High reoperation rate for stoma erosion; frequent gastroesophageal reflux
Roux-en-Y gastric bypass	Sustained results are good; loss of 50%–60% of excess weight can be expected	No long-term metabolic problems identified
Gastric banding	Loss of 38% of excess weight	23% rate of band slippage, resulting in reoperation

Table 50–4
EFFECTS OF SURGERY ON OBESITY COMORBIDITY

Diabetes mellitus	82% of patients cured of type II diabetes at 15-y follow-up
Sleep apnea	Up to 93% of patients have improvement
Hypertension	Success correlated with the amount of weight loss
Serum lipid abnormalities	Successful gastric bypass is associated with a sustained reduction in triglycerides and low-density lipoproteins and increase in high-density lipoproteins

patients receive proper preoperative counseling and undergo modifications in dietary habits and lifestyle.

Comprehension Questions

[50.1] A 23-year-old female is referred for an opinion regarding the advisability of surgical treatment for obesity. The patient is 5 ft in tall and weighs 210 lb. She has no known comorbidities and is free of symptoms. Your best advice would be which of the following?

A. A small pouch gastric bypass
B. A vertical banded gastroplasty
C. A lap band procedure
D. Further efforts at medical therapy

[50.2] A 45-year-old female, the mother of two teen-aged children, presents with long-standing, clinically severe obesity (BMI 50 kg/m^2) that is refractory to medical therapy. Which of the following surgical procedures is most likely to provide the best chance of long-term weight reduction with the least morbidity?

A. Vertical banded gastroplasty
B. Small pouch gastric bypass

C. Adjustable lap band
D. Duodenal switch

[50.3] Gastric restrictive procedures lead to weight loss by

A. Increasing the basal metabolic rate
B. Enhancing maldigestion and absorption
C. Producing early satiety
D. Inducing nausea and vomiting

[50.4] Which of the following is the most common, most serious post-operative complication associated with small pouch gastric bypass?

A. Pneumonia
B. Leakage of intestinal contents from the gastrojejunal anastomosis
C. Intestinal obstruction
D. Pulmonary embolus

[50.5] Late sequelae from gastric restrictive procedures include which of the following?

A. Anemia
B. Osteoporosis
C. Vitamin deficiencies
D. All of the above

Answers

[50.1] **D.** The patient is young, free of comorbid medical problems, and has a BMI of less than 40. Her BMI is calculated as 210 × 704 / 64 × 64 = 36.1 kg/m². Further attempts at medical management should be made; however, if significant complications such as hypertension and diabetes are already present, a surgical approach might be appropriate.

[50.2] **B.** This patient has strong indications for a surgical approach (BMI >50, superobese). A small pouch gastric bypass performed by either an open or a laparoscopic technique will provide the best long-term weight reduction with minimal early and late long-term morbidity.

[50.3] **C.** Gastric restrictive operations help people lose weight by producing early satiety and decreasing their appetite. To be successful, the patient must simultaneously restrict caloric intake.

[50.4] **B.** Leakage from the attachment of the stomach to the intestine can be a devastating complication. It usually is characterized by fever, leukocytosis, and left shoulder pain on postoperative days 3 to 5.

[50.5] **D.** A small pouch gastric bypass can be accompanied by anemia, osteoporosis, and vitamin deficiencies in view of the marked decrease in food intake. Patients need supplemental vitamins, calcium, and oral iron and vitamin B_{12} following the procedure.

CLINICAL PEARLS

◈ The body mass index represented in kilograms per meter squared body surface area is a common tool in assessing obesity.

◈ Many diseases are considered to be obesity-related comorbidities such as hypertension, diabetes, coronary heart disease, gall stones, and sleep apnea.

◈ In general, surgical weight reduction surgeries should be reserved for severe obesity, or those obese individuals with comorbidities.

REFERENCES

National Institutes of Health. Clinical guidelines on the indentification, evaluation, and treatment of overweight and obesity in adults: the evidence report. NIH Publication No. 98-4083. September 1998. National Institutes of Health, Bethesda, MD.

Klein S, Wadden T, Sugerman HJ. AGA technical review on obesity. Gastroenterol-
    ogy 2002;123:882–932.

MacLean LD, Rhode BM, Sampalis J, Forse RA. Results of the surgical treatment
    of obesity. Am J Surg 1993;165:155–162.

National Institutes of Health. Conference on gastrointestinal surgery for severe
    obesity: Consensus Development Conference Panel. Ann Intern Med 1991;
    115:956–961.

Schaver PR, Ikramuddin S, Ramanathan R, Gourash W, Panzak G. Outcomes after
    laparoscopic Roux-en-Y gastric bypass for morbid obesity. Ann Surg
    2000;232:515–529.

A 32 year-old woman complains of bleeding gums while brushing her teeth and easy bruising of several weeks' duration. She has no significant past medical history, has had no previous surgery, and does not take any medication. She denies consumption of alcohol, tobacco, or illicit drugs. On examination, you notice several petechiae on her legs and bruises over the knees. The results from her head and neck, cardiopulmonary, and abdominal examinations are unremarkable. No masses are palpable in the abdomen. The laboratory evaluation reveals a normal white blood cell count and normal hemoglobin and hematocrit values. Results from serum chemistry studies are within the normal range. Her platelet count is 27,000/mm^3. A bone marrow biopsy is performed, demonstrating the presence of numerous megakaryocytes but no evidence of malignancy.

◆ **What is the most likely diagnosis?**

◆ **What is the mechanism associated with this disease process?**

◆ **What is your next step in treatment?**

ANSWERS TO CASE 52: Immune Thrombocytopenia Purpura (Splenic Disease)

Summary: A 32-year-old woman presents with easy bruisability, gum bleeding and petechiae, and thrombocytopenia. The bone marrow aspirate shows an increased number of megakaryocytes.

◆ **Diagnosis:** Immune thrombocytopenia purpura (ITP).

◆ **Mechanism responsible for the process:** ITP is associated with the production of antiplatelet immunoglobulin G (IgG) by the spleen.

◆ **Next step:** The initial treatment is with corticosteroids. Seventy-five percent of patients respond to corticosteriods, but the best long-term results are achieved with splenectomy.

Analysis

Objectives

1. Become familiar with the role of splenectomy in the treatment of ITP.
2. Be familiar with splenic function and the complications associated with the loss of splenic function.
3. Be familiar with indications for splenectomy other than traumatic injuries.

Considerations

This patient exhibits many of the common clinical manifestations of thrombocytopenia, which include ecchymoses, gum bleeding, purpura, excessive vaginal bleeding, and gastrointestinal tract bleeding. Mechanisms producing thrombocytopenia include inadequate production because of primary or secondary bone marrow dysfunction, splenic sequestration (hypersplenism), and increased platelet destruction. ITP is an acquired disorder leading to increased platelet destruction due to the production of antiplatelet IgG by the spleen. The spleen may further contribute to thrombocytopenia by functioning as a primary site of sequestration and destruction of sensitized platelets. ITP is most common in middle-aged women. The diagnosis of ITP is one of exclusion, which requires a careful search for possible precipitating factors such as drugs and infections. **The diagnosis requires demonstration of a normal to hypercellular megakaryocyte count in the bone marrow, a response to the increased peripheral destruction.** Splenomegaly is rare in ITP, and its presence should suggest another source of thrombocytopenia, such as hemolytic disease.

APPROACH TO IMMUNE THROMBOCYTOPENIA PURPURA

The spleen has a number of important functions, particularly its immunologic and phagocytic activities. It removes old erythrocytes (120 days old) and platelets (10 to 14 days old). It also removes abnormal intracellular erythrocyte particles (Howell–Jolly bodies, Heinz bodies, and Pappenheimer bodies) and erythrocytes with abnormal membranes. Immunologically, the spleen produces opsonins (tuftsin and properdin) and antibodies (particularly IgM).

Approach to Immune Thrombocytopenia Purpura

A carefully recorded history and a physical examination are important in the diagnosis of ITP. A bone marrow aspirate is also necessary to confirm the diagnosis. The initial treatment for ITP is corticosteroids, which leads to an increased platelet count in more than 75% of patients. Other medical therapies include administration of intravenous immunoglobulins, plasmapheresis, and chemotherapeutic agents. Splenectomy is recommended for patients who do not respond to steroids, those who require an excessively high steroid dose, and those who require chronic steroid therapy (1 year or longer). The platelet count can be expected to rise shortly after splenectomy, and sustained remissions are seen in more than 80% of cases. The best indication that splenectomy will be of lasting benefit is an increase in the platelet count with corticosteroid therapy. Patients who are refractory to corticosteroid treatment have a lower rate of long-term remission (about 60%). Spontaneous remission occurs in most children (85%), and splenectomy is rarely indicated. When splenectomy is needed, it should be delayed until after the age of 4 years, at which time the risk of post-splenectomy sepsis is decreased. Recently, laparoscopic splenectomy has been shown to be safe and effective. Furthermore, patients undergoing laparoscopic splenectomy tolerate feeding sooner, require less pain medication, and are discharged from the hospital sooner than those undergoing open splenectomy. Generally, platelet transfusions are not required despite low platelet counts unless bleeding is uncontrollable. Platelet transfusion should be withheld intraoperatively until just after the spleen is removed; if given before this time, they are consumed and confer minimal benefit.

Other Indications for Splenectomy

Traumatic injury has been the most common indication for splenectomy. Other common nontraumatic indications for splenectomy include congenital hemolytic anemias, such as hereditary spherocytosis and thalassemia major. Myeloproliferative disorders may lead to massive splenomegaly, which can cause symptoms that are best relieved by splenectomy. Splenectomy for myeloproliferative disorders is performed primarily for symptomatic relief.

Because of the loss of splenic immunologic function following splenectomy, postoperative infectious complications may occur, such as wound infections and intra-abdominal abscesses. **Overwhelming post-splenectomy sepsis (OPSS) is an uncommon but well-recognized potential complication associated with splenectomy.** The risk of OPSS depends on the age of the patient and the reason for splenectomy. It occurs in 0.3% of adults and 0.6% of children and is **more common when splenectomy is performed for hematologic disease compared to splenectomy for trauma.** OPSS most commonly develops within the first 2 years after splenectomy, although it can occur later. The typical onset of this clinical syndrome is often insidious and is marked by nonspecific symptoms of malaise, headache, nausea, and confusion; it can progress rapidly to shock and death. Early medical evaluation at the fist signs of illness is important in decreasing mortality. The mortality of OPSS exceeds 50% in children and is approximately 20% in adults. The most common organisms are encapsulated bacteria such **as *Strep-tococcus pneumoniae, Haemophilus influenzae* B, and *Neisseria meningitidis,*** which are typically killed by the immunologic functions of the spleen. **All patients undergoing planned elective splenectomy should receive a polyvalent pneumococcal vaccination 2 weeks before surgery. Children and all immunosuppressed patients** should be vaccinated against **pneumococcus,** *H. influenzae* **B, and meningococcus.**

Comprehension Questions

[51.1] Which of the following describes the normal function of the adult spleen?

    A. Erythrocyte production
    B. Removal of erythrocytes after 60 days
    C. Production of erythopoietin
    D. Production of antibodies

[51.2] Which of the following is *true* regarding OPSS?

    A. It occurs 20% of the time.
    B. It occurs more commonly in adults than in children.
    C. The most common organism isolated is *Staphylococcus aureus.*
    D. The mortality in children exceeds 50%.

[51.3] A middle-aged woman has ITP *refractory* to corticosteroid therapy. How likely would her condition respond to splenectomy?

    A. 20%
    B. 40%
    C. 60%
    D. 80%

[51.4] Splenectomy for ITP is most likely to provide long-term remission in which of the following patients?

    A. Patients with an enlarged spleen
    B. Patients with a high reticulocyte count
    C. Patients below the age of 4
    D. Patients who respond to corticosteroid therapy

Answers

[51.1] **D.** The spleen produces antibodies. It does not participate in erythrocyte production, it removes erythrocytes after 120 days. The kidney produces erythropoietin.

[51.2] **D.** Overwhelming postsplenectomy sepsis may be associated with a mortality rate of 50%. It is more common in children than in adults.

[51.3] **C.** Approximately 60% of patients with ITP refractory to corticosteroid therapy respond to splenectomy.

[51.4] **D.** The patient group that has the best response to splenectomy consists of patients with ITP who respond to corticosteroid therapy.

CLINICAL PEARLS

◈ Splenomegaly is rare in ITP.
Splenectomy for ITP is most likely to provide long-term remission in patients who respond to corticosteroid therapy.

◈ **Overwhelming postsplenectomy sepsis is an uncommon but well-recognized potential complication associated with splenectomy;** it has a higher incidence in children than in adults.

◈ The typical bone marrow findings in ITP are increased numbers of megakaryocytes.

REFERENCES

Gargiulo NJ III, Zenillman MA. In: Cameron J. Current surgical therapy, 7th ed. St. Louis: Mosby-Year Book, 2001:587–591.

Lefor AT, Phillips EH. In: Norton JA, Bollinger RR, Chang AE, et al, eds. Surgery: basic science and clinical evidence. New York: Springer, 2001:763–785.

A 26-year-old man with 3-year history of Crohn's disease presents to the emergency center with postprandial abdominal pain and vomiting of 2 days' duration. He has been taking prednisone 40 mg/d for the past 2 weeks for treatment of disease exacerbation. Prior to that time, the patient has received Asacol (a 5-aminosalicylate [5-ASA] derivative) 2.4 g/d. The patient reports a 15-lb weight loss over the past 2 months. His past surgical history is significant for an appendectomy 4 years ago. On examination, his temperature is 38.0°C (100.4°F), pulse rate 95/min, and blood pressure 130/70. His abdomen is moderately distended and tender in the right lower quadrant. There are no masses or peritonitis. A rectal examination reveals no perianal disease or abnormalities. The other results from the physical examination are unremarkable. The complete blood count revealed a white blood cell count of 14,000/mm^3, and his hemoglobin level is 10.5 g/dL. The results from serum electrolyte studies and a urinalysis are within the normal range.

◆ **What is the most likely diagnosis?**

◆ **What is the next step?**

ANSWERS TO CASE 52: Crohn's Disease

Summary: A 26-year-old man presents with a history of Crohn's disease with disease exacerbation. Despite high-dose steroid therapy, the patient's symptoms have not improved. Currently, he has nausea, vomiting, abdominal pain and distention, and a low-grade fever and leukocytosis, which are suggestive of chronic small bowel obstruction and low-grade sepsis.

◆ **Diagnosis:** Crohn's disease complicated by obstruction and possible intra-abdominal infection.

◆ **Next step:** The next step is to define the extent of disease involvement, the site of obstruction, and the possible presence of intra-abdominal abscesses. A computed tomography (CT) scan of the abdomen and pelvis, upper gastrointestinal (GI) tract contrast radiography, and colonoscopy are indicated.

Analysis

Objectives

1. Know the clinical features, diagnosis, and natural history of Crohn's disease.
2. Be familiar with the medical therapies and the role of surgery in Crohn's disease.

Considerations

A young man presents with a 3-year history of Crohn's disease which has been refractory to maintenance therapy with a 5-ASA derivative and a recent course of steroid therapy. His lack of response to medical therapy is evidenced by weight loss, GI tract obstructive symptoms, and fever. This patient's bowel obstruction is likely due to chronic fibrotic strictures rather than subacute inflammation. **Obstruction from subacute inflammation can be resolved with anti-inflammatory and**

immunomodulator therapies; in contrast, fibrotic strictures cannot be resolved with medical management and generally require surgical therapy to relieve the obstruction. A CT scan is a useful initial imaging study for assessing the severity and extent of the disease and for detecting intra-abdominal abscesses. **Crohn's disease may involve both the small bowel and colon;** therefore, complete evaluation should include colonoscopy and an upper GI tract contrast study to visualize the location and severity of small bowel disease. **Once the small bowel and colon have been evaluated, this patient should undergo exploratory laparotomy to relieve his bowel obstruction.** Surgical options include resection of the obstructed bowel or stricturoplasty.

APPROACH TO CROHN'S DISEASE

Definitions

Disease activity: Severity can be assessed by histology, endoscopy, radiography, symptoms, or surgical findings. Histologic, endoscopic, radiographic, and surgical criteria frequently do not correlate with clinical criteria and may not accurately reflect the physiologic impact of the disease on the patient. It is more important to know how the disease is affecting the patient.

Disease patterns: Most patients with Crohn's disease have one of three predominant disease patterns: **stricture, perforation,** or **inflammation.**

Medical therapy: Pharmacologic therapy can be generally categorized as maintenance therapy (to maintain disease remission) and therapy for active disease (for acute flare-ups).

Stricturoplasty: A surgical option that may be effective for patients with intestinal strictures from Crohn's disease. This approach may help preserve bowel length and function for patients with a long segment or multiple sites involved by fibrotic strictures.

Clinical Approach

Most patients with Crohn's disease have distinct patterns of disease distribution: in the terminal ileum and right colon (35% to 50%), ileum

(30% to 35%), colon (25% to 35%), or stomach and/or duodenum (0.5% to 4%). **Anorectal involvement** is frequently found in patients with **small bowel Crohn's disease** and may be the **initial manifestation in 10% of patients.** Therefore, **Crohn's disease should be considered whenever recurrent or complex perianal abscesses and fistulas are encountered in young patients.** The other symptoms related to Crohn's disease may be nonspecific, including chronic abdominal pain, postprandial abdominal cramps and weight loss, and **fever due to fistulizing disease.** It is not uncommon for patients with Crohn's disease to have symptoms for months to years before the diagnosis is established. **The goals of management are to relieve symptoms and optimize the patient's quality of life. Medical and surgical options should be viewed as complementary therapeutic options rather than competing modalities.** Thus, when medical therapy becomes ineffective or significantly compromises the patient's quality of life, surgical interventions should be implemented. Similarly, the role of surgery in Crohn's disease is palliative and not curative; therefore, surgical goals should be directed toward symptom relief without exposing patients to excessive short- and long-term morbidity. Whenever an operative procedure is to be implemented, it is vital for the surgeon to coordinate with the gastroenterologist in formulating plans so that the patient will have the best possible outcome.

Medical Therapy

The etiology of Crohn's disease remains unknown, but it is in part caused by stimulation of an intestinal immune cascade in genetically susceptible individuals. **Medical therapy** can be broadly categorized **as nutritional, anti-inflammatory, immunomodulatory, and antimicrobial** (Table 52–1). Nutritional therapies include bowel rest with total parenteral nutrition (TPN), elemental feeding, or omega-3 fatty acid supplementation. Nutritional therapies have been shown to produce improvement and cause remission in patients with active disease; however, because of the impact of nutritional therapy on a patient's lifestyle, nutritional therapy has been limited to the short-term treatment of active disease. Antimicrobial therapy with **metronidazole or ciprofloxacin** has been found to be **effective in the resolution of active intestinal and perineal disease,** and **long-term metronidazole maintenance** therapy has been **found to be effective in preventing disease recurrence.** The mechanisms of antimicrobial therapy are largely unknown and may be in part based on its

Table 52–1
MEDICAL THERAPY FOR CROHN'S DISEASE

AGENTS	INDICATIONS	SIDE EFFECTS/ ADVERSE EFFECTS
Corticosteroids	Active disease	Multiple metabolic side effects
5-Aminosalicylate derivatives (sulfasalazine, Asacol, Pentasa)	Active disease; maintenance treatment	Sperm abnormality, folate malabsorption, nausea, dyspepsia, headache
Metronidazole	Active disease; maintenance treatment	Nausea, metallic taste, peripheral neuropathy, disulfiram-like reaction
Azathioprine and 6-mercaptopurine	Active disease; maintenance treatment (requires 3–6 months to become effective)	Nausea, rash, fever, hepatitis, bone marrow suppression, B-cell lymphoma
Methotrexate	Active disease with fistulas	Nausea, headaches, bone marrow suppression, stomatitis
Cyclosporin A	Severe active disease with fistulas	Hypertension, tremors, opportunistic infections, nephrotoxicity, paresthesias, hepatic abnormalities, gingival hyperplasia
Anti–tumor necrosis factor	Severe active disease with fistulas; maintenance treatment	Abdominal pain, myalgias, nausea, fatigue, delayed hypersensitivity, lymphoma, teratogenic effect

immunosuppressive effects. **Long-term metronidazole therapy is poorly tolerated** because of multiple **side effects including nausea, metallic taste, disulfiram-like reactions, and peripheral neuropathy.** Corticosteroids are nonspecific anti-inflammatory agents that are effective in treating small bowel and ileocolonic disease. **Although effective for active disease, corticosteroids have not been found to be efficacious in maintenance therapy.** Corticosteroids are associated with many major side effects, including **hyperglycemia, fluid retention, fat**

redistribution, acne, mood changes, and growth retardation in children. Budesonide is a newer agent that is more rapidly metabolized than prednisone and may lead to fewer side effects.

Aminosalicylates (5-ASA) are effective in maintenance therapy and in the treatment of active disease. Limitations of 5-ASA derivatives include GI tract and systemic side effects, and hypersensitivity reactions. Several immunomodulators have been used in the treatment of Crohn's disease. Azathioprine and 6-mercaptopurine are two commonly used immunomodulators that are highly effective in inducing remission in patients with active disease and in the prevention of flare-up in patients with inactive disease. The potential toxic effects of azathioprine and 6-mercaptopurine include bone marrow suppression, nausea, fever, rash, hepatitis, and pancreatitis. Although shown to be effective in the treatment of active disease, **methotrexate** is associated with many side effects including **nausea, headache, stomatitis, bone marrow suppression, hepatitis, and pneumonitis.** Cyclosporin A (CSA) has been shown to produce significant improvement in severe disease associated with fistulas; however, controlled trials in patients with moderate disease have not demonstrated significant benefits. CSA use is associated with severe side effects including hypertension, hyperesthesias, tremors, and nephrotoxicity. Anti–tumor necrosis factor (TNF) therapy (infliximab, CDP571, thalidomide) have been shown to be highly effective in the treatment of patients with fistulas that are difficult to manage. There are major drawbacks associated with anti-TNF therapy, including B-cell lymphoma development associated with infliximab and the teratogenic effects of thalidomide.

Surgical Therapy

The roles of surgery are to **relieve symptoms** associated with Crohn's disease (pain, obstructive symptoms, weight loss) **refractory to medical therapy** and to **improve the quality of life of patients who experience severe side effects from medical therapy** (eg, growth retardation from corticosteroid therapy). Surgical options include bowel resection, stricturoplasty, and abscess drainage. One of the potential long-term complications of surgical therapy is the development of malabsorption syndromes. Approximately 30% of patients may require another operation within 5 years after undergoing resection for Crohn's disease. **Repeat resection of the gastrointestinal tract can result in clinical short bowel syndrome requiring permanent TPN therapy** (about 1% of patients with Crohn's disease). Patients with multiple sites of disease involvement have a greater risk for disease recurrence. In addition, nonsteroidal anti-inflammatory agent use and tobacco smoking have been linked to disease recurrences; therefore, patients should be counseled regarding these issues.

Comprehension Questions

[52.1] Medical management may be effective in the treatment of which of the following symptoms associated with Crohn's disease?

    A. Partial bowel obstruction
    B. Enterocolonic fistulas
    C. Abdominal pain due to an inflammatory mass
    D. All of the above

[52.2] A 22-year-old woman is newly diagnosed with Crohn's disease of the terminal ileum. She complains of significant abdominal pain. Her temperature is 98°F, and HR 90/min. Which of the following is the best management for this patient?

    A. Exploratory celiotomy to assess for bowel perforation.
    B. Medical management and reassess
    C. Radionuclide-tagged leukocyte imaging study to assess location of disease
    D. Intravenous morphine for pain control

Answers

[52.1] **D.** Medical management may be effective for all these complications associated with Crohn's disease. They can include obstruction, fistulas, and inflammation. Surgery is also indicated for all these complications if a patient does not respond to medications or if medications produce unacceptable side effects.

[52.2] **B.** Medical management is the appropriate choice in a patient with uncomplicated newly diagnosed Crohn's disease. A CT-scan of the abdomen should be performed to rule-out the possibility of intraabdominal abscess associated with Crohn's disease and rule-out alternative pathology such as appendicitis.

CLINICAL PEARLS

◈ With the exception of the treatment of toxic colitis, there is virtually no indication for emergency (unplanned) operative treatment for patients with Crohn's disease.

◈ Fibrotic strictures cannot be resolved with medical management and generally require operative therapy to relieve the obstruction.

◈ Crohn's disease may involve both the small bowel and the colon; therefore, a complete evaluation should include colonoscopy and an upper GI tract contrast study to visualize the location and severity of the small bowel disease.

◈ Repeated resection of the gastrointestinal tract can result in clinical short bowel syndrome requiring **permanent TPN therapy** in about 1% of patients with Crohn's disease.

◈ In general, the roles of surgery in Crohn's disease are to relieve symptoms refractory to medical therapy (pain, obstructive symptoms, weight loss) and to improve the quality of life of patients who experience severe medication side effects.

REFERENCES

Delaney CP, Fazio VW. Crohn's disease of the small bowel. Surg Clin North Am 2001;81:137–158.

Schraut WH, Medich DS. Crohn's disease surgery: scientific principles and practice, 2nd ed. Philadelphia: Lippincott-Raven, 1997.

Stein RB, Lichtenstein GR. Medical therapy for Crohn's disease. Surg Clin North Am 2001;81:71–101.

A 35-year-old man with a 15-year history of ulcerative colitis (UC) is evaluated in the outpatient office with chronic bloody diarrhea over the past 6 weeks. The patient's vital signs are unremarkable. His hemoglobin level is 11.0 g/dL. His current medications consist of prednisone and mesalamine (a 5-aminosalycilate derivative), and he recently completed a course of cyclosporine therapy 2 months ago for another bout of disease flare-up. The patient has been unable to maintain full time employment over the past year because of UC. Previous colonoscopy has shown that his disease extends from the rectum to the cecum.

◆ **What should be your next step?**

◆ **What is the best therapy?**

ANSWERS TO CASE 53: Ulcerative Colitis

Summary: A 35-year-old man has pancolonic chronic UC that is refractory to medical management and causes significant disability.

◆ **Next step:** The option of surgical therapy should be presented to this patient. The discussion should explain the benefits and limitations of surgery versus those of continued medical therapy.

◆ **Best therapy:** Proctocolectomy with ileal pouch-anus anastomosis.

Analysis

Objectives

1. Become familiar with the clinical presentation, natural history, medical management, and complications of UC.
2. Become familiar with the indications for urgent and elective operations for the treatment of UC.
3. Be aware of the surgical options and their outcomes for the treatment of UC.

Considerations

Ulcerative colitis is a chronic disease with variable disease severity. The symptoms associated with this disease generally respond to medicated enemas or systemic therapy. When a 35-year-old man presents with a 15-year history of pancolitis and disabling symptoms that have been refractory to medical management, the discussion regarding treatment should explain medical as well as surgical options. **Surgical excision of the diseased colon and rectum would lead to resolution of the gastrointestinal (GI) symptoms** associated with UC. However, the operation would result in permanent changes in bowel function and body image. It is essential to convey to the patient that **surgical excision will not resolve the extraintestinal manifestation of UC** and that ongoing medical therapy for these symptoms will more than likely be required. Another important consideration for this patient is **cancer risk in the setting of chronic UC,** as this risk is increased with disease extent and duration. Proctocolectomy with ileal reservoir reconstruction can improve the quality of life and virtually eliminate the colorectal cancer risk in properly selected patients.

APPROACH TO ULCERATIVE COLITIS

Definitions

Toxic fulminant colitis (megacolon):   A condition characterized by abdominal pain, distension, fever, and sepsis that most commonly develops in the setting of UC but occasionally occurs in the settings of Crohn colitis and pseudomembranous colitis. Patients with toxic megacolon can **become extremely ill with clinical signs of sepsis, and this clinical entity can be highly lethal** if not promptly recognized and treated. When identified with this condition, patients require prompt fluid resuscitation and the initiation of broad-spectrum antibiotic therapy, with maximal medical treatment. Colectomy is indicated if the patient fails to respond to medical therapy, and generally one-third of patients go on to require colectomy for this complication.

Dysplasia: Premalignant transformation of the mucosa due to chronic UC. The risk of cancer associated with dysplasia varies depending on the severity of the dysplastic changes. Roughly 40% of patients with high-grade dysplasia harbor synchronous cancer, and 20% of patients with low-grade dysplasia harbor synchronous cancer.

Dysplasia-associated lesion or mass: A sessile pseudopolyp arising from dysplastic mucosa affected by chronic UC. **Fifty percent of patients with these lesions have carcinoma.** Patients with this finding should undergo colorectal resection.

Pancolitis: Ulcerative colitis that involves the rectum and the entire colon. Patients with this pattern of disease have a significant risk for the development of subsequent colorectal cancers.

Pouchitis: Idiopathic inflammation of the ileal pouch that can develop following ileal reservoir reconstruction. Patients can present with any number of symptoms including increased stool frequency, fecal urgency, incontinence, watery diarrhea, bleeding, abdominal cramps, fever, and malaise. Bacterial overgrowth can be a contributing factor for pouchitis, and therefore some patients respond to antibiotic therapy.

Clinical Approach

Ulcerative colitis is an inflammatory condition of unknown etiology. The disease involvement is limited to the mucosa, and the distribution begins in the rectum and extends to the proximal colon, with occasional extension to the terminal ileum (backwash ileitis). With **chronic inflammation of the colonic mucosa,** there is **loss of water reabsorption and normal motility, leading to watery diarrhea, cramplike pain, tenesmus, and urgency.** A number of **extraintestinal manifestations** are associated with UC, including **ankylosing spondylitis, uveitis, scleroderma, sclerosing cholangitis, arthritis, dermatomyositis, and hypercoagulable states.** Surgical therapy has been shown to virtually eliminate the symptoms related to the diseased colon and rectum; however, the benefits of surgery for the extraintestinal manifestations have not been established (Table 53–1). In fact, **some reports have suggested that extraintestinal disease can be aggravated by removal of the colon and rectum.**

The medical management of UC consists of anti-inflammatory therapies of escalating intensity coupled with the administration of antibiotics. When antibiotics and anti-inflammatory agents fail, steroid agents are the next line of therapy. The long-term use of steroids can be effective in reducing the symptoms associated with UC but can lead to immunosuppression, accelerated bone loss, hirsutism, masculinization, osteoporosis, aseptic necrosis, glucose intolerance, and loss of muscle mass. Short- and long-term steroid use has been shown to increase the morbidity associated with surgical treatment.

The **three main indications for surgical therapy in UC are toxic colitis, dysplasia or cancer, and intractable disease.** The most commonly performed operation for toxic colitis is total abdominal colectomy with ileostomy. As the colorectal cancer risk increases with

Table 53-1

SURGICAL OPTIONS FOR ULCERATIVE COLITIS

SURGICAL PROCEDURE	INDICATION	ADVANTAGES	DISADVANTAGES
Abdominal colectomy with ileostomy	Acute toxic colitis; less frequently for other indications	Less morbidity under urgent settings	Cancer risk in rectum up to 15%–20% at 25–30 y
Abdominal colectomy with ileorectal anastomosis	For intractability or cancer or dysplasia	Preservation of bowel functions with acceptable results in patients with limited rectal disease	Cancer risk in rectum up to 15%–20% at 25–30 y; patients can have continued symptoms
Total proctocolectomy with permanent ileostomy	For intractability or cancer or dysplasia	All colorectal disease removed with symptom resolution	Permanent ileostomy
Total proctocolectomy with ileal pouch–anus anastomosis	For intractability or cancer or dysplasia	All colorectal disease removed with symptom resolution and maintenance of transanal continence	4–12 bowel movements per day; some have day or nighttime incontinence; pouchitis (7%–40%)
Total proctocolectomy with continent ileostomy	For intractability or cancer or dysplasia	All colorectal disease removed with symptom resolution; patients do not require external stoma appliance	High malfunction rate associated with the nipple valve requiring revision or urgent cannulation for drainage

chronic UC, **patients with a UC duration greater than 7 to 9 years should undergo annual or biannual surveillance colonoscopy with biopsies or be considered for proctocolectomy if a surveillance program is not instituted.** The majority of patients with UC undergoing surgery do so because of disease intractability. This is determined on the basis of disease symptomatology and tolerance to medical therapy. In the nonurgent setting, surgical options include total abdominal colectomy with ileorectal anastomosis or ileostomy, total proctocolectomy with standard ileostomy or continent ileostomy, or total proctocolectomy with ileal reservoir reconstruction.

Comprehension Questions

[53.1] A 35-year-old woman with ulcerative colitis underwent a colonoscopy revealing an area of colonic dysplasia described as high grade. Which of the following is the best management for this patient?

    A. Surgical resection of colon
    B. Intensive medical therapy and reevaluate with colonoscopy in 3 months
    C. Increase to surveillance every 6 months
    D. Add a immunosuppressive agent to the medical therapy

[53.2] A 40-year-old woman with a 15-year history of chronic diarrhea and a diagnosis of UC is referred for consideration for total proctocolectomy with ileal pouch-anus anastomosis to eliminate future cancer risks. During the colonoscopy, you notice that the disease involves the entire colon and terminal ileum, with sparing of the rectum. What is the most appropriate treatment?

    A. Proctocolectomy with ileal pouch-anus anastomosis
    B. Total abdominal colectomy with ileal-rectal anastomosis
    C. Repeated biopsy of the rectum and involved portions of the colon and ileum
    D. Total proctocolectomy with the construction of continent ileostomy

Answers

[53.1] **A.** High grade dysplasia found on colonic surveillance in a patient with ulcerative colitis is usually treated with total colectomy to avoid the development of cancer.

[53.2] **C.** Noninvolvement of the rectum should raise a suspicion of possible Crohn's disease, which is a contraindication to performing total proctocolectomy and ileal pouch-anus reconstruction. Repeated colonoscopy and biopsy are indicated in this case.

CLINICAL PEARLS

◈ A definitive diagnosis of UC must be confirmed prior to performing proctocolectomy and a reconstruction procedure.

◈ The three main indications for surgical therapy in UC are toxic colitis, dysplasia or cancer, and intractable disease.

◈ Extraintestinal manifestations of UC include ankylosing spondylitis, uveitis, scleroderma, sclerosing cholangitis, arthritis, dermatomyositis, and hypercoagulable states, for which surgery is not effective.

◈ Surgical and medical treatments for UC are complementary and not competing modalities.

◈ The term "refractory to medical therapy" is not strictly defined and should also refer to the failure of appropriate medical therapy as well as patient intolerance to the adverse effects of medical therapy.

REFERENCES

Sitzmann JV. Surgical alternative for ulcerative colitis. Probl Gen Surg 1999; 16:115–123.

Welton ML, Varma MG, Amerhauser A. Colon, rectum, and anus. In Norton JA, Bollinger RR, Chang AE, Lowery SF, Mulvihill SJ, Pass HI, Thompson RW, eds. Surgery: basic science and clinical evidence. New York: Springer, 2001: 667–762.

CASE 54

A 55-year-old male complains of a 4-month history of lower back pain that is worsened by walking and relieved by lying down. He denies back trauma, heavy lifting, or urologic abnormalities. He states that at times the pain radiates to the back of his right leg. On examination, his blood pressure is 130/84 and his pulse rate 80/min; he is afebrile. He is slightly overweight. The findings from his heart and lung examinations show no abnormalities. The back is without scoliosis. Raising either leg reproduces the pain, which radiates to the right leg. The results from the neurologic examination are normal.

◆ **What is the most likely diagnosis?**

◆ **What is the best test to confirm the diagnosis?**

ANSWERS TO CASE 54: Lumbar Prolapsed Nucleus Pulposus

Summary: A 55-year-old male complains of a 4-month history of lower back pain radiating to the right leg, which is worsened by walking and relieved by lying down. He denies trauma to the back, heavy lifting, or urologic abnormalities. He is slightly overweight. The back is without scoliosis. Raising either leg reproduces the pain, which radiates to the right leg. The neurologic examination is normal.

◆ **Most likely diagnosis:** Lumbar prolapsed nucleus pulposus.

◆ **Best diagnostic step:** Magnetic resonance imaging (MRI) or myelography.

Analysis

Objectives

1. Know the differential diagnosis for lower back pain.
2. Know the typical clinical presentation of lumbar prolapsed nucleus pulposus.
3. Understand that MRI and myelography are the imaging tests that confirm the diagnosis.

Considerations

This 55-year-old male complains of lower back pain with radiation to the right leg. The pain is worse when walking and during straight leg raising. This is typical of herniated lumbar pulposus due to compression of the intervertebral disk causing impingement of the nerve root, typically at the L4-5 level. There is usually paresthesia or radiation of the pain in the leg, usually posterior and/or lateral. MRI is a very accurate test for evaluating the spinal cord and nerve roots.

APPROACH TO LOWER BACK PAIN

Definitions

Mechanical backache: Usually chronic and may result in a long-term debilitating illness without any definite or demonstrable cause. Back sprains are usually associated with minor trauma producing ligamentous or muscular injury.

Entrapment neuropathies: Involve compression of a nerve, such as that produced in sciatica, when a prolapsed intervertebral disk applies pressure to an adjacent nerve in the lumbosacral plexus.

Cauda equina syndrome: Compression of the sacral nerve bundle, which forms the end of the spinal cord, with symptoms of bladder or bowel dysfunction and/or pain or weakness in the legs. This disorder should be diagnosed at an early stage to avoid permanent injury.

Clinical Approach

As low back pain is so common, it is of fundamental importance to differentiate significant from insignificant pain and thus to prevent the onset of chronicity. Spinal pain can be local or referred or can occur along the distribution of nerves. Osteoarthritis and rheumatoid arthritis are associated with conditions such as spinal stenosis, spondylolisthesis or ankylosing spondylitis which may cause chronic back pain.

Herniation of the nucleus pulposus, the softer inner part of an intervertebral disk, through the outer tough annulus fibrosus causes **compression of adjacent nerves** emanating from the spinal canal. On occasion, fragmentation of the disk may occur without protrusion of the nucleus pulposus; the annulus itself then protrudes. This condition may cause severe pain, weakness, and sensory loss. The problem may also be caused by the protrusion of osteophytes; bony spurs that occur in osteoarthrosis of the spine. Ultimately, **spinal stenosis** may develop.

With disk prolapse, the severity of symptoms may vary from mild, localized back pain to **urgent cauda equina compression resulting in the loss of motor and sensory function. The L4-5 and L5-S1 intervertebral disks are the most commonly involved; thus, pain down**

the posterior or lateral leg is characteristic (sciatica). Back pain frequently radiates into the buttock, posterior thigh, or calf. Coughing, sneezing, or straining tends to increase the pain. Other exacerbating factors are bending, sitting, and getting in and out of a vehicle, whereas **lying flat characteristically relieves pain.** Caudal equina compression may affect **bladder and bowel function,** and spinal stenosis may produce pain that radiates down both legs.

The paravertebral muscles are often in spasm, and there is loss of the normal lumbar lordosis. Straight leg raising is limited on the side of the lesion, and dorsiflexion of the foot at the limit of straight leg raising often exacerbates the discomfort. There may be tenderness to palpation of the central back or buttock. Sensory loss and muscular weakness may be present along the appropriate dermatomes; ankle or knee reflexes may be absent. The differential diagnosis includes fracture; joint subluxation; tumors of the bone, joint, or meninges; abscess; arachnoiditis; ankylosing spondylitis; rheumatoid arthritis; aortic occlusion; and peripheral neuropathies. Magnetic resonance imaging may demonstrate the disk protrusion, and plain radiographs of the lumbosacral spine may show narrowing of the intervertebral space, but these modalities cannot establish a definitive diagnosis.

Bed rest, the application of either heated pads or ice packs, administration of nonsteroidal anti-inflammatory drugs and muscle relaxants, and/or physical therapy represent the first line of conservative management. A back brace or corset may help the patient through the early stages of mobilization. **The indications for surgical decompression are the development of an acute disabling neurologic deficit (bladder dysfunction) or intractable severe pain.**

After the site of the disk prolapse is precisely identified, surgery involves laminectomy and removal of the protruding disk. The overlying stretched nerve may show erythema and narrowing, and great care must be exercised in removing the offending protruding disk from underneath this nerve. If several disk spaces are involved, posterior spinal fusion in addition to removal of the disks may be indicated. This form of surgery has been performed with increasing frequency in recent years, using a minimally invasive approach with short incisions, meticulous and specific removal of the disk, and early mobilization. The results of surgery are excellent. Techniques under review are dissolution of the disk by the injection of chemicals, and sometimes steroid injections in the region of the disk may be helpful in the short term.

Comprehension Questions

[54.1] Which of the following describes the most common location of herniated disks in the lumbar spine region?

    A. L1-2
    B. L2-3
    C. L3-4
    D. L4-5

[54.2] A 47-year-old woman complains of lower back pain with radiation to the right leg, and she is treated with ibuprofen and bed rest. Over the next 3 weeks, the patient's pain worsens, and she complains of difficulty with voiding and bowel movements. Which of the following is the most likely diagnosis?

    A. Spinal stenosis
    B. Lumbar neoplasm
    C. Cauda equina syndrome
    D. Tuberculosis of the spine (Pott disease)

[54.3] A 56-year-old mailman is diagnosed with probable lumbar prolapsed nucleus pulposis. Which of the following is most consistent with his diagnosis?

    A. Pain in the lower back radiating down the anterior thigh
    B. Decreased patellar deep tendon reflex
    C. Pain worsened with valsalva
    D. Decreased sensation in the medial thigh and weakness of the adductor muscles of the lower leg.

Answers

[54.1] **D.** The L4-5 interspace is most commonly affected.

[54.2] **C.** The bowel and bladder complaints are typical of cauda equina syndrome.

[54.3] **C.** Pain of lumbar disc disease is worse with valsalva, straight leg raising, and the sitting position. The pain typically radiates from the back to the posterior or lateral leg.

CLINICAL PEARLS

◆ The most common locations of herniated lumbar disk disease are at the L4-5 and L5-S1 levels.

◆ Bowel and bladder complaints with lower back pain are suggestive of cauda equina syndrome, which must be diagnosed early to avoid permanent damage.

◆ The initial treatment for herniated lumbar pulposus is bedrest and the administration of nonsteroidal anti-inflammatory agents.

REFERENCE

Hoff JT, Boland MF. Neurosurgery. In: Schwarz SI, Shires GT, Spencer FC, et al, eds. Principles of surgery, 7th ed. New York: McGraw-Hill, 1999:1896–1899.

A 1-month-old girl is evaluated for persistent jaundice. The infant was born at 39-weeks' gestation to a healthy 28-year-old woman with no family history of medical problems. The delivery was by cesarean after premature rupture of membranes with a birth weight of 3200 grams and Apgar scores of 9 and 9 at one/five minutes. She had passage of meconium on the first day of life, and she was mildly jaundiced at the time of discharge from the hospital on day 2 of life. During the past several days, the patient has been having acholic stools and darkly stained urine. On examination, she is deeply jaundiced; the cardiopulmonary examination is unremarkable. The liver is palpable and firm. No other abdominal masses are identified. The laboratory evaluations reveal a normal CBC, total bilirubin and direct bilirubin levels of 28mg/dL and 24mg/dL, and serum levels of AST/ALT and alkaline phosphatase of 300/ 250 U/L and 950 IU/L respectively.

◆ **What are the differential diagnoses?**

◆ **What is your next step(s)?**

◆ **Should this be urgently evaluated or electively and definitively diagnosed?**

ANSWERS TO CASE 15: Neonatal Jaundice (Persistent)

◆ **Differential Diagnoses:** Neonatal hepatitis, TORCH infections, metabolic diseases (alpha-1-antitrypsin deficiency, cystic fibrosis, and others), biliary atresia, and choledochal cyst.

◆ **Next Steps:** After the initial laboratory studies are performed, the evaluation should simultaneously include TORCH/metabolic studies (as listed in Table 15–1), abdominal ultrasound, and HIDA scan (^{99m}Tc-labelled iminodiacetic acid).

◆ **Timing:** Hyperbilirubinemia in the neonate that persists beyond 2 weeks of age is rarely physiologic, particularly when it is predominantly conjugated bilirubin. Because surgical correction of biliary atresia is optimally performed before 8 weeks of age (12 weeks maximum), urgent evaluation and potentially preoperative preparation is warranted over 5-6 days.

Analysis

Considerations

This patient is fairly typical of those referred for surgical consultation in the evaluation of neonatal jaundice. Usually, the infant has no specific symptoms. Physical findings include acholic stools and occasionally, a palpable, firm liver. The onset of jaundice can give some clues as to the diagnosis (e.g., hemolytic diseases often present early and are more progressive/severe). The degree of conjugated hyperbilirubinemia offers a key distinguishing direction as to how to approach the work-up. Table 55–1 lists the causes of neonatal hyperbilirubinemia and some of their distinguishing characteristics. Metabolic and infectious causes should be investigated. A prompt evaluation includes an abdominal ultrasound and HIDA scan ± percutaneous liver biopsy. If the imaging studies do not rule out biliary atresia, then operative exploration with intraoperative cholangiogram is indicated. Surgical reconstruction for

Table 55–1

CLINICAL MANAGEMENT OF PERSISTENT
JAUNDICE IN CHILDREN

DISEASE	CLINICAL FINDINGS	STUDIES	TREATMENT
UNCONJUGATED HYPERBILIRUBINEMIA			
Hemolytic diseases	Early, severe jaundice	Coombs positive	Phototherapy; exchange transfusion
Metabolic diseases	Disease specific	Disease specific	Disease specific
Physiologic jaundice	Nonspecific	Fractionated bilirubin	Phototherapy
CONJUGATED HYPERBILIRUBINEMIA			
Biliary Atresia	Nonspecific	US; HIDA; liver biopsy; IOC	Portoenterostomy
Choledochal cyst	Abdominal mass Rarely, cholangitis	US; HIDA	Cyst excision and hepaticojejunostomy
Biliary hypoplasia (Alagille's Syndrome)	Cardiovascular, spinal, eye abnormalities & jaundice common	US; HIDA; liver biopsy; IOC; investigate other organ systems	Choleretics
Total parenteral nutrition	Short bowel syndrome (anatomic or functional)	US; HIDA/ liver biopsy if diagnosis in question	Enteral feeding
Inspissated bile syndrome	Hemolytic diseases or cystic fibrosis	US	IOC may be diagnostic and therapeutic
Sepsis/infection	Clinically ill	TORCH screen, blood culture	Supportive/specific to disease

US-ultrasound; IOC-intraoperative cholangiogram.

biliary atresia is a Kasai portoenterostomy, and hepatico-jejunostomy for choledochal cyst.

Objectives

1. Be familiar with the differential diagnosis for neonatal jaundice.
2. Be familiar with the diagnostic approach and initial supportive management of patients with neonatal jaundice.
3. Be familiar with the treatment for biliary atresia and chole-dochal cyst.

APPROACH TO NEONATAL OBSTRUCTIVE JAUNDICE

Pathophysiology: Biliary atresia—the precise etiology of biliary atresia is unknown. Various theories include viral infections and autoimmune processes. Microscopically, the biliary tracts contain inflammatory cells surrounding obliterated ductules. The liver shows signs of cholestasis, and in later stages fibrosis. Grossly, the most common finding is fibrosis of the entire extrahepatic biliary tree, followed by proximal duct fibrosis with distal duct patency.

Choledochal cyst: Similar to biliary atresia, the exact etiology of choledochal cysts is unknown. A widely held theory is that the common bile duct and pancreatic duct share a common channel leading to retrograde reflux of pancreatic juice into the choledochus with subsequent cystic dilation. There are 5 types of choledochal cysts, but the fusiform or Type I comprises 90% of all lesions.

Preoperative management and surgical treatment of biliary atresia and choledochal cysts: Prior to surgical intervention, these patients must be evaluated for coagulation abnormalities, anemia, and hypoproteinemia. Correction of coagulopathy usually requires both vitamin K and fresh frozen plasma. Anemia may be of moderate severity requiring the availability of cross-matched blood. Parents should be made aware of the prognosis of biliary atresia preoperatively. Conversely, the surgical management of choledochal cyst carries an excellent prognosis.

Surgical Treatment: The surgical management of biliary atresia consists of operative exploration of the porta hepatis with intraoperative cholangiogram. If dye does not enter the duodenum, then the limited right upper quadrant incision is extended and the extrahepatic biliary tree is dissected up to the level of the portal plate. The portal plate is transected flush with but not into the liver. This exposes the biliary ductules that drain bile. A Roux-en-Y limb of jejunum is attached to the porta in a retrocolic manner. Previously, jejunal valves, stomas, and other approaches were used, but these have fallen out of favor due to complexity and lack of improved outcomes with the more complex procedures. Similarly, choledochal cysts are excised, but instead of fashioning the limb of jejunum to the porta, it is attached to the bifurcating hepatic ducts at their confluence.

Complications: The **three main complications of the surgical management of biliary atresia** are: **cholangitis, cessation of bile flow, and portal hypertension. Cholangitis is the most frequent complication** occurring **after portoenterostomy** and is manifest by **fever, leukocytosis, and elevations in the bilirubin. Treatment** includes intravenous **antibiotics** against gram-negative organisms and **steroids.** Cessation of bile flow can be related to progression of the disease, cholangitis, or Roux limb obstruction (rare). Treatment is based on steroids and other choleretic agents. Portal hypertension is a late complication of portoenterostomy, and it occurs even in those that are successful in terms of bile flow. The complications of variceal bleeding can usually be managed, and the symptoms progress if the degreee of cirrhosis worsens.

Outcome: Biliary atresia—before the introduction of the **Kasai procedure,** the survival rates were less than 5% at 12 months. Approximately 50% of patients have good long-term results. Ultimately, **only 20% of patients undergoing portoenterostomy survive into adulthood without transplantation.** Factors that affect early bile flow after operation are: age, immediate bile flow (technically sound operation), and degree of parenchymal disease at diagnosis. The presence and size of ductules in the hilum are of controversial prognostic significance. Choledochal cyst—the prognosis for patients undergoing excision of choledochal cyst and Roux-en-Y hepaticojejunostomy is excellent.

Comprehension Questions

[55.1] Which imaging study is most definitive in its ability to diagnose biliary atresia?

   A. Abdominal ultrasound
   B. HIDA scan
   C. Intraoperative cholangiogram
   D. Magnetic resonance cholangiopancreatography

[55.2] A 140-day-old infant with a mixed hyperbilirubinemia undergoes a percutaneous liver biopsy, HIDA scan, and abdominal sonography that are consistent with biliary atresia. Metabolic and infectious evaluations are negative. Which of the following is the best management for this patient?

   A. Kasai procedure (portoenterostomy)
   B. Listing for liver transplantation
   C. Open liver biopsy and cholangiogram
   D. Tube cholecystostomy

[55.3] An 18-month-old infant who underwent a successful Kasai procedure as an infant returns with fever, leukocytosis, and a new hyperbilirubinemia. What is the best initial management?

   A. Revision of portoenterostomy
   B. Corticosteroids and antibiotics
   C. Corticosteroids alone
   D. Antibiotics alone

Answers

[55.1] **C.** While abdominal ultrasound and HIDA scan are used as suggestive evidence of biliary atresia, they do not definitively rule it in or out. For example, approximately 10%-15% of biliary atresia cases have visible, normally distended gallbladders. It is not uncommon for patients with biliary hypoplasia (Alagille's syndrome) to have no excretion of tracer into the duodenum on HIDA scan. The only definitive way to diagnose biliary atresia is by operative exploration and intraoperative cholangiogram. Magnetic resonance cholangiopancreatography is not routinely used to evaluate the neonatal biliary tract.

[55.2] **B.** After 120 days of life, portoenterostomy is rarely indicated. While there have been occasional successful procedures, these are the overwhelming exception. A cholangiogram and liver biopsy may be useful, they will not alter the therapy—meaning that a finding of biliary atresia would not prompt a portoenterostomy. Therefore, a standard approach to these infants is referral for liver transplantation after 120 days of life.

[55.3] **B.** The child described has a classic clinical presentation of post-Kasai cholangitis. This is a frequent complication of portoenterostomy. Revision of the portoenterostomy is rarely indicated. Occasionally this is done for the functioning Kasai that acutely fails—usually in the immediate post-op period. The findings of fever, leukocytosis, and rising bilirubin suggest cholangitis. Standard management include supportive measures, blood cultures, antibiotics against gram-negative organisms, and steroids (function as choleretic and anti-inflammatory).

CLINICAL PEARLS

◆ Jaundice in the neonate beyond 2 weeks of age is rarely physiologic, especially when involving mainly conjugated bilirubin.

◆ The most common complication after portoenterostomy is cholangitis.

◆ Neonates with biliary atresia or choledochal cysts should be assessed for coagulopathy prior to surgery.

REFERENCES

Tagge DU, Tagge EP, Drongowski RA, Oldham KT, Coran AG. A long term experience with biliary atresia. *Ann Surg* 1991: 214: 590–598.

Lally KP, Kenegaye J, Matsumura M, Rosenthal P, Sinatra F, Atkinson JB. Perioperative repair of biliary atresia. *Pediatrics* 1989; 83: 723–726.

Valayer J. Conventional treatment of biliary atresia: Long term results. *J Pediatr Surg* 1996; 31: 1546–1551.

Miyano T, Yamataka A, Kato Y, et al., Hepaticoenterostomy after excision of choledochal cyst in children: A 30 year experience with 180 cases. *J Pediatr Surg* 1996; 31: 1417–1421.

Listing
of
Cases

LISTING BY CASE NUMBER

LISTING BY DISORDER (ALPHABETICAL)

Index

Note: Page numbers followed by f indicate figures; those followed by t indicate tables.